DR. J. J. PYSH

ADVANCES IN NEUROLOGY
VOLUME 12

DR. J. J. PYSH

Advances in Neurology

Advances in Neurology
Volume 12

Physiology and Pathology
of Dendrites

Editor:

Georg W. Kreutzberg, M.D.
Chief, Section of Experimental Neuropathology
Max Planck Institute for Psychiatry
Munich, Federal Republic of Germany

Raven Press, Publishers ▪ New York

Made in the United States of America

International Standard Book Number 0–911216–99–5
Library of Congress Catalog Card Number 74–14474

ISBN outside North and South America only: 0–7204–7544–9

Advances in Neurology Series

Preface

The dendrites of nerve cells were discovered during the classical period of neurohistology following the introduction of a new staining technique by Camillo Golgi in 1873. In the hands of Santiago Ramon y Cajal this method became an effective instrument for the anatomical investigation of the brain and for the elaboration of the neuron doctrine. For many years this doctrine remained highly controversial and was the basis for fierce disagreements over the functional significance of the new and beautiful dendrite histology. In the field of neuropathology, Spielmeier's negative verdict on the usefulness of studying dendritic abnormalities with the Golgi technique discouraged the systematic investigations of this important neuronal structure. Indeed, it took 50 more years and required the electron microscope to reawaken the neuropathologist's interest in the dendrite.

In recent years, the investigation of dendritic structure and phenomena has undergone a considerable acceleration. This neuronal segment is now being studied with a great variety of methods by researchers operating with different and even divergent concepts and approaches. It therefore appeared timely to bring together an interdisciplinary group of researchers for the purpose of determining the state of sophistication of present investigative endeavors and of establishing appropriate goals for future research.

This volume contains contributions to the international symposium on the physiology and pathology of dendrites held at the Max Planck Institute for Psychiatry, Munich, in September 1974. It was hoped that the attending physiologists, anatomists, and pathologists would benefit from an exchange of information and ideas and would be stimulated to formulate new concepts and experimental approaches in dendritology.

Among the topics covered we find signal propagation in dendrites and new insights into the cable properties of dendrites with their capability of spiking, electrical coupling, and signal amplification. These functions will probably assume a central role in neuronal information processing. Emphasis was also given to dendro-dendritic interaction in the developing and adult nervous system, to intradendritic transport, and to the release of substances from the dendritic membrane. Is the latter mechanism involved in the regulation of the neuron's microenvironment and its local blood supply? What happens to the dendrites if specific input is taken away? How vulnerable are dendrites to therapeutic interventions or pathological interactions? Dendritic abnormalities were found in developmental disorders as well as in senile diseases. To what degree are these the morphological correlates of mental malfunction? Although these questions have not been answered completely it appears that solutions can be expected in the near future.

Georg W. Kreutzberg, M.D.

Contents

Advances in Neurology, Vol. 12, edited by
G. W. Kreutzberg, Raven Press, New York
© 1975.

Electroresponsive Properties of Dendrites in Central Neurons

Rodolfo Llinás

*Division of Neurobiology, Department of Physiology and Biophysics, University of Iowa,
Oakdale, Iowa 52319*

The ability of dendrites to generate spikes has been a matter of controversy for the last two decades. The basis for the controversy has been the implicit hypothesis that in order to have integration in a Sherringtonian sense (Sherrington, 1906), the receiving pole of the neuron – the dendrites – must be able to sum the graded excitatory and inhibitory influences algebraically. If dendrites were to fire action potentials too readily, it would be correctly assumed that neurons could be regarded simply as relay devices, rather than as a site for integration. In fact, temporal summation would hardly occur if a high percentage of afferent inputs were individually capable of generating a full action potential.[1] Conversely, if dendrites combine excitatory and inhibitory potentials algebraically without being capable of generating spikes themselves, the dendrites would be used for neuronal integration at maximal capacity (Lorente de Nó and Condouris, 1959). In order to complete the hypothesis, it must then be assumed that action potentials are always initiated at the same site (the axon hillock), and that any depolarization having the necessary amplitude and rate of rise at that site will generate an action potential in the neuron. This view received very strong support from the early motoneuronal studies (Brock, Coombs, and Eccles, 1952; Coombs, Eccles, and Fatt, 1955; Fuortes, Frank and Becker, 1957), which showed that the action potential in the spinal motoneurons is initiated at the axon hillock level, and that normally dendritic spikes are not present in these cells (but cf. Nelson and Burke, 1967). At first approximation, therefore, integration appeared to be produced by the algebraic summation of excitatory and inhibitory inputs to the somadendritic surface. This useful model of neuronal integration was then further elaborated by research on the different functional properties of axodendritic versus axosomatic synapses in motoneurons of different vertebrates. Experimental work by Fadiga and Brookhart (1962) provided evidence that in the frog synaptic inputs that terminated in dendrites had functional properties different from those terminating in the soma- and proximal dendrites. Similar

---

[1] This may occur following the activation of single Ia afferents in chromatolyzed motoneurons (Kuno and Llinás, 1970).

conclusions were reached experimentally in the cat by Llinás and Terzuolo (1964, 1965), Terzuolo and Llinás (1966), Burke (1967), Smith, Wuerker, and Frank (1967), Kuno and Miyahara (1969), and Jack et al. (1971). Theoretical studies of motoneuron models by Rall (1959, 1962, 1964, 1967) had emphasized some of the functional implications of dendritic morphology prior to their encounter by the experimentalists. Many of these concepts have since been demonstrated and studied amply in papers such as those by Lux (1967), Nelson and Lux (1970), Lux, Schubert, and Kreutzberg (1970), Burke and Bruggencate (1971), Jack and Redman (1971), and Barrett and Crill (1974).

The basic postulate is that synaptic inputs occurring near the soma have a faster and more decisive depolarizing action at the level of the initial segment, and thus are more apt to produce activation of motoneurons. In contrast, the distal axodendritic synapses have a slower-rising and to a certain extent longer-lasting depolarization, which may serve more as a modulatory influence on neurons. It appears reasonable, therefore, that spinal reflexes (especially those of segmental origin) are distributed mainly in the proximal dendrosomatic area, and that less specific inputs, such as the reticulospinal system, are distributed on the dendrites (Llinás and Terzuolo, 1965; Terzuolo and Llinás, 1966; Kuno and Llinás, 1970). This latter site of termination could thus exercise a wider and rather unspecific action in what could be analogous to the so-called "central excitatory and central inhibitory states." This state of affairs was further modified by description of dendritic spikes with intracellular recording, first reported by Spencer and Kandel (1961) in hippocampal neurons. This demonstration at the intracellular level was followed by a series of papers on this subject, which were summarized by Purpura in 1967. However, even before this time, it had been observed that spinal motoneurons could generate dendritic spikes if their axons were transected (Eccles, Libet, and Young, 1958; McIntyre, Bradley, and Brock, 1959). These findings were confirmed and enlarged upon by Lux and Winter (1968), Shapovalov and Grantyn (1968), and Kuno and Llinás (1970). More recently, Baker and Precht (1972) have demonstrated possible dendritic spikes in normal trochlear motoneurons, and Czeh (1972) and Precht et al. (1974) in the frog spinal motoneurons and vestibular neurons, respectively.

Controversy still remained, however, as to whether the prepotentials observed by Spencer and Kandel (1961) or the fast depolarization observed in chromatolyzed motoneurons indeed represented dendritic spikes rather than local responses of a decremental nature. In theory, these could be evoked by an injured portion of membrane in the somadendritic area or in the axon or axon collaterals. The most recent confrontation between the proponents of dendritic spikes and those opposing this concept occurred following the publication of Llinás, Nicholson, Freeman, and Hillman (1968), in which the authors proposed that reptilian Purkinje cell dendrites had electroresponsive properties as measured by field potentials and current-density analysis (Llinás and Nicholson, 1969). In a series of communications, Calvin (1969), Calvin and Hellerstein (1969), and Zucker (1969) discussed the various pros and cons regarding the interpretation of these fields. Final clarification of the point was obtained by intradendritic recording from Purkinje cells (Llinás and Nicholson, 1971) and by verification of the conclusion reached by field-potential analysis. This verification was made possible through the development of a mathematical model for field-potential analysis (Nicholson and Llinás, 1971; Nicholson, 1973; cf. Werman, 1972).

Assuming, therefore, that the question of dendritic spike generation has been settled, one may question their functional significance. It is clear that the presence of dendritic spikes in some ways complicates our early view of integration as a simple algebraic summation of synaptic inputs. However, the presence of dendritic spikes does not modify the view that integration must be subserved by temporal and spatial summation. It simply states that summation to the point of spike generation may occur in more than one site in a given neuron. From this finding it follows that if integration is defined as the summation of graded depolarization to the level of an action potential,[2] then the unit of integration does not necessarily represent a "confederation" of such integrative segments. Based on this hypothesis of partial independence of dendritic integration (Llinás and Nicholson, 1969, 1971), several functional properties of dendritic spikes in neurons may be postulated.

DENDRITIC SPIKES

Independence of Dendritic Spike Generation in Neurons

Several examples are now available to illustrate independence of dendritic spike generation in neurons. In chromatolyzed motoneurons, Kuno and Llinás (1970) have shown that a given neuron may generate several distinct all-or-none potentials following afferent fiber stimulation. A close scrutiny of these action potentials demonstrated that they are a rather stereotyped group of events. Based on their amplitude and duration, it is possible to recognize, in a given cell, two, three, or more repeating patterns of electro-responsive activation. For instance, in Fig. 1 (A, a to e) it is obvious that the all-or-none potential indicated by a dot has the same amplitude and time course in all the traces, and that the potential indicated by an asterisk has a very distinct and repeated waveform as well, but very different from the one indicated by a dot. The obvious conclusion would be that these two spikes

---

[2] This point is particularly relevant since the discovery of dendrodendritic synapses (Rall, Shepherd, Reese, and Brightman, 1966). It is theoretically possible to have a dendritic segment generating a spike and acting upon other neurons without the generation of an axonal spike.

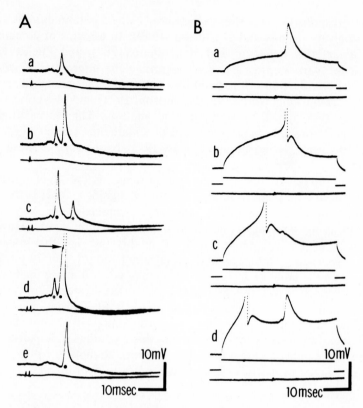

FIG. 1. (A) Responses of a chromatolyzed motoneuron to muscle afferent volleys from the quadriceps; 18 days after axotomy. (Upper traces) Intracellular potentials; (lower traces) afferent volleys recorded from the cord surface. (a,b) Responses to single afferent stimulation; (c–e) responses to two successive afferent stimuli. Arrow in (d) indicates an inflection between the partial response and the action potential (the action potential retouched by dots). (B) Responses of a chromatolyzed motoneuron to muscle afferent volleys from the triceps surae during postsynaptic depolarization, 19 days after axotomy. (Upper traces) Intracellular potentials; middle traces, recordings of currents applied; (lower traces) afferent volleys recorded from the cord surface. Note elimination of partial response at a short interval following directly evoked action potential (c). Ten-mV calibration also indicates current of 10 nA. Spikes retouched by dots. (Modified from Kuno and Llinás, 1970.)

represent activations generated at different portions of the neuron, probably from different dendritic branches. This conclusion is readily acceptable for motoneurons for it is well known that five to seven main dendrites branch off directly from their soma. The demonstration that these spikes are generated in different dendritic segments is illustrated in Fig. 1A,d. Here the generation of one action potential does not impede generation of the other, which suggests that they are summing at the somatic level, as they are not mutually refractory. The most parsimonious conclusion, therefore, is that in chromatolyzed motoneurons each dendrite may generate an action potential that is conducted in a decremental manner to the soma, the soma itself being the site of summation of spikes coming from the different dendritic segments. An example of summation of these dendritic inputs is shown in Fig. 1A,d. Other examples of the property of independence of the dendritic spike have been discussed at length for Purkinje cells in the alligator (Llinás and Nicholson, 1969, 1971; Nicholson and Llinás, 1971).

Uni- and Bidirectional Conduction of Dendritic Spikes

One of the most salient of the basic postulates of neuronal function introduced by Ramón y Cajal (1911) was that of "dynamic polarization." He viewed the "directions of nervous currents" as traveling via afferents onto the dendrites, the acceptor pole of the neurons. From the acceptor poles the current was then visualized as moving into the soma and out through the axon. This "dynamic polarization" ensured that brain circuits be utilized in only one direction. This unidirectionality of nervous flow was assumed by Sherrington (1906) to occur at the synaptic level, for it was shown that central synapses can conduct only in one direction (however, cf. Decima and Goldberg, 1970). The electrophysiology of nerve cells, especially in motoneurons, has emphasized the fact that following the activation of the axon and somadendritic components of the action potentials, the dendrites

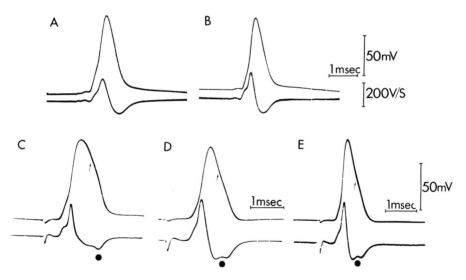

FIG. 2. Antidromic invasion of normal and of chromatolyzed motoneurons 9 days after axotomy. (A,B) Normal motoneurons; (C–E) chromatolyzed motoneurons showing a third component in the falling phase of the action potential (arrow). Differentiated records accentuate the distinguishing features of normal motoneurons (lower traces in A and B) and chromatolyzed neurons (lower traces in C–E). The third potential found in the falling phase of the action potentials is demonstrated by an upward deflection in the differentiated record (dots). (Llinás and Alley, *unpublished results.*)

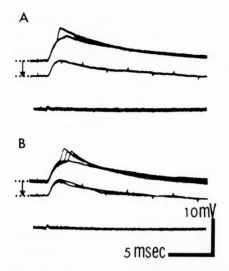

FIG. 3. Responses of a chromatolyzed motoneuron to muscle afferent volleys from the biceps semitendinosus, 18 days after axotomy. (A,B) Lower traces, monosynaptic excitatory postsynaptic potentials (EPSP's) with reticular inhibitory stimulation; upper traces, without reticular inhibitory stimulation. Note elimination of partial responses by reticular stimulation. (Modified from Kuno and Llinás, 1970.)

may be invaded. This antidromic invasion into dendrites has an erasing action on the integrative activity for a period lasting many milliseconds (Coombs, Eccles, and Fatt, 1955). In fact, antidromic invasion of dendrites in motoneurons was postulated by Fatt (1957) and was recorded by Terzuolo and Araki (1961). A different demonstration of antidromic invasion of dendrites was recently produced in chromatolyzed neurons (Kuno and Llinás, 1970). Among the distinctive changes in waveform generated by chromatolysis is the appearance of a third large component in the intracellularly recorded action potential. Thus, besides the initial segment (IS) and somadendritic (SD) potentials described by Coombs, Eccles, and Fatt (1955), a third depolarization (Fig. 2, arrow) is present in chromatolyzed motoneurons; this most probably represents the antidromic invasion of the dendritic tree, which in chromatolyzed motoneurons has electroresponsive properties. This particular dendritic component may be powerful enough to generate a total reactivation of the neuron (Llinás and Alley, *unpublished observations*). Furthermore, inhibition known to be distributed mainly in motoneuron dendrites, such as in the reticular inhibitory system (Llinás and Terzuolo, 1965; Kuno and Llinás, 1970), is able to block specifically the orthodromically evoked dendritic spikes (Kuno and Llinás, 1970) (Fig. 3). The actual demonstration that action potentials do invade antidromically was provided by Kuno and Llinás (1970), who showed that orthodromic dendritic spikes have a refractory period of approximately 6 msec following either antidromic invasion or direct stimulation through the recording intrasomatic microelectrode (Fig. 1B,a–d).

A different situation, however, appears to occur in Purkinje cells. Here the antidromic invasion of the cell seems to be blocked at the level of the main dendrites as demonstrated by field potential analysis (Nicholson and Llinás, 1971). Whereas orthodromic activation of Purkinje cells can give field potentials with large sinks at the superficial level, such types of potentials cannot be obtained following antidromic invasion. These results together with those from intradendritic recordings strongly support the view that, in these rather complex cells, dendritic spikes may be unidirectionally conducted in a somatopetal direction. Somatofugal spikes cannot actively invade the dendritic tree because of the heavy load imposed by the dendritic tree on the ascending action current and by possible impedance mismatch (Llinás and Nicholson, 1969, 1971; Nicholson and Llinás, 1971). In this manner, a type of "dynamic polarization" may be achieved, caused by the electrical properties of the neuron in question. The conduction of dendritic spikes in this case is envisaged as a type of pseudosaltatory conduction. A local stimulation evokes a large depolarization in a given dendrite (Fig. 4A). If the dendrite is hyperpolarized to different levels during the generation of the dendritic spikes, several all-or-none components may be observed (arrows in Fig. 4A). A reconstruction of the potential produced by the addition of the all-or-none components (Fig. 4B) gives an exact analogue of the intradendritic spike recorded in this Purkinje dendrite. The mode of generation and conduction of the dendritic spikes is diagrammed in Fig. 4C.

A similar conclusion regarding unidirectional dendritic spike conduction was reached by Kidokoro (1969) in the oculomotor neurons of fish where dendritic spiking appeared to be readily conducted orthodromically, but antidromic dendritic invasion was shown to be lacking in many instances.

Dendritic Spikes in Conjunction with Electrotonic Coupling

In the last few years a series of papers on teleost oculomotor neurons (Kidokoro, 1969; Kriebel, Bennett, Waxman, and Pappas, 1969; Korn and Bennett, 1971, 1972) have shown that these neurons are electrotonically coupled. The actual coupling appears to occur by means of electrotonic junctions between vestibular afferents and the somas of the oculomotor neurons (Kidokoro, 1969; Kriebel et al., 1969). The functional implication of the somasomatic coupling, however, became clear only when a mechanism of nystagmus was studied in these fish (Korn and Bennett, 1971, 1972). Whereas the somatic input is amply capable of activating these motoneurons, the coupling that occurs through common afferents ensures a synchronous activation of the motoneurons. This form of activation appears to be the underlying mechanism for generation of the rapid (saccadic) eye movement during nystagmus. Although it is evident that the electrotonic coupling between neurons is not very great, it would tend to facilitate synchronous activation of the oculomotor pool. The authors go on to demonstrate that during the slow eye movements following a saccade, oculomotor neurons are activated through dendritic inputs that are able to generate dendritic spikes of sufficient magnitude to generate full spike initiation at the axon hillock. From a functional point of view, therefore, the same set of

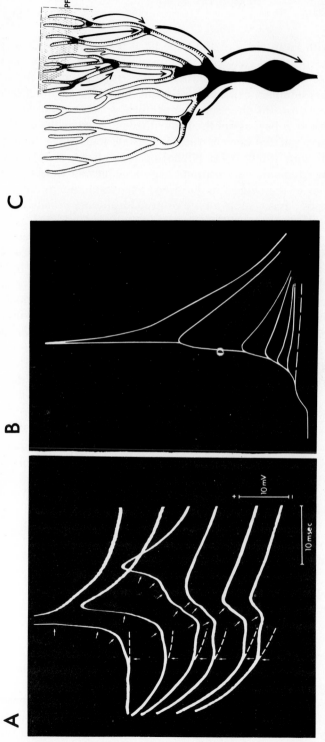

FIG. 4. Intracellular recording in alligator Purkinje cells. (A) Action potentials recorded in Purkinje cells. (A) Action potentials recorded in Purkinje cell dendrite 200 μm from the surface. Succes- sive hyperpolarizing current injected through the recording electrode revealed that the large dendritic spike shown on the first trace is actually produced by the addition of all-or-none components (arrows). This dendritic spike was generated by a dendritic EPSP produced by parallel fiber stimulation (upward arrow). As the hyperpolarization is increased, the different all-or-none depolarizing potentials are blocked in a sequential manner. (B) Reconstruction of the intradendritic action potential showing the six all-or-none components shown in (A). (C) Diagram of mechanism of dendritic spike generation. Each all-or-none component is taken to be generated by a different hot spot (shown as a dark area) at or near den- dritic bifurcation. The action potential is produced by the summation of all-or-none local responses that finally reach the soma and generate a full outgoing action potential. (Modified from Llinás and Nicholson, 1971.)

neurons can, in principle, be utilized synchronously to generate a rapid movement, and asynchronously to produce a more protracted motion. Because the coupling between somas is feeble, action potentials in given neurons do not necessarily activate neighboring cells. This view of neuronal integration differs from that which supposes dendritic inputs as establishing a tonic modulation of neuronal firing and somatic inputs as having a more decisive type of action. In contrast, it is very much in keeping with the view that dendritic segments may serve as integrational subunits.

DENDRITIC INHIBITION

The classic view of inhibition has assumed that inhibition occurs for the most part at the somatic level (Eccles, 1957; Eccles, 1964; Andersen and Eccles, 1965). However, electrophysiologic data have been accumulating which demonstrate that inhibition can also occur at the dendritic level and that it may have a rather decisive role in neuronal integration (Llinás and Terzuolo, 1965; Diamond, 1968; Kidokoro et al., 1968; Llinás and Nicholson, 1969, 1971; Kuno and Llinás, 1970; Burke, Fedina, and Lundberg, 1971; Nicholson and Llinás, 1971; Cook and Cangiano, 1972). The apparent conclusions are that dendritic inhibition may have a rather tonic action on the neuronal system by hyperpolarizing the neuron without significantly changing the resistive properties of the soma or initial dendrites (Llinás and Terzuolo, 1965). In this manner, a tonic depression in some ways similar to the "central inhibitory state" can be obtained without a grave shunting of the synaptic inputs terminating in the somatic and proximal dendritic region. It would thus be once again a modulatory effect.

Another advantage of dendritic inhibition, especially in neurons capable of initiating dendritic spikes, is that of functional amputation of the activity of certain dendritic segments (Llinás and Nicholson, 1969). Their importance is especially clear when coupled with the view that dendrites can generate action potentials independently from the activity of other dendrites or the soma. Morphologic studies of cerebellum (Llinás and Hillman, 1969; Chan-Palay and Palay, 1972) and of cortical structures (Gottlieb and Cowan, 1972) favor the view of dendritic location of inhibitory synapses in remote dendrites. In the case of Purkinje cells, this distinction is rather significant given that excitatory terminals tend to establish contact with spines in the dendrites. This form of termination may be visualized as serving a "current-limiting resistor" function (Llinás and Hillman, 1969), which allows a more linear summation of synaptic potentials at the expense of a reduced efficacy for any particular synapse. However, direct synaptic contact of inhibitory boutons with the smooth portion of dendrites would ensure that the shunt produced by the activation of this synapse completely annihilates all currents arising from related dendritic branches peripheral to that particular junctional location (Llinás and Hillman, 1969). This rather critical placement of synapses suggests that the strategic location of inhibitory synapses may have the function of specifically shunting out particular portions of afferent inputs to a given neuron.

In this respect a very elegant set of experiments by Spira and Bennett (1972) further strengthens the case. In the invertebrate *Navanax*, these authors have demonstrated that activation of the inhibitory system produced a marked reduction of the potentials generated by electrotonic coupling between these neurons without greatly affecting the overall input resistance of the cell. As in the case of the reticular formation projection onto motoneurons and of the stellate inhibition on the dendrites of Purkinje cells, it is thus implied that inhibitory terminals can be strategically located to modify the integrative properties, either (1) by modulating the activity in the neuron, or (2) by shunting in a more or less specific manner the coupling between cells, without greatly modifying the activity generated by other inputs onto other portions of the same cell. It must be concluded, therefore, that inhibition should be understood not only as a mechanism capable of preventing spike initiation in a global sense, but also as a mechanism capable of changing the integrative properties of neurons by their strategic spatial distribution in the somadendritic area. (See note added in proof.)

SUMMARY

A brief sketch of the historic development of the concept of neuronal integration is given. Some of the properties of dendritic spikes in chromatolyzed motoneurons, alligator Purkinje cells, and fish oculomotor neurons are reviewed, as well as the various ways in which the generation of dendritic spikes has altered our basic concept of neuronal integration. The principles of dendritic inhibition are elaborated, both as a "tonic modulatory action" and as a "functional amputating system" for dendrites that generate spikes.

ACKNOWLEDGMENT

This research was supported by USPHS research grant NS-09116 from the National Institute of Neurological Diseases and Stroke.

REFERENCES

Andersen, P., and Eccles, J. C. (1965): Locating and identifying postsynaptic inhibitory synapses by the correlation of physiological and histological data. *Symp. Biol. Hung.*, 5:219–242.

Baker, R., and Precht, W. (1972): Electrophysiological properties of trochlear motoneurons as revealed by IVth nerve stimulation. *Exp. Brain Res.*, 14:127–157.

Barrett, J. N., and Crill, W. E. (1974): Influence of dendritic location and membrane properties on the effectiveness of synapses on cat motoneurones. *J. Physiol.*, 239:325–345.

Brock, L. G., Coombs, J. S., and Eccles, J. C. (1952): The recording of potentials from motoneurones with an intracellular electrode. *J. Physiol.* 117:431–460.

Burke, R. E. (1967): Composite nature of the monosynaptic excitatory postsynaptic potential. *J. Neurophysiol.,* 30:1114–1137.

Burke, R. E., and ten Bruggencate, G. (1971): Electrotonic characteristics of alpha motoneurones of varying size. *J. Physiol.,* 212:1–20.

Burke, R. E., Fedina, L., and Lundberg, A. (1971): Spatial synaptic distribution of recurrent and group Ia inhibitory systems in cat spinal motoneurones. *J. Physiol.,* 214:305–326.

Calvin, W. H. (1969). Dendritic spikes revisited. *Science,* 166:637–638.

Calvin, W. H., and Hellerstein, D. (1969). Dendritic spikes vs cable properties. *Science,* 163:96–97.

Chan-Palay, V., and Palay, S. L. (1970): Interrelations of basket cell axons and climbing fibers in the cerebellar cortex of the rat. *Z. Anat. Entwicklungsgesch.,* 132:191–227.

Cook, W. A., Jr., and Cangiano, A. (1972): Presynaptic and postsynaptic inhibition of spinal motoneurons. *J. Neurophysiol.,* 35:389–403.

Coombs, J. S., Eccles, J. C., and Fatt, P. (1955): Excitatory synaptic action in motoneurons. *J. Physiol.,* 130:374–395.

Czéh, G. (1972): The role of dendritic events in the initiation of monosynaptic spikes in frog motoneurons. *Brain Res.,* 39:505–509.

Decima, E. E., and Goldberg, L. J. (1970): Centrifugal dorsal root discharges induced by motoneurone activation. *J. Physiol.,* 207:103–118.

Diamond, J. (1968): The activation and distribution of GABA and L-glutamate receptors on goldfish Mauthner neurons: An analysis of dendritic remote inhibition (with appendix by A. F. Huxley). *J. Physiol.,* 194:669–723.

Eccles, J. C. (1957): *The Physiology of Nerve Cells.* Johns Hopkins Press, Baltimore, Maryland.

Eccles, J. C. (1964): *The Physiology of Synapses.* Springer-Verlag, Berlin, Gottingen, and Heidelberg.

Eccles, J. C., Libet, B., and Young, R. R. (1958): The behaviour of chromatolysed motoneurones studied by intracellular recording. *J. Physiol.,* 143:11–40.

Fadiga, E., and Brookhart, J. M. (1962): Interactions of excitatory postsynaptic potentials generated at different sites on the frog motoneurons. *J. Neurophysiol.,* 25:790–804.

Fuortes, M. G. F., Frank, K., and Becker, M. C. (1957): Steps in the production of motoneuron spikes. *J. Gen. Physiol.,* 40:735–752.

Gottlieb, D. I., and Cowan, W. M. (1972): Distribution of axonal terminals containing spheroidal and flattened synaptic vesicles in hippocampus and dentate gyrus of rat and cat. *Z. Zellforsch. Mikrosk. Anat.,* 129:413–429.

Jack, J. J. B., Miller, S., Porter, R., and Redman, S. J. (1971): The time course of minimal excitatory postsynaptic potentials evoked in spinal motoneurones by group Ia afferent fibres. *J. Physiol.,* 215:353–380.

Jack, J. J. B., and Redman, S. J. (1971): An electrical description of the motoneurone and its application to the analysis of synaptic potentials. *J. Physiol.,* 215:321–352.

Kidokoro, Y. (1969): Cerebellar and vestibular control of fish oculomotor neurones. In: *Neurobiology of Cerebellar Evolution and Development,* edited by R. Llinás, pp. 257–276. American Medical Association, Chicago, Illinois.

Kidokoro, Y., Kubota, K., Shuto, S., and Sumino, R. (1968): Reflex organization of cat masticatory muscles. *J. Neurophysiol.,* 31:695–708.

Korn, H., and Bennett, M. V. L. (1971): Dendritic and somatic impulse initiation in fish oculomotor neurons during vestibular nystagmus. *Brain Res.,* 27:169–175.

Korn, H., and Bennett, M. V. L. (1972): Electrotonic coupling between teleost oculomotor neurons: Restriction to somatic regions and relation to function of somatic and dendritic sites of impulse initiation. *Brain Res.,* 38:433–439.

Kriebel, M. E., Bennett, M. V. L., Waxman, S. G., and Pappas, G. D. (1969): Oculomotor neurons in fish: Electrotonic coupling and multiple sites of impulse initiation. *Science,* 166:520–523.

Kuno, M., and Llinás, R. (1970): Enhancement of synaptic transmission by dendritic potentials in chromatolysed motoneurones of the cat. *J. Physiol.,* 210:807–821.

Kuno, M., and Miyahara, J. T. (1969): Non-linear summation of unit synaptic potentials in spinal motoneurones of the cat. *J. Physiol.,* 201:465–477.

Llinás, R., and Hillman, D. E. (1969): Physiological and morphological organization of the cerebellar circuits of various vertebrates. In: *Neurobiology of Cerebellar Evolution and Development,* edited by R. Llinás, pp. 43–73. American Medical Association, Chicago, Illinois.

Llinás, R., and Nicholson, C. (1969): Electrophysiological analysis of alligator cerebellum: A study on dendritic spikes. In: *Neurobiology of Cerebellar Evolution and Development,* edited by R. Llinás, pp. 431–465. American Medical Association, Chicago, Illinois.

Llinás, R., and Nicholson, C. (1971): Electrophysiological properties of dendrites and somata in alligator Purkinje cells. *J. Neurophysiol.,* 33:532–551.

Llinás, R., Nicholson, C., Freeman, J., and Hillman, D. E. (1968): Dendritic spikes and their inhibition in alligator Purkinje cells. *Science,* 160:1132–1135.

Llinás, R., and Terzuolo, C. A. (1964): Mechanisms of supraspinal actions upon spinal cord activities. Reticular inhibitory mechanism on alpha-extensor motoneurons. *J. Neurophysiol.,* 27:579–591.

Llinás, R., and Terzuolo, C. A. (1965): Mechanisms of supraspinal actions upon spinal cord activities. Reticular inhibitory mechanisms upon flexor motoneurons. *J. Neurophysiol.,* 28:413–422.

Lorente de Nó, R., and Condouris, G. A. (1959): Decremental conduction in peripheral nerve. Integration of stimuli in the neuron. *Proc. Natl. Acad. Sci. USA,* 45:592–617.

Lux, H. D. (1967): Eigenschaften eines Neuron-Modells mit Dendriten begrenzter Länge. *Pfluegers Arch.,* 297:238–255.

Lux, H. D., and Winter, P. (1968): Studies on EPSPs in normal and retrograde reacting facial motoneurones. *Proc. Int. Union Physiol. Sci.,* 7: Abst. 818.

Lux, H. D., Schubert, P., and Kreutzberg, S. W. (1970): Direct matching of morphological and electrophysiological data in cat spinal motoneurons. In: *Excitatory Synaptic Mechanisms,* edited by P. Andersen and J. K. S. Jansen. Universitetsforlaget, Oslo.

McIntyre, A. K., Bradley, K., and Brock, L. G. (1959): Responses of motoneurones undergoing chromatolysis. *J. Gen. Physiol.,* 42:931–958.

Nelson, P. G., and Burke, R. E. (1967): Delayed depolarization in cat spinal motoneurones. *Exp. Neurol.,* 17:16–26.

Nelson, P. G., and Lux, H. D. (1970): Some electrical measurements of motoneuron parameters. *Biophys. J.,* 10:55–73.

Nicholson, C. (1973): Theoretical analysis of field potentials in anisotropic ensembles of neuronal elements. *IEEE Trans. Biomed. Eng.,* BME-20:278–288.

Nicholson, C., and Llinás, R. (1971): Field potentials in the alligator cerebellum and theory of their relationship to Purkinje cell dendritic spikes. *J. Neurophysiol.,* 34:509–531.

Precht, W., Richter, A., Ozawa, S., and Shimazu, H. (1974): Intracellular study of frog's vestibular neurons in relation to the labyrinth and spinal cord. *Exp. Brain Res.,* 19:377–393.

Purpura, D. P. (1967): Comparative physiology of dendrites. In: *The Neurosciences: A Study Program,* edited by G. C. Quarton, T. Melnechuk, and F. O. Schmitt, pp. 372–393. Rockefeller Univ. Press, New York.

Rall, W. (1959): Branching dendritic trees and motoneuron membrane resistivity. *Exp. Neurol.,* 1:491–527.

Rall, W. (1962): Electrophysiology of a dendritic neuron model. *Biophys. J.,* 2 (No. 2, Pt. 2): 145–167.

Rall, W. (1964): Theoretical significance of dendritic trees for neuronal input–output relations. In: *Neural Theory and Modelling,* edited by R. F. Reiss, pp. 73–97. Stanford Univ. Press, Stanford, California.

Rall, W. (1967): Distinguishing theoretical synaptic potentials computed for different soma-dendritic distributions of synaptic input. *J. Neurophysiol.,* 30:1138–1168.

Rall, W. (1971): Cable properties of dendrites and effects of synaptic location. In: *Excitatory Synaptic Mechanisms,* edited by P. Andersen and J. K. S. Jansen, pp. 175–187. Universitetsforlaget, Oslo.

Rall, W., Burke, R. E., Smith, T. G., Nelson, P. G., and Frank, K. (1967): Dendritic location of synapses and possible mechanisms for the monosynaptic EPSP in motoneurons. *J. Neurophysiol.,* 30:1170–1193.

Rall, W., Shepherd, G. M., Reese, T. S., and Brightman, M. W. (1966): Dendro-dendritic synaptic pathway for inhibition in the olfactory bulb. *Exp. Neurol.,* 14:44–56.

Ramón y Cajal, S. (1911): *Histologie du système nerveux de l'homme et des vertébrés.* Maloine, Paris.

Shapovalov, A. I., and Grantyn, A. A. (1968): Nadsegmentarnye sinapticheskie vliianiia na khromatolizirovannye motoneurony. *Biofizika,* 13:260–269.

Sherrington, C. S. (1906): *The Integrative Action of the Nervous System,* p. 18. Yale Univ. Press, New Haven and London.

Smith, T. G., Wuerker, R. B., and Frank, K. (1967): Membrane impedance changes during synaptic transmission in cat spinal motoneurones. *J. Neurophysiol.,* 30:1072–1096.

Spencer, W. A., and Kandel, E. R. (1961): Electrophysiology of hippocampal neurons. IV. Fast prepotentials. *J. Neurophysiol.,* 24:272–285.

Spira, M. E., and Bennett, M. V. L. (1972): Synaptic control of electrotonic coupling between neurons. *Brain Res.,* 37:294–300.

Terzuolo, C. A., and Araki, T. (1961): An analysis of intra- versus extracellular potential changes associated with activity of single spinal motoneurones. *Ann. NY Acad. Sci.,* 94:547–558.

Terzuolo, C. A., and Llinás, R. (1966): Distribution of synaptic inputs in the spinal motoneurone and its functional significance. In: *Nobel Symposium I. Muscular Afferents and Motor Control,* edited by R. Granit, pp. 373–384. Almqvist and Wiksell, Stockholm.

Werman, R. (1972): CNS cellular level: Membranes. *Ann. Rev. Physiol.,* 34:337–374.

Zucker, R. S. (1969): Field potentials generated by dendritic spikes and synaptic potentials. *Science,* 165:409–413.

Note: The possibility that chemical synapses may modulate electrotonic coupling at the cat inferior olive has recently been suggested (Llinás et al., and Sotelo et al., 1974: *J. Neurophysiol.,* 37:541–571).

Advances in Neurology, Vol. 12, edited by
G. W. Kreutzberg, Raven Press, New York
© 1975.

Some Dendritic Properties of Amphibian Neurons

Wolfgang Precht

Neurobiologische Abteilung, Max-Planck-Institut für Hirnforschung, Frankfurt am Main, Germany

Since the classic work of Araki and Otani (1955), Araki, Otani, and Furukawa (1953), Brookhart and Fadiga (1960), Fadiga and Brookhart (1960, 1962), and Washizu (1960), amphibian spinal motoneurons have played an important role in the investigation of electrical and functional properties of different areas of central neurons. Two findings are of particular interest in the context of this chapter: (1) motoneurons appear to be electrotonically coupled with each other, presumably through their dendrites; and (2) functionally different inputs (lateral column and dorsal root pathways) connect with a spatially different area of the motoneuron membrane (soma and dendrites, respectively). Because there was no evidence to suggest electrically excitable dendrites it was assumed that—as in motoneurons of higher vertebrates—distal dendritic inputs influence the level of polarization at the soma by electrotonic propagation of the excitatory postsynaptic potential (EPSP).

The results presented in this chapter deal with a comparison of some characteristics of amphibian vestibular, ocular motor, and spinal motoneurons. They strongly suggest that vestibular neurons, in particular, are capable of generating dendritic spikes in response to various inputs including electrical transmission. Such dendritic responses were, however, only occasionally observed in ocular and spinal motoneurons. In addition the dendrites of vestibular and spinal motoneurons appear to play a role in the electrical coupling between neurons or between afferents and neurons.

METHODS

Experiments were performed on *Rana esculenta* or *R. temporaria* at room temperature (20° to 22°C). Dissecting procedures were carried out under MS 222 anesthesia. For recording the animals were unanesthetized and immobilized by i.p. injection of *d*-tubocurarine (0.5 mg/kg). Responses of vestibular neurons were studied following their activation by ipsi- and contralateral VIIIth nerve stimulation as well as by electrical stimulation of the spinal cord (for methods see Precht, Richter, Ozawa, and Shimazu, 1974). Ocular motoneurons of the VIth and IIIrd nuclei were investigated after their antidromic and synaptic activation by both the motor nerves and the VIIIth nerves (Magherini, Precht, and Schwindt, 1974). Studies on hind-limb motoneurons were performed in the *in situ* spinal cord. Antidromic and synaptic activation of motoneurons was produced by electrical stimulation of ventral roots or sciatic nerve (dorsal roots 8 to 11 cut) and dorsal roots, respectively (for details see Magherini, Precht, and Schwindt, 1975*a*). Intracellular potentials from these three types of neurons were recorded with glass micropipettes filled with 3 M KCl or 2 M potassium citrate.

VESTIBULAR NEURONS

Following stimulation of the ipsi- and contralateral vestibular nerves, spike-like partial responses were superimposed on the EPSP's in most vestibular neurons (Fig. 1A–C,E,F,I,J,H). EPSP's were evoked only occasionally without the partial responses superimposed on them (Fig. 1D). The generation of partial spikes had no direct relationship with the level of depolarization measured presumably at the cell body of the vestibular neuron (Fig. 1B,I,J). Full action potentials were evoked in most cells. When the intensity of vestibular nerve stimulation was increased they appeared to be generated from partial spikes of different amplitudes (Fig. 1E,F,I). When hyperpolarizing currents were applied across the cell membrane through the intracellular electrode, the full action potentials evoked by VIIIth nerve stimulation were easily blocked, whereas the partial spikes were little affected (Fig. 1I,J). Application of depolarizing current pulses through the intracellular electrode as well as postanodal rebound events failed to evoke the partial spikes. In contrast, partial spikes often occurred spontaneously (Fig. 1G).

In some neurons the EPSP's were preceded by early depolarizing potentials (EDP's) (latencies 0.5 to 1.1 msec), even at very low stimulus intensities (Fig. 2). It was previously postulated that the vestibular EDP's were generated by electrical transmission, which may occur between primary afferent and vestibular neurons, and/or by electrotonic coupling between secondary vestibular neurons and efferent vestibular neurons (Precht, Richter, Ozawa, and Shimazu, 1974). The vestibular EDP's consisted of graded small potentials (Fig. 2A–C,F–K,L–O) at low intensities; and all-or-none partial spike responses similar to the ones described above were superimposed on the graded potential with higher intensities of stimulation (Fig. 2B,L–N). A further increase in stimulus intensity generated full action potentials (Fig. 2B,I,N). Whereas the full action potentials were easily blocked by the application of hyperpolarizing currents through the micropipette, the EDP's generally were not affected by polarizing currents (Fig. 2O). Occasionally, small EDP's showed no refractoriness when they followed a full spike with a short interval (Fig. 2E). These EDP's are for the most part the graded component of the early depolarizations and represent the true coupling potentials.

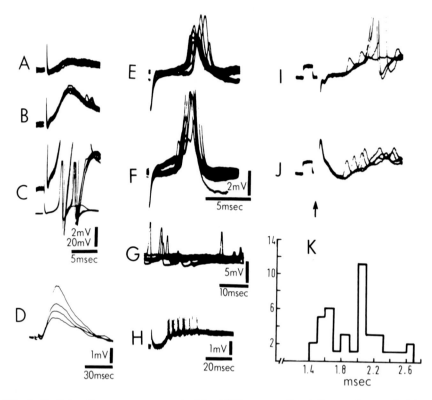

FIG. 1. Partial spike responses evoked by VIIIth nerve stimulation and recorded from vestibular neurons. (A–C)EPSP's evoked at different intensities of ipsilateral VIIIth nerve stimulation. (D) Superposition of EPSP's evoked at four different intensities of contralateral VIIIth nerve stimulation (each trace consists of 16 computer-averaged responses). (E,F) Partial spikes evoked from vestibular neuron by ipsilateral VIIIth nerve stimulation. (G) Spontaneously occurring dendritic spikes. (H) EPSP and dendritic spikes evoked by contralateral VIIIth nerve stimulation. (I,J) Another neuron showing dendritic spikes and full spikes after ipsilateral VIIIth nerve stimulation. (I) Control; (J) blockage of full spike by hyperpolarizing current injection; (K) frequency histogram of ipsilaterally evoked EPSP's recorded in vestibular neurons. Time and voltage calibrations as indicated; pulses in I,J indicate 1 msec, 1 mV.

All-or-none partial spikes of very short latencies (Fig. 3O) (time to peak: 0.85 ± 0.3 msec; half-decay time: 0.5 ± 0.2 msec) were also evoked in many vestibular neurons following stimulation of the spinal cord in the region of the vestibulospinal tract (Precht, Richter, Ozawa, and Shimazu, 1974). EPSP's and partial spikes of longer latencies were evoked in vestibular neurons with strong stimulation of the cord. Because the latencies of the early partial spikes overlapped with those of the antidromic action potentials (Fig. 3O), and because they were never evoked by peripheral nerve stimulation, it was concluded that they were caused by electrotonic transmission between neighboring neurons (Precht, Richter, Ozawa, and Shimazu, 1974). In individual neurons partial spikes occasionally preceded the

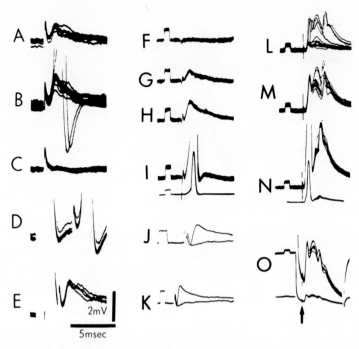

FIG. 2. Early EDP's recorded in vestibular neurons after ipsilateral VIIIth nerve stimulation. (A,B) EDP's and action potentials evoked with weak and stronger stimulation. (C) Extracellular control; (D) vestibular evoked spike (second response) was preceded by action potential evoked by a depolarizing pulse applied across the membrane at longer (D) and shorter intervals (E). (F–K) EDP's in another neuron evoked with increasing strength of stimulation (F–I); (J,K) Superposition of computer-averaged (16 responses) intra- and extracellular traces. (L–O) EDP's of graded and all-or-none nature evoked in vestibular neuron with increasing stimulus strengths (L–N). (O) Effect of hyperpolarizing pulse (40 nA) on spike and EDP's. Note blockage of full spike and survival of EDP's. Time and voltage calibrations as indicated; pulses give 1 msec, 1 mV except for lower trace in I (10 mV); (I) also applies for low gain traces in (N) and (O).

antidromic activation of the neuron (Fig. 3C) or had a higher threshold than the antidromic firing (Fig. 3A,B). These true antidromic activations of vestibulospinal tract neurons were used to construct the lower histogram of Fig. 3O. As with the vestibular evoked EDP's the spinal evoked EDP's consisted of graded and all-or-none components of different amplitudes (Fig. 3C,D–H) and were recruited by increasing stimulus intensities. Full spikes were evoked when the EDP's reached the firing level of the neuron (Fig. 3G,H,I,J,L). As shown in Fig. 3I–K, application of hyperpolarizing currents across the cell membrane blocked the full spikes, thereby revealing EDP's (Fig. 3J). With stronger hyperpolarizing currents (40 nA) some components were blocked but the EDP's still were not entirely abolished (Fig. 3K). In Fig. 3L–N the full action potentials (Fig. 3L) were preceded

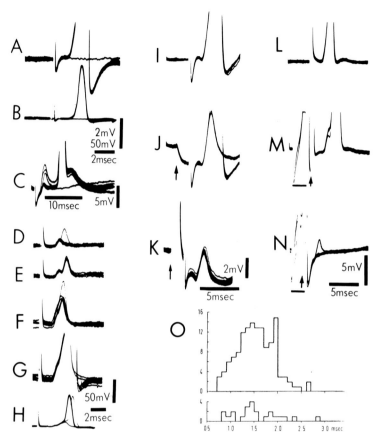

FIG. 3. EDP's recorded in vestibular neurons after stimulation of the spinal cord. (A,B) Antidromic activation of vestibulospinal tract cell. Note absence of prepotential at this intensity. (C) Antidromic activation of vestibulospinal tract cell, and preceding EDP's. (D–H) Spinal EDP's taken in the same neuron as in (A) and (B) with increasing intensities of stimulation. Stimulation site in (D–H) was more caudal than in (A,B). (I–K) Effects of hyperpolarizing current pulses of different magnitudes applied across the membrane. (I) control; (J) 10 nA; (K) 40 nA. (L–N) shows postspike refractoriness for spinal EDP's. (L) Control; M,N, direct activation of the neuron by applying a depolarizing pulse through the microelectrode precedes stimulation of the spinal cord at different intervals. Durations of depolarizing current pulses are shown by horizontal bars below the potential traces. (O) Upper and lower diagrams show frequency distribution of latencies of EDP's and antidromic action potentials following spinal cord stimulation (latencies were normalized with respect to the latencies for conduction distance of 15 mm). Voltage calibration in (D–G) as in (A).

at various time intervals by intracellularly applied depolarizing pulses evoking full spikes (Fig. 3M–N). As the intervals between the two stimuli became shorter, the latency of the full spike increased, thus revealing EDP's (Fig. 3M). As the conduction time from the spinal cord to the site of the impaled neuron was 1.9 msec (Fig. 3L), and EDP's were evoked when spinal shocks were applied 1.4 msec after the onset of the directly evoked spikes, EDP's should have been mediated by axons different from that of the impaled cell. With shorter intervals (Fig. 3N) EDP's were abolished in all but one trial, indicating that some components of the EDP's were affected by refractoriness, which was intrinsic in the impaled cell. Refractoriness of EDP's was also shown with double shock stimulation of the spinal cord.

To summarize the above results it may be stated that central vestibular neurons are characterized by the presence of all-or-none partial spikes that occur spontaneously in response to ipsilateral and contralateral vestibular nerve stimulation, and in response to stimulation of the spinal cord. Partial spikes of different amplitudes were superimposed on the EPSP's, but their generation had no direct relationship with the level of depolarization measured at the cell body. In addition, partial spikes may be evoked in vestibular neurons by electrotonic coupling potentials evoked by ipsilateral VIIIth nerve or spinal cord stimulation. Finally, partial spikes were often superimposed on the humplike positive spike afterpotential. All of these partial spike responses evoked by different stimuli have similar time courses and amplitudes. In most cases hyperpolarizing currents applied across the membrane did not abolish partial spikes, and depolarizing current pulses or postanodal rebound events never evoked them. These findings suggest that the sites of origin of these spike-like partial responses are located at some distance from the soma, presumably in the dendrites. Therefore the dendritic membrane of frog vestibular neurons appears to be electrically excitable, and the various all-or-none components of the partial responses may represent spike responses generated in particular active dendritic areas. These active areas probably do not extend to the soma, so that a passive membrane region is interposed. Intracellular recordings from dendrites of Purkinje cells provided direct evidence for this assumption (Llinás and Nicholson, 1971). Partial responses similar to those described here were never seen in cat vestibular neurons but were observed in a variety of mammalian neurons. The mechanism for the generation of partial spikes postulated in this chapter is in keeping with the interpretation given by previous authors (Eccles, Libet, and Young, 1958; Spencer and Kandel, 1961; Kuno, Llinás, 1970; Llinás and Nicholson, 1971). One of the functional implications of dendritic spikes may be that they increase the efficacy of synaptic excitation occurring at distal regions of neurons that would otherwise be too small to influence the firing level of the neurons. Another important aspect of dendritic spike generation is related to the integrative properties, which become much more complex in the presence of the all-or-none events occurring in different segments and branches of dendritic trees. It cannot presently be explained why some neurons (e.g., vestibular neurons of amphibia) can electrically excite dendrites whereas others [e.g., spinal and ocular motoneurons of amphibia (see below) or vestibular neurons of higher vertebrates] lack this property.

OCULAR MOTONEURONS

In contrast with vestibular neurons, motoneurons of the oculomotor system generally did not show partial spikes on activation by various stimuli (Magherini, Precht, and Schwindt, 1974). As with many other neurons in the central nervous system these cells generated EPSP's that on increasing strength of VIIIth nerve stimulation gradually increased in amplitudes until firing level was reached. Only in very few cases were partial spike responses observed in conjunction with EPSP's or with the positive after-potential of the action potentials. Unlike their amphibian counterparts fish ocular motoneurons were characterized by the frequent occurrence of dendritic spikes in response to VIIIth nerve stimulation (Korn and Bennett, 1971).

SPINAL MOTONEURONS

As in the cat, spinal motoneurons of amphibia are large enough to permit stable intracellular recordings for periods long enough to study the electrical properties of the neuronal membrane. Some of the data relevant to the present subject will be briefly described. Morphologic studies of amphibian motoneurons have shown that their dendritic trees can be at least as extensive as those of cat motoneurons (Silver, 1942; Kennard, 1959; Stensaas and Stensaas, 1971). Because the extent of the dendritic tree is the main geometric factor governing input resistance in cat motoneurons (Rall, 1959; Nelson and Lux, 1970; Burke and ten Bruggencate, 1971; Barrett and Crill, 1974a) frog motoneurons might be expected to have a similar resistance. This assumption based on morphologic grounds has been confirmed in recent physiologic studies (Magherini, Precht, Schwindt, 1975a). It was found that the input resistance values obtained by the injected current pulse method in the *in situ* preparation ranges from 0.4 to 3 MΩ, which is almost identical to the range reported for cat spinal motoneurons (Coombs, Eccles, and Fatt, 1955). It should be pointed out, however, that the resistance values measured in frog motoneurons have to be interpreted with care because some of these neurons are electrically coupled (see below).

Previous studies have suggested that monosynaptic activation of different areas of the motoneuron membrane may be obtained by stimulating different inputs. Therefore in the anesthetized frog, stimulation of the dorsal roots and lateral column generated dendritic and somatic EPSP's, respectively (Fadiga and Brookhart, 1960). If the motoneurons behave like infinitely long cables, EPSP's occurring in distal dendrites would not be seen at the soma. In contrast, if motoneurons have a finite electrotonic length of one or two space constants, even the most remote dendritic input can have an important effect on the membrane potential at the soma (Barrett and Crill, 1974*b*). The electrotonic length of the motoneurons in terms of electrically equivalent uniform cables can be estimated by analyzing the responses of a neuron to the injection of subthreshold current pulses and by combining the measurements with a theory developed by Rall (1969). The responses of motoneurons to subthreshold hyperpolarizing and depolarizing currents were composed of two or more exponentials (Magherini, Precht, and Schwindt, 1975*a*). The long time constants ranged from 12.5 to 28 msec (mean 20 ± 4.7 msec SD), and the short time constants ranged from 1.5 to 3.6 msec (mean 2.5 ± 0.6 msec SD). These values are significantly longer than the time constants found in cat motoneurons (Nelson and Lux, 1970). Using the short and long time constants from frog motoneurons in the equation for a "sealed end" equivalent cylinder (Rall, 1969) resulted in electrotonic lengths of 1.0 to 1.5 space constants (mean 1.2 ± 0.2 SD), which suggests that the dendritic input may still have an important effect on the soma. It is necessary to mention again that the frog motoneuron time constants must be interpreted with caution as electric coupling between motoneurons would tend to make the time constant longer than the values resulting from membrane properties alone.

Spike afterpotentials have been used frequently to deduce conductance properties of the somadendritic membrane. In a recent study afterpotentials of frog motoneurons in the *in situ* preparation have been analyzed in detail (Magherini, Precht, and Schwindt, 1975*a*). Some points of interest in the context of dendritic properties will be mentioned here. It is generally believed that the positive afterpotential or delayed depolarization (DD) seen in many neurons after the spike potentials represents invasion of the dendrites by the full spike (Kernell, 1964; Nelson, Burke, 1967). The pronounced humplike DD generally recorded from frog motoneurons (Fig. 4A) differs somewhat in form from the DD in cat motoneurons (Kernell, 1964). In the cat, spike and hump form a continuous waveform, whereas in the frog, spike and hump are separated by the short afterhyperpolarization. The frog DD has the following characteristics: it is associated only with somadendritic invasion; it increases with hyperpolarization and decreases with depolarization; it shows summation when two action potentials are evoked in close succession; it summates with PSP's; and it can sometimes generate all-or-none potentials. Because the above characteristics of frog motoneurons DD's are similar to those recorded in cat, it may be assumed that the DD's recorded in frog motoneurons are also generated by dendritic invasion. However, the fact that even large DD's do not occlude but rather summate with dorsal root EPSP's (Fig. 4B,C), which presumably are generated in dendrites (Fadiga and Brookhart, 1960), indicates that dendritic invasion must be mainly passive or electrotonic. Therefore the motoneuronal dendrites are for the most part electrically nonexcitable as is the case in cat motoneurons. This notion is supported by the rare occurrence of partial-spike responses or dendritic spikes in frog motoneurons in

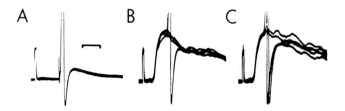

FIG. 4. Interaction of spikes and afterpotential components of spinal motoneurons with postsynaptic potentials. (A) Control antidromic action potential. (B) Antidromic spikes evoked on top of a dorsal-root-evoked EPSP. (C) Orthodromic spike from dorsal-root EPSP. Note summation of DD and long afterhyperpolarization with EPSP. Calibration: 10 mV pulse and 10 msec bar in (A) apply for (B) and (C).

response to dorsal-root stimulation (Czeh, 1972; Magherini, Precht, and Schwindt, 1975*a*). Thus, the dendrites of the spinal motoneurons appear to have different electrical properties than the vestibular neurons. In the frog no attempts have been made to study dendritic properties of chromatolyzed motoneurons, which are known to become electrically excitable in the cat (Eccles, Libet, Young, 1958; and Kuno and Llinás, 1970).

Finally, recurrent excitation of motoneurons should be discussed in relationship to the dendrites. The assumption that short latency recurrent excitation of frog motoneurons upon antidromic stimulation occurs at remote dendritic sites (Washizu, 1960; Katz and Miledi, 1963; Kubota and Brookhart, 1963; Grinnell, 1966) was based on several findings: (1) the existence of a long period of occlusion of the recurrent depolarization after spike initiation (Grinnell, 1966); (2) changes in shape of antidromic field potentials after conditioning stimuli (Grinnell, 1966); (3) differences in shape and size of the spikes evoked by stimulation of two different ventral roots (Washizu, 1960); (4) lack of effects of current injections on the amplitude of the recurrent depolarization (Kubota and Brookhart, 1963). Furthermore, pharmacologic studies have strongly suggested that recurrent excitation is caused by electrical transmission between motoneurons (Grinnell, 1966). Morphologic studies lend some support to this assumption as frog motoneuron dendrites are known to have large areas of close membrane apposition (Stensaas and Stensaas, 1971), and some dendrodendritic gap junctions have also been observed (Sotelo and Taxi, 1970). Recent physiologic studies of the *in situ* spinal cord by Magherini, Precht, and Schwindt (1975*b*) fully support the previous notion that recurrent excitation is caused by electrical transmission between motoneurons, but partly disagree with the assumption that electrical coupling occurs between remote dendrites exclusively. The evidence will be briefly summarized here (for details see Magherini, Precht, and Schwindt, 1975*b*).

As shown in Fig. 5A strong antidromic stimulation resulted in recurrent action potentials that followed the normal antidromically evoked action potentials. When the intensity of stimulation was subthreshold for anti-

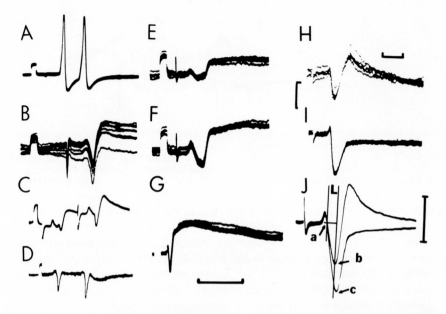

FIG. 5. Electrotonic coupling in spinal motoneurons. (A) Antidromic and recurrent action potentials evoked in spinal motoneuron after peripheral nerve stimulation (all dorsal roots cut). (B) Same neuron shows coupling potential on weak stimulation. (C,D) Facilitation of coupling potentials (C) and antidromic field potentials (D) by conditioning antidromic stimulation. (E–G) Coupling potentials evoked with increasing stimulus strengths (E,F) and displayed with slow sweep speed (G). (H–J) Intracellular (H) and extracellular traces (I) and superposition of 16 computer-averaged traces of both types of records (J). The two vertical lines in (J) indicate the points (a,b) taken for latency measurements. Calibrations: pulse in (A) 10 mV, 1 msec; (B–F) 1 mV, 1 msec; (G) voltage calibration as in (F); bar indicates 20 msec; (H–J) vertical bars, 1 mV; 2-msec horizontal bar in (H) applies to (H–J).

dromic excitation (Fig. 5B) a negatively directed antidromic field potential was observed intracellularly from which the recurrent depolarization arises. The recurrent depolarization appears to be a true PSP rather than an active response because its amplitude is graded and it exhibits neither all-or-none behavior nor refractoriness (Fig. 5E–G). Its latency (L) was measured by superposition of intra- and extracellular records (Fig. 5J). In spite of these conservative measurements, the latencies were 0.5 ± 0.1 msec SD ($n = 22$), which is significantly shorter than the 1.1 ± 0.08-msec synaptic delay of the chemically mediated EPSP evoked by lateral column stimulation (Fadiga and Brookhart, 1960). These data further strengthen the evidence for electrical transmission between motoneurons. When two antidromic stimuli were applied or when antidromic stimuli were preceded by dorsal-root stimulation the coupling potentials recorded from motoneurons were facilitated (Fig. 5C). Similarly, the antidromic field potentials were facilitated by antidromic (Fig. 5D) or dorsal-root conditioning. The latter findings indicate that more of the somadendritic membranes of the motoneuron population are being antidromically invaded as a result of conditioning. The facilitation of presumed coupling potentials was observed only when the antidromic fields were also facilitated by conditioning. This finding strongly suggests that coupling potentials are transmitted in the soma-dendritic region of the motoneurons rather than by axon collaterals. The question, however, remains as to where electrotonic transmission occurs in a given neuron.

As mentioned above various authors have put forth arguments favoring transmission between dendrites. Our recent studies, however, indicate that this is not the only site for transmission. One of the arguments suggesting dendritic coupling was based on the facilitation of antidromic fields and coupling potentials by conditioning. Because the shape of the conditioned antidromic field differed from that of the controls, it was assumed that the increase in amplitudes of these potentials may best be explained by an increase of dendritic invasion by antidromic action potentials. In our recent study we were unable to confirm marked changes in antidromic field configuration and/or changes of the antidromic spike superimposed on the dorsal-root EPSP's or coupling potentials. We found, however, that many motoneurons were not fully invaded, but that they exhibited only m-spikes upon antidromic stimulation. Therefore the above facilitation by conditioning can be explained simply by an increase in the number of motoneurons invaded. If the total number of invaded neurons increases, coupling potentials are also enhanced. Another point in favor of dendritic coupling has been the observation of a long period of occlusion of the coupling potential by a preceding action potential in the *in vitro* preparation at 5° to 10°C (Grinnell, 1966). The *in situ* preparation at room temperature did not confirm Grinnell's findings. Coupling potentials showed no refractoriness following motoneuron spike components. There is yet another experimental finding suggesting that dendrites are not the only site for electrotonic transmission. The peaking times of the coupling potentials (1.3 ± 0.2 msec, SD) is much less than in either the somatic lateral column or in dendritic dorsal-root EPSP's seen by Fadiga and Brookhart (1960). Given that both rise- and decay times of EPSP's increase the more dendritically or decrease the more somatically they are generated (Rall, 1969). The above values suggest the occurrence of electrical coupling at more proximal sites than was previously assumed. The very slow decay times of coupling potentials that were occasionally noted (Fig. 5G) may be considered as evidence for the additional involvement of distal dendrites. If one accepts the view that electrotonic transmission has its morphologic substrate in the so-called "gap" junction (Bennett, 1972), then the rare observation of this junction in the spinal cord of the frog where electrical coupling is a frequent event is somewhat disappointing (Sotelo and Taxi, 1970). As suggested by Sotelo and Taxi (1970) and by Stensaas and Stensaas (1971), electrotonic coupling between frog motoneurons may also occur to some extent by means of large appositions between dendrites (dendritic thickets) found in the spinal cord. The frog motoneuron appears to be a good model for further studies of functional meaning of dendritic appositions.

ACKNOWLEDGMENTS

The results reported here were obtained in collaboration with Drs. P. C. Magherini, S. Ozawa, A. Richter, P. C. Schwindt, and H. Shimazu.

REFERENCES

Araki, T., and Otani, T. (1955): Response of single motoneurons to direct stimulation in toad's spinal cord. *J. Neurophysiol.,* 18:472–485.

Araki, T., Otani, T., and Furukawa, T. (1953): The electrical activities of single motoneurones in toad's spinal cord, recorded with intracellular electrodes. *Jap. J. Physiol.,* 3:254–267.

Barrett, J. N., and Crill, W. E. (1974a): Specific membrane properties of cat motoneurons. *J. Physiol.,* 239:301–324.

Barrett, J. N., and Crill, W. E. (1974b): Influence of dendritic location and membrane properties on the effectiveness of synapses in cat motoneurons. *J. Physiol.,* 239:325–346.

Bennett, M. V. L. (1972): A comparison of electrically and chemically mediated transmission. In: *Structure and Function of Synapses,* edited by G. D. Pappas and D. P. Purpura, pp. 221–256. Raven Press, New York.

Brookhart, J. M., and Fadiga, E. (1960): Potential fields initiated during monosynaptic activation of frog motoneurones. *J. Physiol.,* 150:633–655.

Burke, R. E., and ten Bruggencate, G. (1971): Electrotonic characteristics of alpha motoneurones of varying size. *J. Physiol.,* 212:1–20.

Coombs, J. S., Eccles, J. C., and Fatt, P. (1955): The electrical properties of the motoneurone membrane. *J. Physiol.,* 130:291–325.

Czéh, G. (1972): The role of dendritic events in the initiation of monosynaptic spikes in frog motoneurons. *Brain Res.,* 39:505–509.

Eccles, J. C., Libet, B., and Young, R. R. (1958): The behavior of chromatolysed motoneurones studied by intracellular recording. *J. Physiol.,* 143:11–40.

Fadiga, E., and Brookhart, J. M. (1960): Monosynaptic activation of different portions of the motor neuron membrane. *Am. J. Physiol.,* 198:693–703.

Fadiga, E., and Brookhart, J. M. (1962): Interactions of excitatory postsynaptic potentials generated at different sites on the frog motoneuron. *J. Neurophysiol.,* 25:790–804.

Grinnell, A. D. (1966): A study of the interaction between motoneurons in the frog spinal cord. *J. Physiol.,* 182:612–648.

Katz, B., and Miledi, R. (1963): A study of spontaneous miniature potentials in spinal motoneurons. *J. Physiol.,* 168:389–422.

Kennard, D. W. (1959): The anatomical organization of neurons in the lumbar region of the spinal cord of the frog (*Rana temporaria*). *J. Comp. Neurol.,* 111:447–567.

Kernell, D. (1964): The delayed depolarization in cat and rat motoneurones. *Progr. Brain Res.,* 12:42–55.

Korn, H., and Bennett, M. V. L. (1971): Dendritic and somatic impulse initiation in fish oculomotor neurons during vestibular nystagmus. *Brain Res.,* 27:169–175.

Kubota, K., and Brookhart, J. M. (1963): Recurrent facilitation of frog motoneurons. *J. Neurophysiol.,* 26:877–893.

Kuno, M., and Llinás, R. (1970): Enhancement of synaptic transmission by dendritic potentials in chromatolysed motoneurones of the cat. *J. Physiol.,* 210:807–821.

Llinás, R., and Nicholson, C. (1971): Electrophysiological properties of dendrites and somata in alligator Purkinje cells. *J. Neurophysiol.,* 34:532–551.

Magherini, P. C., Precht, W., and Schwindt, P. C. (1974): Functional organization of the vestibular input to ocular motoneurons of the frog. *Pfluegers Arch.,* 349:149–158.

Magherini, P. C., Precht, W., and Schwindt, P. C. (1975a): Properties of frog spinal moto-neurones. (*in preparation*).

Magherini, P. C., Precht, W., and Schwindt, P. C. (1975b): Evidence for electric coupling between frog spinal motoneurones. (*in preparation*).

Nelson, P. G., and Burke, R. E. (1967): Delayed depolarization in cat spinal motoneurons. *Exp. Neurol.*, 17:16–26.

Nelson, P. G., and Lux, H. D. (1970): Some electrical measurements of motoneuron parameters. *Biophys. J.*, 10:55–73.

Precht, W., Richter, A., Ozawa, S., and Shimazu, H. (1974): Intracellular study of frog's vestibular neurons in relation to the labyrinth and spinal cord. *Exp. Brain Res.*, 19:377–393.

Rall, W. (1959): Branching dendritic trees and motoneuron membrane resistivity. *Exp. Neurol.*, 1:491–527.

Rall, W. (1969): Time constants and electrotonic lengths of membrane cylinders and neurons. *Biophys. J.*, 9:1483–1508.

Silver, M. L. (1942): The motoneurons of the frog spinal cord. *J. Comp. Neurol.*, 77:1–39.

Sotelo, C., and Taxi, J. (1970): Ultrastructural aspects of electrotonic junctions in the spinal cord of the frog. *Brain Res.*, 17:137–141.

Spencer, W. A., and Kandel, E. R. (1961): Electrophysiology of hippocampal neurons. IV. Fast prepotentials. *J. Neurophysiol.*, 24:272–285.

Stensaas, L. J., and Stensaas, S. S. (1971): Light and electron microscopy of motoneurons and neuropile in the amphibian spinal cord. *Brain Res.*, 31:67–84.

Washizu, Y. (1960): Single spinal motoneurons excitable from two different antidromic pathways. *Jap. J. Physiol.*, 10:121–131.

Advances in Neurology, Vol. 12, edited by
G. W. Kreutzberg, Raven Press, New York
© 1975.

Some Aspects of the Electroanatomy of Dendrites

Hans Dieter Lux and Peter Schubert

Max-Planck-Institute for Psychiatry, D-8000 Munich 40, Federal Republic of Germany

A clear concept of synaptic transmission in mammalian nerve cells can evolve only through prior knowledge of the specific role of the dendritic structure. The dissipation of charge into dendritic processes from currents passing through the soma surface membrane will determine the amount and the time course of potentials at this central site. Junctional innervation in central neurons probably acts often at dendritic locations that are remote from the somatic and axonal areas. To describe the distortions that affect the synaptic signal during its transmission along the dendritic pathway, a neuron model is required that sufficiently reproduces the essential geometric features as well as the electrical membrane parameters of the neuron. It is apparent that these properties cannot be determined separately in a neuron of complex geometry. An analytic separation depends on the availability of a reasonably comprehensive neuron model for which simplifying assumptions are necessary, e.g., uniformity of dendritic and soma membrane properties and homogeneity of intra- and extracellular conducting media, which are summarized and described in detail by Rall (1959, 1960). Dendrites are represented as cylindric cables with a surface membrane, which at small enough voltages, behaves as a capacitor shunted by a leak conductance. This classic concept was extended when the principle of impedance-matching within branching dendritic trees was elegantly concluded by Rall (1959) and supported through anatomic measurements on available Golgi preparations of cat spinal motoneurons. These studies have extended and rectified the earlier concept of a standard motoneuron of Coombs, Eccles, and Fatt (1955), which, however insufficiently, considered the possible effects of dendritic processes.

ELECTROANATOMIC PARAMETERS OF MOTONEURONAL DENDRITES

The finding that the diameters of successive dendritic branches scale in a fortunately simple way, with the sum of the $^3/_2$ power of all branch diameters at any distances being constant, was further supported by measurements on histologic preparations from *in vivo* studies that combined electrophysiologic studies with subsequent staining techniques (Lux, Schubert,

Kreutzberg, 1970; Barrett and Crill, 1971). If a change in diameter between branch points is absent the entire tree can be transformed into an equivalent dendritic cylinder, the length of which is measured in units of the length constant.

Electrophysiologic and anatomic data were obtained from the same neurons. Following the determination of their input resistance predominantly with hyperpolarizing pulses, the neurons were intracellularly injected with ^{3}H-glycine. At different times after injection (usually between 1 and 6 hr) the cats were perfused with phosphate-buffered Formalin (pH 7.3), the spinal cords were embedded in paraplast, and autoradiographs were prepared from 6-μm serial sections. Needle marks set stereotactically at 20 mm distance allowed the determination of the linear tissue shrinkage during the histologic procedure and the relocation of the neurons studied by their stereotactic coordinates. Linear shrinkage was found to be between 12 and 16% and is taken into consideration in all subsequent calculations. Because the intracellularly injected ^{3}H-glycine is incorporated into proteins and is transported with a fast intradendritic transport system from the soma up to the peripheral branches, the dendritic tree is filled within 20 min after injection with radioactive proteins and can be visualized by autoradiography. (Fig. 1, for details see Schubert and Kreutzberg, this volume.)

Intraneuronal transport and therefore the labeling of the dendritic tree occurs under physiologic conditions as is indicated by the recording of stable neuronal resting and action potential during the postinjection period. The extension of the labeled dendritic tree was reconstructed from serial section autoradiographs by projecting the labeled dendrites found in each of the sections on translucent folia, marking them, and by superimposing the folia. The diameters of the labeled dendritic branches were measured within the individual sections by high-power magnification. Full dendritic cross and oblique sections were used. When determining the real dimensions of a structure by measuring the extension of its labeling, a systematic overestimation has to be accounted for, which is brought about by the limited autoradiographic resolution caused by the spread of radiation. The resolution defined as the distance from the radiation source at which the grain density falls to one-half that directly over the source, is reported to be 0.5 to 1 μm for tritium (Rogers, 1967). This area of decreased grain density considered to represent label outside the border of the labeled structure could be identified easily in our material and was excluded from the measurements. Usually the dendritic labeling was rather confined, which allowed for identification of differences down to branches of an apparent thickness of 1 μm.

The validity of the $3/2$ power rule was checked in four completely reconstructed large motoneurons on 127 bifurcations. Because dendrites show a circumscribed inflation before and at the branching region, the dendritic diameters were measured outside this area. The mean of multiple measure-

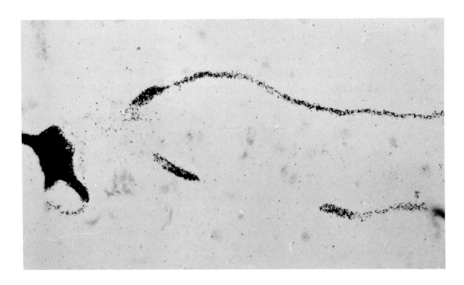

FIG. 1. One of the serial section autoradiographs of the completely reconstructed spinal motoneuron 110/4 which has been intracellularly injected with ^{3}H-glycine, about 4 hr before Formalin perfusion. Radioactive material is found transported from the nerve cell soma far into the dendrites where labeling appears well confined. Autoradiography counterstained with toluidine blue. (×340.)

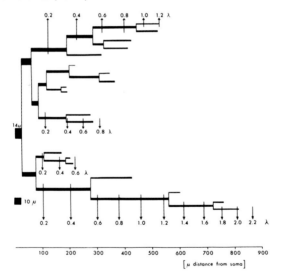

FIG. 2. Arborization of one of the stem dendrites of the neuron shown in Fig. 1. The diameters of the schematically displayed dendritic branches represent average diameters determined by several measurements along the whole length and corrected for shrinkage. The ordinate gives the overall extension in microns from the nerve cell soma. The numbers below the arrows give the lengths in units of the length constant λ of the particular intersected branches. Notice the reduction of electrotonic lengths with the thickness of the branches. The dendritic branching occurs largely according to the $^3/_2$ power rule.

ments at intervals of about 50 μm along the length of the dendritic branches
was taken to be the representative diameters of these dendrites. The present
estimates, which were intended to incorporate the presence of dendritic
taper, resulted in a mean ratio of the combined dendritic parameters of
daughter and parent branches ($\Sigma d^{3/2}/D^{3/2}$) of 0.95 ± 0.16 (SD). This is not
statistically different from the previous evaluation of Lux et al. (1970) (see
also Barrett and Crill, 1971). For a more direct determination of dendritic
tapering, the combined dendritic parameters ($\Sigma d^{3/2}$) of all dendrites were
measured at distances of 80 and 300 μm from their origin at the soma. Over
this interval, $\Sigma d^{3/2}$ was reduced on the average by $34 \pm 13.5\%$ (SD). Disappearance of terminal branches had attributed by $22.6 \pm 8.8\%$. The remaining loss of $11.4 \pm 6.4\%$ is obviously brought about mainly by dendritic
thinning within the arborizations. The possibility that fine terminal branches
have been missed would even make this value an overestimate of tapering.
This pattern of dendritic reduction seems to proceed into the periphery,
although accurate differentiation of the reduction within the region of the
fine dendrites is difficult.

The overall reduction of $\Sigma d^{3/2}$ is very similar to that found by Barrett
and Crill (1971). However, their conclusion that almost all of the loss is
caused by dendritic tapering is not supported by our data (see also Lux
et al., 1970). This discrepancy cannot be explained by the different procedure of histologic processing, as structural preservation of the material
selected for analysis was ensured to be of high quality. Therefore, we expected to find the resolution of this discrepancy with the different process
of marking the dendritic tree. However, comparable material with procion
yellow-injected motoneurons, which was kindly provided to us by Dr.
Zieglgänsberger, did not show the kind of continuous dendritic thinning
described by Barrett and Crill (1971) and revealed a ratio of 0.92 ± 0.17 of
combined daughter branch diameters (to the $^3/_2$ power) to that of the parent
branch. The time before perfusion which is significant for the intracellular
distribution of the dye was less than 3 hr in this procion yellow material
and evidently shorter than in the material of Barrett and Crill (1971). Hence,
the possibility remains that this alkylating dye is not fully inert intravitally
and causes a smooth dendritic shrinkage over longer periods of time.

The appropriate length parameter for the description of the functional
properties of dendrites in a linear cable model is the length constant $\lambda = \sqrt{(d/4)R_M/R_i}$, following the definition of Rall (1959). The electrotonic
lengths $L = X/\lambda$ (X is the real length) are thus inversely related to the
square root of the dendritic diameters and the ratio of membrane resistance
R_M to the internal resistance R_i. It becomes necessary to have a joint estimate of both quantities.

The quantities d and X should be known for every dendrite branch because it determines the dendritic input conductance, which, in the simple
case of a finite equivalent dendritic cylinder, is given by $G_f = G_\infty$ tanh L

(Rall, 1970; Lux et al., 1970; Jack and Redman, 1971), with G_∞ being the input conductance of an infinitely extended dendritic cable of the same diameter defined by $(\pi/2)D^{3/2}/\sqrt{R_M R_i}$ (Rall, 1959). Owing to the intrasomal location of the electrodes, the neuronal input conductance G_N is basically available. This consists of the sum of the difference G_f of the proximal dendritic trunks and of the apparently smaller G_{soma}. G_f and G_∞ are of the same order, as tanh L is between zero and unity. Starting with an estimate of R_M from $G_{N\infty}$ (by assuming infinite dendritic length) and correcting the resulting overestimation with G_{Nf}, a sufficient R_M estimate is achieved within a few steps to match the experimental value of G_N when R_M is applied to the entire membrane of the dendritic tree and of the soma surface. This is the easiest way to determine R_M because explicit solutions are different for the individual dendritic trees.

The many arborizations of dendrites obviously have different electrotonic lengths. It is therefore advisable to apply the core conductor equation for the finite cylinder first to the end terminals and to proceed proximately by relating the input conductances of lower-order branches to that of bifurcating branches [in the manner described by Rall, 1959, Eq. (21)].

An example of L estimates for four arborizations of a motoneuronal dendrite ranging from about 0.5 to 2 length constants is given in Fig. 2. The estimates represent the extreme case with a mean dendrite length of 1.15 ± 0.52 λ weighted for the different trunk input conductances. Electrotonic lengths of major branches usually vary by about 20% (Lux et al., 1970; see also Barrett and Crill, 1971). However, proximal side branches of small diameter are usually found, which terminate at short electrotonic distances from the soma, although their overall contribution to the average length of the dendritic tree is rather small. No functional meaning of this variability or correlation with motoneuronal type is as yet obvious.

Estimates of motoneuronal electrotonic lengths can be obtained in principle by pure analysis of voltage transients during step current application (Lux, 1967; Nelson and Lux, 1970; Burke and ten Bruggencate, 1971; Lux et al., 1970) as substantiated and discussed in detail by Rall (1969) for different terminal boundary conditions and for combinations of dendrites of unequal lengths. A range of dendritic cable lengths was obtained also by Jack and Redman (1971) from the analysis of the time courses of unitary excitatory postsynaptic potentials (EPSP's). In all these investigations the most frequently occurring values for $L_{transient}$ were located between 1 and 2λ similarly, as determined from the combined estimates based on cell morphology. Table 1 summarizes the geometric and derived data on cat spinal motoneurons. The values incorporate the previous estimates of Lux et al. (1970) and are quite similar to those from the dye-injected motoneurons in the work of Barrett and Crill (1971).

Their lower values of R_M determinations can be considered a virtual difference because R_M appears predominantly in conjunction with R_i in the

TABLE 1. *Geometric and derived data on cat spinal motoneurons*

Condition	Parameter	Mean value
Combined dendritic trunk parameter, 80 μm from soma	$\Sigma D^{3/2}$	320 $\pm$ 150 (10^{-6} cm$^{3/2}$)
Specific membrane resistance for uniform somadendritic membrane	R_M	2,700 $\pm$ 920 (Ωcm^2)
Input resistance, ratio of membrane potential change (< 10 mV) in steady state during hyperpolarizing currents	R_N	1.1 $\pm$ 0.5 (MΩ)
Assumed specific resistivity of the internal medium	R_i	100 (Ωcm)
Dendritic to soma conductance ratio for finite equivalent dendritic cable	ρ_{finite}	20.8 $\pm$ 4.0
Electrotonic length, determined from morphologic data and neuronal input resistance	L_{geom}	1.5 $\pm$ 0.3
Electrotonic length, determined by comparing early and late time constant of voltage transients during current steps	$L_{transient}$	1.5 $\pm$ 0.3
Final time constant from measurements of voltage transients during current steps	τ_m	5.3 $\pm$ 1.0 (msec)

Soma area	10,500 $\pm$ 3,700 (μm^2)
Dendritic area	217,900 $\pm$ 137,000 (μm^2)
Soma volume	109,000 $\pm$ 51,600 (μm^3)
Dendritic volume	298,000 $\pm$ 184,400 (μm^3)
Dendritic to somatic area ratio	20.4 $\pm$ 5.7
Dendritic to somatic volume ratio	2.6 $\pm$ 0.5

ratio R_M/R_i. Considerable uncertainties are involved in measuring the resistivity of the intracellular medium of mammalian nerve cells *in vivo*. Experience with motoneurons and other nerve cells as well as *in vitro* studies in extruded plasma of neuronal tissue led us to suggest that a value of 100 Ωcm or more, but significantly higher than that of cerebral spinal fluid (62 Ωcm), is appropriate. A mean value of 2.350 $\pm$ 545 Ωcm^2 for R_M results from the data of Barrett and Crill, if allowance is made for an R_i of 100 Ωcm as used in our estimates.

There is some arbitrariness in distinguishing the border between soma and the beginning of its dendritic trunks. We included in the area of the soma the strongly tapering part of the proximal trunks. The somal surface area was calculated from measurements with the Leitz-Classimat (Fig. 3). These resulted in greater estimates than were previously given when approximation to the surface of an ellipsoid was used. Even these favorable estimates of soma surfaces are by far exceeded by that of the dendritic trees by a factor of 20 $\pm$ 5.7 (SD). Evidently the major receptive area of junctional innervation of the neuron is provided by dendrites (see also Aitkin and Bridger, 1961; Schadé, 1964; Gelfan, Kao, and Ruchkin, 1970).

In the motoneuronal model with uniform R_M the dendritic input con-

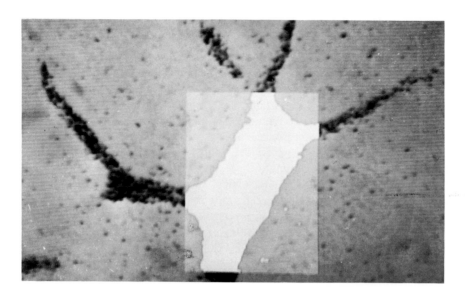

FIG. 3. Quantitative determination of the somal surface area by means of the Leitz-Classimat, used as an areal densitometer. The microscopic picture of the autoradiograph is displayed on a television screen. The parts of the labeled neuron to be measured, the soma and the proximal segments of the stem dendrites, are covered by the adjustable measuring area (the brightly illuminated rectangular field). The labeled parts are electronically identified and appear white. Measurement of the areas of the marked structures within the individual subsequent 6-μm serial sections determines their circumference and thus the total surface area of the nerve cell soma.

duction would dominate to an extent that the soma membrane would merely represent a high resistance barrier for the axial dendritic currents as already envisaged by Rall (1959, 1964). However, many papers have questioned the uniformity of membrane resistance and suggested, from different points of view, that the somal membrane resistance may be considerably lower than that of the dendritic tree (Fatt, 1957; Rall, 1960; Katz and Miledi, 1963; Lux et al., 1970).

A practical measure of the dendritic loading on the soma is the ratio ρ of the dendritic to soma conductance for direct currents (Rall, 1959). Extending Rall's treatment, Jack and Redman (1971) have succeeded in establishing equations for, and applying explicit solutions to, a continuous nerve cell model consisting of a finite cable connected to a lumped soma. It could be shown in detail equivalent to the different analysis of Rall (1969) how the neuronal parameters (dendritic unit membrane resistance and time constant, dendritic to soma conductance ratio, dendritic length), the form, and location of injected current, all determine the time course of voltage transients recorded at the soma. It turned out to be a difficult task to measure ρ, which quantitizes the coupling between the soma and the combined dendritic cable. However, the conditions under which ρ can be estimated even in conjunction with dendritic lengths have become clear. The most successful procedure for the estimation of ρ was to use brief current pulses or synaptic currents (Jack and Redman, 1971; Iansek and Redman, 1973). A current pulse that is short compared with the membrane time constant, injected into or near the soma, is primarily used to load the somal capacitance. This capacitance discharges through the somal resistance and into the dendrites. The component of the voltage transient attributable to the soma is largest at the instant the current pulse is removed. The changes during the early part of the decaying slope can be used quantitatively to estimate ρ. From the analysis of the shape of minimal group Ia EPSP's, Jack, Miller, Porter, and Redman, (1971) concluded for ρ a lower limit of 4.

Most of the analyses of these transients revealed ρ to be valued between 2.5 and 25 with the majority in excess of 6 (Jack and Redman, 1971; Iansek and Redman, 1973). Curve-fitting of current responses for which a value of ρ could not be assessed by assuming a uniform somadendritic R_M was facilitated by the use of a lumped soma with a considerably reduced somal unit membrane resistance. These results indicate that the specific resistance of the soma could likely be lower than that of the dendrites by a factor of 3. This would explain that many of the electrical ρ estimates are somewhat lower than a consideration of neuron geometry would suggest. Although the need might arise for certain cells to correct the data obtained from using the simpler uniform circuit model of the dendritic neuron, these findings do not seriously impair the concept of dendritic predominance.

ISOLATED DENDRITIC POSTSYNAPTIC POTENTIALS

The propagation of postsynaptic potentials in dendrites depends upon the electrical and geometric properties of the dendritic and somatic membrane, the location of the synapses, and the postsynaptic conductance change. The electrical distance over which transmission occurs is the most relevant parameter and should be signified by the increase of the time course of the synaptic transients. Rise-times (times to peak potential) and half-widths (duration at one-half of peak amplitude) are the most useful shape indices of synaptic potentials (see Rall, Burke, Smith, Nelson, and Frank, 1967). Unfortunately, their attenuation along the dendritic membrane cannot be assessed experimentally.

Dendritic synaptic potentials can be observed in some isolation (Lux and Winter, 1968; Kuno and Llinás, 1970b) during the initial period of chromatolysis of about 1 week after axonal transection (Fig. 4). During the process of retrograde reaction the synapses are peeled off from the soma by microglial cells (Blinzinger and Kreutzberg, 1968). This can be shown even at the light-microscopic level when the sections are stained according to Armstrong and Stephens (1960), a rather specific staining technique for demonstrating synapses (Fig. 4A, page 38).

The view that EPSP's with short rise-times are to be allocated a region near or at the soma is supported by the observation that the frequency of occurrence of this variety of postsynaptic transients is largely reduced in retrograde reacting neurons (Fig. 4B,C). Rise-times greater than 0.2 of the membrane time constants of 3.5 to 6 msec dominate in transient spontaneous voltage changes in these motoneurons. Also natural or electric stimulation of facial skin afferents fails to evoke sharply rising EPSP's (Fig. 4B), although composite synaptic activity during which single, always slowly rising EPSP's can be distinguished is quite effective in depolarizing the axotomized neurons. This was observed to hold for continuous stimulation, which resulted in a sustained reduction of the membrane potential and in cell firing as well as for single electrical volleys, which were able to elicit large EPSP's with rise-times of more than 0.5 msec. Dendritic lengths of facial motoneurons probably are not much different from those of spinal motoneurons as some analyses of voltage transients indicate (by the use of the "peeling off" procedure of exponential components during current steps; Rall, 1969). The possibility exists that proximal parts of dendrites are also affected by synaptic loss. However, a reasonable alignment of dendritic location depends upon the condition that all synaptic activity is brought about by similar synaptic currents or conductance changes of a duration that is short compared with that of the voltage transients. The argument of a similar synaptic action of short duration is stronger for the case of EPSP's from a homogeneous class of afferent fibers. Kuno and Llinás (1970a) have investigated the distribution of minimal EPSP's from group Ia afferents in the normal and in the retrograde-reacting spinal motoneurons. They also found that in the latter neurons juxtasomatic EPSP's were largely absent as concluded from determinations of shape indices. It is also notable that inhibitory postsynaptic action elicited from muscle antagonists was more reduced than that from other pathways, e.g., antidromic and reticular, which appear to terminate predominantly on dendrites. Chromatolytic motoneurons are also characterized by their ability to develop partial action potentials in response to afferent stimulation (Eccles, Libet, and Young, 1958; Kuno and Llinás, 1970a). Large EPSP's are often suprathreshold for these spikes, which were allocated to possible circumscribed dendritic regions by Kuno and Llinás. This phenomenon would create considerable difficulties in any quantitative assessment of its obvious role in dendritic transmission comparable to that of minimal EPSP's.

SOME LIMITS OF THE APPLICABILITY OF THE LINEAR CABLE MODEL

It is notable that the linear cable approximation of the dendritic neuron model has proved its virtue in the analysis of comparable small distortions in a narrow region of membrane potential at the soma, in which a constant membrane resistance can be assumed. Caution against the extension of the linear cable assumptions to larger voltage excursions was already advised by Jack and Redman (1971), as some minimal EPSP's of probably dendritic origin showed slope deviations that were not fitted by a linear cable model, in contrast to EPSP's in the same motoneuron from different Ia afferents. Characteristic for the deviating EPSP's are the delayed decays (prolonged half-widths) and sometimes smooth hyperpolarizing afterreactions.

Nonlinearities of membrane resistance can be observed in many motoneurons. Most obvious is a phenomenon termed anomalous rectification (Nelson and Frank, 1967). It is usually defined as a relative decline of the membrane potential displacement in response to hyperpolarizing direct currents, i.e., a decrease of the apparent membrane resistance with hyperpolarization. Anomalous rectification was first observed in ganglionic cells of the land snail *Helix aspersa* by Kandel and Tauc (1966). From recent analyses on a similar *Helix* preparation (Eckert and Lux, 1975; Lux and Eckert, 1974) it appears more appropriate to describe this phenomenon as an increase of the apparent membrane resistance by changing from hyper- to depolarization. It is strongly suggested that the anomalous rectification is brought about by the appearance of a slow or noninactivating inward current, probably carried by calcium ions, which sums with the steady-state outward current. Because the net current decreases strongly or is seen in certain cells to invert under a voltage-clamp condition, a drastic increase of the apparent membrane resistance or even a negative resistance slope results. The current develops in a voltage region near resting potential and subthreshold for the early inward current of the action potential.

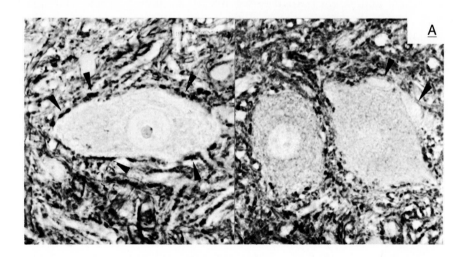

FIG. 4. (A) Removal of the somal synapses during retrograde reaction in cat facial motoneurons. Left, The soma of a normal facial neuron at the control side appears densely covered by synapses demonstrated here by the black reaction product (*arrow*). Right, Four days after nerve transection, the facial neuron of the operated side is surrounded by an

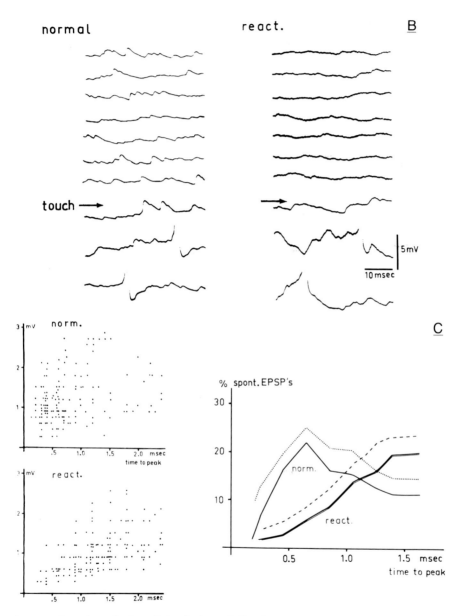

increased number of microglial cells (*arrow*). Nearly no staining is seen at the surface of the nerve cell soma indicating the disappearance of somal synapses. Stained according to Armstrong and Stephens. (×700.) (B) Spontaneous synaptic potentials of a normal (left) and a chromatolytic facial motoneuron (right) from the same experiment. Touch is applied to the whiskers. (C) Frequency of occurrence of spontaneous EPSP's with rise-times below 2.5 msec during the recording time of 1 min versus individual amplitude (left side) and in percent of the overall frequency with average frequency (continuous line) and standard deviation (dotted line) of spontaneous EPSP's of five cells each in two experiments (right side).

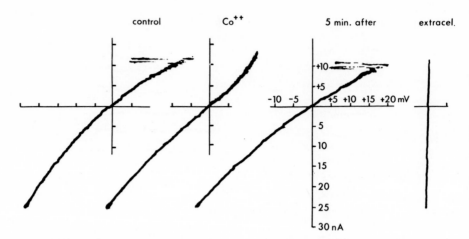

FIG. 5. Current-voltage relation of a spinal motoneuron *before, during* (iontophoretic current temporarily off), and about 5 min *after* extracellular injection of Co ions. Current was applied in sawtooth mode from hyper- to depolarizing direction. Neuronal potential is displayed by the *X* deflection and current strength by *Y* deflection. Slow frequency (of 1.4/sec) was used to minimize contribution of membrane time constant. Curves show the increase of the ratio membrane potential to current (R_N) from 0.95 (control) and 1.20 (after Co^{2+}) to 1.70 and 1.75 $M\Omega$, respectively, during depolarizing currents. A decrease of apparent R_N is displayed under Co^{2+} and neuron potential fails to reach threshold for spikes for this range of current. At the right border the same measurement performed in extracellular location of the electrode. Calibration applies for all curves.

Agents that affect this slow inward current have been investigated in experiments with L. Liebl for their possible action on anomalous rectification in spinal motoneurons (see Fig. 5). Cobalt ions applied extracellularly by electrophoresis from a micropipette, located about 100 μm from the intracellular electrode, reversibly change the anomalous slope of the voltage–current relation to a more monotonous slope of normal rectification which is usually found in the nerve fiber membrane. Barium ions extracellularly applied slightly enhanced "anomalous rectification," whereas injection of the calcium antagonist D 600 changed it toward the "normal" slope. Unfortunately, a direct demonstration of the current that may underlie anomalous rectification is as yet not possible in the spinal motoneuron.

Whether or not it is caused by a slow inward current, the increase in membrane resistance with depolarization is of considerable interest for postsynaptic transmission. Because anomalous rectification and the slow inward current was observed at the somal membrane of snail neurons it should be asked whether anomalous rectification may be restricted to the membrane of the motoneuronal soma. In the presence of a largely dominating dendritic input conductance, even an infinite membrane resistance, if restricted to the soma, could hardly increase the overall neuron input resistance by the observed amount of 50 to 150% maximally (Nelson and Frank, 1967).

Such an assumption also contrasts with the conclusion of a smaller somatic than dendritic unit membrane impedance.

Alternatively, a considerable net inward current should be present at the soma to balance the loss across the passive dendritic input conductances and result in anomalous rectification of the somadendritic input. In this case an abrupt increase of the early decay of the voltage transients of EPSP's and of a short current pulse applied at the soma should be observable during hyperpolarization, which removes the inward current. However, the observed changes of EPSP transients with variations of the membrane potential appear to be smooth and comparable with the overall change of apparent membrane resistance. This suggests that anomalous rectification can also be allocated to the dendritic membrane.

An apparent increase in dendritic membrane resistance will shorten their electrotonic length. However, if it is caused by a time and voltage depending inward current, similar to that of *Helix* neurons, it will become difficult to derive conclusions from shape indices about the dendritic locations of the synaptic action as well as of the region in which the hypothetical slow inward current is produced. During the active support or amplification of synaptic currents a change in the time course is to be expected, particularly a prolongation of the time course but not necessarily a shortening of rise-times of the postsynaptic potentials. EPSP varieties of prolonged durations (halfwidths) to which the rise-time did not correspond for any set of dendritic location or synaptic distribution have already been described (Iansek and Redman, 1973; see also Jack et al., 1971). It is also notable that minimal EPSP's of peripheral dendritic allocation (in the passive dendritic neuron model) showed amplitudes comparable to those of juxtasomatic EPSP's. Synaptic activity within the dendritic periphery of small branches should produce large potential deflections at the points of origin. They may lead into a membrane voltage region in which the current-voltage relation can no longer be considered linear. Considering the attenuation in the dendritic arborization during transmission toward the soma and the probable number of synaptic contacts of single group Ia fibers, Iansek and Redman were led to conclude that in the periphery synaptic currents per synapse should be far greater (by a factor of 10) than in the vicinity of the soma. An alternative explanation for this surprising observation would be that dendritic postsynaptic action is actively supported, a possibility which was mentioned already by Jack et al. (1971). A major difference to the spike-like intradendritic propagation (see Llinás, this volume) should be a nearly complete absence of refractoriness since an effective time-dependent inactivation of the supposed slow inward current is unlikely. Although there is no evidence, it is tempting to speculate that the development of spike discharges in the retrograde reacting neuron results from a transformation of the same sites at which the smoothly graded electrogenesis is produced in the normal neuron.

SUMMARY

An understanding of the neuronal function requires the knowledge of the electroanatomy of dendrites, which comprise the major area and receive the main input in most neurons. Some simplifying assumptions are necessary to describe the electrical characteristics of the dendritic tree. The applicability of the simplified model of a combined equivalent dendritic cylinder proposed by Rall, was tested and verified by a combined analysis of anatomic and electrical data from the same spinal motoneurons. Assuming a uniform somadendritic membrane, estimates of the specific membrane resistance (R_M: $2,700 \pm 920 \, \Omega\text{cm}^2$) were made by relating the neuronal input resistance with the combined dendritic trunk parameter ($\Sigma D^{3/2}$: $320 \pm 150 \cdot 10^{-6} \, \text{cm}^{3/2}$). From these combined anatomic and electrical data the dendritic electrotonic lengths (L_{geom}: 1.5 ± 0.3 times the length constant) were derived. Comparable L values (L_{trans}: 1.5 ± 0.3) resulted independently from analysis of membrane voltage transients during current steps. The linear dendritic cable model has proved its applicability for the analysis of small voltage deflections during current step applications at the soma as well as for the analysis of the majority of minimal postsynaptic potentials (PSP's).

During the transmission along the dendritic cable the PSP undergoes changes in shape. These changes often permit a determination of the distance of the dendritic input from the soma. Unfortunately, the attenuation of the dendritic signal cannot be directly assessed. Dendritic synaptic transmission can be observed in isolation in chromatolytic motoneurons because the somal synapses are peeled off from the soma by proliferating glial cells in the course of retrograde reaction. These observations support the prediction that the PSP's with relatively short rise-times and duration originate from synapses near the soma.

It may be questioned as to whether the linear dendritic cable approximation also applies to the larger voltage displacements during excitatory synaptic action. Particularly interesting is an increase of the apparent membrane resistance during depolarization known as anomalous rectification. The anomalous rectification could be reversibly eliminated and turned into a normal rectification by the application of cobalt ions or other calcium antagonists. Therefore, it appears likely that this phenomenon is caused by a voltage- (and time-) dependent reaction of the membrane, consisting of a smoothly increased calcium conductance during depolarizations that are even subthreshold for eliciting action potentials. Such a process would result in a shortening of the dendritic electrotonic length and in facilitating the postsynaptic excitatory transmission.

REFERENCES

Aitkin, J. T., and Bridger, J. E. (1961): Neuron size and population density in lumbosacral region of the cat's spinal cord. *J. Anat.*, 95:38–53.

Armstrong, J., and Stephens, P. R. (1960): A modified chrome–silver paraffin wax technique for staining neural end feet. *Stain Technol.,* 35:71–75.

Barrett, J. N., and Crill, W. E. (1971): Specific membrane resistivity of dye injected cat motoneurons. *Brain Res.,* 28:556–561.

Blinzinger, K., and Kreutzberg, G. W. (1968): Displacement of synaptic terminals from regenerating motoneurons by microglial cells. *Z. Zellforsch. Mikrosk. Anat.,* 85:145–157.

Burke, R. E., and ten Bruggencate, G. (1971): Electrotonic characteristics of alpha motoneurones of varying size. *J. Physiol. (Lond.),* 212:1–20.

Coombs, J. S., Eccles, J. C., and Fatt, P. (1955): The electrical properties of the motoneurone membrane. *J. Physiol. (Lond.),* 130:291–325.

Eccles, J. C., Libet, B., and Young, R. R. (1958): The behaviour of chromatolyzed motoneurones studied by intracellular recording. *J. Physiol. (Lond.),* 143:11–40.

Eckert, R., and Lux, H. D. (1975): A non-inactivating inward current recorded during small depolarizing voltage steps in snail neurons. *Brain Res.,* 83:486–489.

Fatt, P. (1957): Sequence of events in synaptic activation of a motoneurone. *J. Neurophysiol.,* 20:61–80.

Gelfan, S., Kao, G., and Ruchkin, D. S. (1970): The dendritic tree of spinal neurons. *J. Comp. Neurol.,* 139:385–411.

Iansek, R., and Redman, S. J. (1973): The amplitude, time course and charge of unitary excitatory post-synaptic potentials evoked in spinal motoneurone dendrites. *J. Physiol. (Lond.),* 234:665–688.

Jack, J. J. B., Miller, S., Porter, R., and Redman, S. J. (1971): The time course of minimal excitatory post-synaptic potentials evoked in spinal motoneurones by group Ia afferent fibers. *J. Physiol. (Lond.),* 215:353–380.

Jack, J. J. B. and Redman, S. J. (1971): An electrical description of the motoneurone and its application to the analysis of synaptic potentials. *J. Physiol. (Lond.),* 215:321–352.

Kandel, E. R. and Tauc, L. (1966): Anomalous rectification in the metacerebral giant cells and its consequences for synaptic transmission. *J. Physiol. (Lond.),* 183:287–304.

Katz, B., and Miledi, R. (1963): A study of spontaneous miniature potentials in spinal motoneurones. *J. Physiol. (Lond.),* 168:389–422.

Kuno, M., and Llinas, R. (1970a): Enhancement of synaptic transmission by dendritic potentials in chromatolysed motoneurones of the cat. *J. Physiol. (Lond.),* 210:807–821.

Kuno, M., and Llinas, R. (1970b): Alterations of synaptic action in chromatolysed motoneurones of the cat. *J. Physiol. (Lond.),* 210:823–838.

Lux, H. D. (1967): Eigenschaften eines Neuron-Modells mit Dendriten begrenzter Länge. *Pfluegers Arch.,* 297:238–255.

Lux, H. D., and Eckert, R. (1974): Inferred slow inward current in snail neurones. *Nature,* 250:574–576.

Lux, H. D., Schubert, P., and Kreutzberg, G. W. (1970): Direct matching of morphological and electrophysiological data in cat spinal motoneurones. In: *Excitatory Synaptic Mechanisms,* edited by P. Andersen and J. K. S. Jansen, pp. 189–198. Universitetsforlaget, Oslo.

Lux, H. D., and Winter, P. (1968): Studies on EPSPs in normal and retrograde reacting facial motoneurones. *Proc. Int. Union Physiol. Sci.,* 7:Abst. 818

Nelson, P. G., and Frank, K. (1967): Anomalous rectification in cat spinal motoneurons and the effect of polarizing currents on the excitatory postsynaptic potential. *J. Neurophysiol.,* 130:1097–1113.

Nelson, P. G., and Lux, H. D. (1970): Some electrical measurements of motoneuron parameters. *Biophys. J.,* 10:55–73.

Rall, W. (1959): Branching dendritic trees and motoneurone membrane resistivity. *Exp. Neurol.,* 1:491–527.

Rall, W. (1960): Membrane potential transients and membrane time constants of motoneurones. *Exp. Neurol.,* 2:503–532.

Rall, W. (1964): Theoretical significance of dendritic trees for neuronal input–output relations. In: *Neural Theory and Modelling,* edited by R. F. Reiss, pp. 73–79. Stanford Univ. Press, Stanford, California.

Rall, W. (1969): Time constants and electrotonic length of membrane cylinders and neurons. *Biophys. J.,* 9:1483–1508.

Rall, W. (1970): Cable properties of dendrites and effects of synaptic location. In: *Excitatory*

Synaptic Mechanisms, edited by P. Andersen and J. K. S. Jansen, pp. 175–187. Universitetsforlaget, Oslo.

Rall, W., Burke, R. E., Smith, T. G., Nelson, P. G., and Frank, K. (1967): Dendritic location of synapses and possible mechanisms for the monosynaptic EPSP in motoneurons. *J. Neurophysiol.,* 30:1169–1193.

Rogers, A. W. (1967): *Techniques of Autoradiography,* pp. 49–57. Elsevier, Amsterdam.

Schadé, J. P. (1964): On the volume and surface area of spinal neurons. In: *Organization of the Spinal Cord.* In: *Progress in Brain Research,* edited by J. C. Eccles and J. P. Schadé, vol. 11, pp. 261–277. Elsevier, Amsterdam.

Advances in Neurology, Vol. 12, edited by
G. W. Kreutzberg, Raven Press, New York
© 1975.

Glutamic Acid Sensitivity of Dendrites in Hippocampal Slices *In Vitro*

P. A. Schwartzkroin and P. Andersen

The Institute of Neurophysiology, University of Oslo, Oslo 1, Norway

The morphology in the hippocampal formation facilitates the study of dendritic properties. The basis for this is the histologically well-known structure with a monolayered cortex and the stratified arrangement of the input fibers and their synapses. Based on field-potential studies, particularly recording of large population spikes, Andersen, Blackstad, and Lømo, (1966) identified four excitatory afferent pathways to the CA3 and CA1 regions in the rabbit hippocampus. A combination of Golgi impregnation and experimental interruption of the same pathways showed the majority of these excitatory synapses to be located on dendritic spines; none were on the cell bodies.

Delivery of putative transmitter substances (Curtis and Johnston, 1974) to dendritic synapses is made difficult by the considerable distance between the synapses and the cell body, where the electrodes are usually located. However, in the transverse hippocampal slice (Skrede and Westgaard, 1971) it is possible to place both recording and ejection electrodes in any part of the dendritic tree under direct visual inspection. With this technique we wanted to deliver L-glutamic acid to various dendritic territories to see whether this substance could mimic the effect of the natural occurring excitatory transmitter substance at these synapses.

METHODS

The recording was made from pyramidal cells in the CA1 region, identified by antidromic invasion, following alveus stimulation. Iontophoretic electrodes (1–2 μm) were filled with 2 mol L-glutamic acid and titrated to pH 8.0 with NaOH. All electrodes were carried by manipulators and placed under direct visual control under transillumination. Extra- and intracellular recording was made with potassium acetate electrodes (10 to 50 MΩ). Slices were maintained in the interphase between artificial cerebrospinal fluid (134 mM NaCl, 5mM KCl, 1.24 mM KH_2PO_4, 2.0 mM $MgSO_4$, 2.0 mM $CaCl_2$, 16 mM $NaHCO_3$, and 10 mM glucose), and a flow of moist gas, a mixture of oxygen (95%) and carbon dioxide (5%). The temperature was maintained between 35° and 37°C.

RESULTS

When appropriately placed, L-glutamate excited cells with short latency (10 to 200 msec) and in small doses (down to 1 nA for 100 msec). The responsive area had a shape of a double cone, the tips of which corresponded to the soma of the cell recorded from, with the bases toward the alveus and hippocampal fissure, respectively, corresponding to the apical dendritic and basal dendritic trees. A typical discharge pattern is seen in Fig. 1. The cell discharged following currents down to 1 nA. A backing current of 20 nA ran continuously. Two nA (B) gave a clear depolarization and a relatively regular discharge; with 5 nA (C) the frequency of discharge increased and took off from a depolarization level ~ 10 mV. With moderate currents the glutamate effect was remarkably constant even with long pulses (D). Repeated pulses gave no indication of a reduced sensitivity, irrespective of the duration of the glutamate ejection. With stronger doses there was a clear pause after the excitation. However, this also occurred after spontaneous discharges and was closely related to the number of spikes fired and not to the length or size of the depolarization induced by glutamate per se.

The pattern of discharge was typically an initial depolarization leading up to a burst discharge followed by a pause and thereafter a relatively regular discharge (Fig. 2A). In some cases the burst developed a series of inactivated spikes. In such cases the pause following the burst was of longer duration (Fig. 2B). In both experiments illustrated in Figs. 1 and 2 the glutamate electrodes were located 200 μm from the cell body.

During the regular discharge the spike took off from a slow depolarizing wave, lasting from 10 to 20 msec. Immediately preceding the spike, there

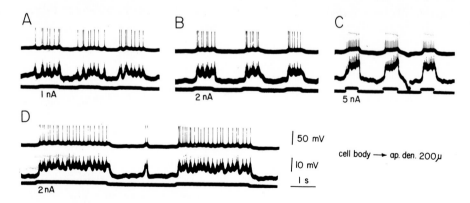

FIG. 1. Excitatory effect of glutamate on CA1 pyramidal cell. (A) Low-gain (upper trace) and high-gain (middle trace) records of response to three pulses of 1 nA glutamate (lower trace) delivered in the apical dendritic region, 200 μm from the pyramidal layer. (B,C) Same as (A), but glutamate pulses of 2 and 5 nA, respectively. (D) Response to two longer pulses of 2 nA.

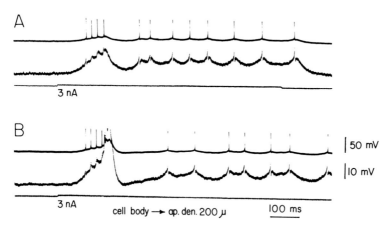

FIG. 2. Pattern of glutamate-induced discharge. (A,B) Responses to glutamate pulses of 3 nA delivered in the apical dendritic tree, 200 μm from the pyramidal layer (cell body). Note longer pause after the initial burst in (B) compared to (A).

was a prepotential. In some cells the size, polarity, and time course were similar to those of the fast prepotential described by Spencer and Kandel (1961). Following the action potential, the depolarizing wave subsided and a hyperpolarization of a few millivolts occurred. The duration of this hyperpolarization was dependent on the dose of glutamate. After cessation of the glutamate ejection the membrane potential repolarized within 0.1 to 1.5 sec, depending upon the dose. In some cases, the glutamate was able to elicit full action potentials for awhile, after which the full spike was blocked and only the prepotentials appeared (Fig. 3). In this case, both the distal (about 250 μm from the soma) and the proximate electrodes (about 100 μm from the soma) gave large depolarizations and triggered depolarizing waves and a series of prepotentials. However, both response types started at different membrane potentials following the two ejections, an indication that neither is a direct function of the soma membrane potential.

The glutamate effect was critically dependent on the location of the iontophoretic electrodes. They had to be located roughly along a line normal to the pyramidal layer, i.e., along the direction of the apical dendritic axis. Effective points were localized both in the stratum oriens and in the

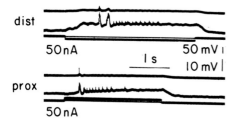

FIG. 3. Isolated prepotentials elicited by glutamate. Low- and high-gain records (upper and middle traces) of response to 50 nA glutamate about 100 μm (upper half) and 250 μm (lower half) from the pyramidal layer. Note train of prepotentials after the large depolarizations.

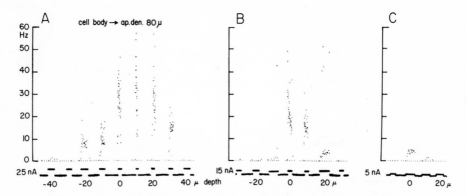

FIG. 4. Transverse distribution of glutaminergic receptors. (A) Discharge frequency (ordinate) of CA1 pyramidal cell to pulses of 25 nA delivered at the indicated depths along a track transverse to the apical dendritic axis. (B) Same as (A), but glutamate pulses of 15 nA. C, Same as (A), but pulses now 5 nA.

stratum radiatum, corresponding to the basal and apical dendrites, respectively. Moving the glutamate electrode vertically through the slice, thus passing through the dendritic tree of the recording cell, the placement was highly critical. In Fig. 4A glutamate was delivered with pulses of 25 nA at the indicated depths. Each dot represents a spike and the ordinate gives the instantaneous frequency. Zero indicates the depth giving the most regular high-frequency activity. At more superficial levels (negative numbers) the discharge fell off rapidly. Similarly, the activity disappeared when the glutamate electrode was 40 μm below the best depth. In Fig. 4B the ejection current was reduced to 15 nA, and the sensitive depths were 0 and 10 μm, with only a late and low-frequency discharge at 20 μm. With the ejection current reduced to 5 nA there was only a moderate discharge at 0 and very weak discharge at 10 μm. As the electrode approached a sensitive spot in parallel to an increased discharge, the latency showed a marked reduction. Because the effect could fall markedly by a movement of 10 μm in a direction transverse to the apical dendritic axis, a possible explanation is that the electrode passes a branch or group of branches of the dendritic tree with associated glutaminergic receptors.

During such a traverse the frequency/depth plots showed several peaks. Such records were commonly obtained and suggest the involvement of several branches of the dendritic tree approached and passed by the glutamate electrode.

The distribution of the excitatory synapses suggested to us that the dendritic area could be more sensitive to the glutamate than the cell body region. However, in spite of a careful search with pairs of iontophoretic electrodes, it was not possible to detect a systematically lower threshold at the cell body region, as compared with dendritic areas.

When a large dose of glutamate is delivered very close to its most sensitive

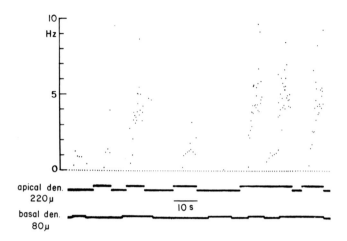

FIG. 5. Summation of two local glutamate ejections. The two lines under the graph indicate the glutamate pulses delivered to the apical dendrites and the basal dendrites at points 220 and 80 μm from the cell body, respectively. In the three periods with ejection from both electrodes the discharge frequency is higher than the sum of the frequency to either electrode ejection alone.

spot, responses very similar to the paroxysmal depolarization shift observed in experimental epileptical foci can be seen (Matsumoto and Marsan, 1964).

Because of the localized effect of the glutamate ejection it was possible to test whether the local dendritic effects could sum to change the discharge pattern of the cell. In Fig. 5 the frequency of discharge to 10 nA glutamate in the basal dendritic area 80 μm from the cell body ranged around 1 per second and the response to 23 nA in the apical dendritic field 220 μm from the cell body was just at threshold. The discharge to this pulse alone was erratic and had a long latency when it occurred. Coupling of the two ejections gave a definite, short-latency discharge between 3 and 10 impulses per second with a mean around 5 per second. In this case, the summation must have taken place in the cell body membrane or close to this as the frequency of the summed effect is very much higher than the sum of the frequencies caused by the individual iontophoretic ejections.

DISCUSSION

The data indicate that very low doses of L-glutamate in regions known to contain excitatory synapses discharge hippocampal pyramidal cells very effectively. Remarkably, the depolarization seen at the cell body in cells with a good membrane potential was considerable, indicating that the space constant of the apical dendritic tree of these cells may be considerably longer than that supposed until now. Therefore moderate glutamate ejections more than half-way along the apical dendritic tree were able to depolarize the cell up to 10 to 15 mV and give rise to a discharge of 25 to 30/sec, which is at least as high as the physiologic range.

Concerning the mechanism of action, the frequent occurrence of prepotentials was striking. The prepotentials were not elicited at a special membrane potential of the soma, they could be initiated both from the apical and basal dendrites; and they had an all-or-none character and occurred with clearly different size and rise-times. All features indicate that these potentials may arise as unitary events generated at different distances from the cell body, possibly in different parts of the dendritic tree. These generation sites are probably located not only at a single bifurcation (Spencer and Kandel, 1961) but may occur at many of the dendritic branching points.

The prepotentials and the spike occurred on top of the slow depolarizing wave, which could vary both in amplitude and slope. These waves may be remote EPSP's grossly attenuated by the cable properties of the dendritic tree. A possible mechanism of action is that the glutamate excites the synaptic area of the membrane, the spine heads, which in turn sum their influence on the initial portion of secondary or tertiary dendrites. Local spikes in this region may travel toward the main apical dendritic shaft but are often blocked at this position, thus giving rise to the prepotential seen by the somatic electrode. If the prepotential in the small dendritic branches reaches an apical dendritic membrane that is already slightly depolarized as a result of other simultaneously active dendritic branches, a full spike travels down the dendritic shaft and into the soma.

The hyperpolarization that occurs after a spike may be either an afterhyperpolarization or an electrogenic pump effect. The available data cannot differentiate these possibilities. One should note that the hyperpolarization has a very long time course and that it increases with the number and the frequency of the spikes in the previous discharges.

The remarkably sharp localization of the glutamic acid receptors when an electrode went transversely to the nominal axis of the cell indicates that the depolarization is of relatively local nature. Therefore any effect cannot be ascribed to diffusion to more central portions of the cell. This suggests that full-blown activity can be triggered by depolarization as far away as two-thirds of the apical dendritic tree. Preliminary investigation indicates that depolarization in the outer third also can be effective.

The experiments with double ejection indicate that local depolarization in the dendritic tree may sum where the spike emerges, probably by summating the effect of the local depolarizations at an area of confluence.

Because summation was also seen when glutamate electrodes were located in the apical and basal dendrites, respectively, the distance precluding any direct effect, the summation resulted from depolarization of the soma membrane itself.

Finally, the data suggest that the transverse hippocampal slice preparation might give useful clues in studying the interaction between synaptic mechanisms and various physiologic and pharmacologic neurochemical agents.

REFERENCES

Andersen, P., Blackstad, T. W., and Lømo, T. (1966): Location and identification of excitatory synapses on hippocampal pyramidal cells. *Exp. Brain Res.,* 1:236–248.

Curtis, D. R., and Johnston, G. A. R. (1974): Amino acid transmitters in the mammalian central nervous system. *Ergeb. Physiol.,* 69:97–188.

Matsumoto, H., and Ajmone-Marsan, C. (1964): Cortical cellular phenomena in experimental epilepsy: Interictal manifestations. *Exp. Neurol.,* 9:286–304.

Skrede, K. K., and Westgaard, R. H. (1971): The transverse hippocampal slice: A well-defined cortical structure maintained *in vitro. Brain Res.* 35:589–593.

Spencer, W. A., and Kandel, E. R. (1961): Electrophysiology of hippocampal neurons. IV. Fast prepotentials. *J. Neurophysiol.,* 24:272–285.

Advances in Neurology, Vol. 12, edited by
G. W. Kreutzberg, Raven Press, New York
© 1975.

The Possible Role of Dendrites in EEG Synchronization

H. Petsche, O. Prohaska, P. Rappelsberger, and R. Vollmer

Institute of Neurophysiology, University of Vienna, and Brain Research Institute of the Austrian Academy of Sciences, A1090 Vienna, Austria

This study is part of an extensive research project with the scope of describing the spatiotemporal characteristics of seizure activities and their possible morphologic background. This chapter is concerned almost exclusively with studies in the vertical dimension of the cortex. The final aim was to understand in which way synchronization may be achieved within the cortex during seizure activities. The word "synchronization," although in use among most electroencephalographers, is not well defined. According to the proposal made by Petsche, Rappelsberger, and Frey (1972) "synchronized activity" may be termed every EEG activity appearing with almost equal shape in large regions of the cortex. However, this property of seizure patterns would be more appropriately termed "synmorphism" or "isomorphism." The word "synchronization" may be misleading for still another reason, as these potentials, if recorded from different electrodes, are usually not at all synchronous, but are shifted in time by tens of milliseconds.

The main problem covered in this chapter is to define the size of those cortical compartments that—during a "synchronized" pattern—actually are synchronously active, and to determine their morphologic background. These zones of uniform electrical activity may be considered as the "generator zones" of the corresponding graphoelements.

Studies since 1970 (Petsche and Rappelsberger, 1970, 1972, 1973; Petsche et al., 1971, 1972) have produced overwhelming evidence that, during seizures, the deep cortical layers differ in several ways in their electrogenesis from the upper cortical layers: the voltage and the content of higher frequencies are several times larger and the degree of coherence—if measured parallel to the cortex surface by equidistant electrodes—is slower than at the surface. These features are the reason why epicortical activity looks as if it had passed through a low-pass filter. This behavior, characteristic for deep recordings down to the pyramidal layer, changes abruptly at about 200 μm below surface; at about this level the apical dendrites of the pyramidal cells turn horizontally to become merged in the fiber feltwork of the two uppermost cortical layers.

Such findings suggested that the authors consider the hypothesis of a columnar organization of the cortex with compartments in the order of 50 μm width. These columns were thought not to reach the cortical surface (Petsche et al., 1972). Fleischhauer experimented with this hypothesis and found the apical dendrites to be combined to bundles that are in close contact to each other (Fleischhauer, Petsche, and Wittkowski, 1972; Massing and Fleischhauer, 1973; Fleischhauer, 1974).

In the context of this chapter, the question as to the physiologic significance of these bundles with respect to seizure activities is examined. For this purpose, intracortical studies with closely spaced horizontally arranged semimicroelectrodes have been performed in order to define the possible size of the generator zones underlying different graphoelements and their possible spatial relationship to the position of the dendritic bundles within the cortex.

MATERIAL AND METHODS

The experiments were performed on unanesthetized, curarized, and artificially respirated rabbits. The pressure points and the tracheotomy wounds were carefully and repeatedly infiltrated by a 2% procaine solution. Because of the geometry of its cortex, the lissencephalic rabbit was chosen as the experimental animal. Seizures were elicited by topical application of penicillin. Used as recording devices were 3 M NaCl double semimicroelectrodes (tip diameters between 1 and 5 μm, 5 to 10 M) arranged horizontally at distances between 120 and 2,000 μm. These microelectrodes were introduced into the cortex through an Ag–AgCl ring electrode (2-mm i.d.) for surface recording. To prevent exsiccation the cortex was covered with 3% agar saline. Recordings were made from different depths at steps of 250 and 500 μm. The penicillin spikes and seizure activities were stored by an Ampex 7-channel analogue-type tape recorder. After impedance transformation they were recorded uni- and bipolarly on a Schwarzer-16-channel EEG machine. Surface recordings from the contralateral hemisphere were also made as a control.

Power spectra, coherence, and phase functions were computed by an IBM 360/44 and 370/155 (programmed by P. Rappelsberger). The coherence estimates were calculated to supply information about the possible size of the generator zones of graphoelements, because as soon as the coherence between two electrodes becomes 100%, the size of the generator zone of this activity approximately equals the distance between these electrodes or is even larger. For the naked eye, a less exact but useful method was applied to visualize differences already during the recording: the comparison between unipolar and bipolar records. A bipolar record, representing the difference between the two unipolarly recorded potentials, contains information about both the amplitude and the shape of the potentials (phase). As soon as the voltages of the two potentials recorded from closely spaced electrodes become equal any deviation of the bipolar record from zero indicates differences in shape or phase or both. This simple method proved a valuable instrument to visualize changes of the size of the generator zones of single graphoelements and to show their variation in certain intracortical lamina.

RESULTS

When recorded from two closely spaced electrodes the cortex was shown to be electrically anisotropic. This is shown in Figs. 1 and 2, both of which demonstrate power spectra and coherence of seizures elicited by locally applied penicillin. In Fig. 1, the seizure activities were recorded epicortically (upper row of power spectra) and intracortically (lower row of power spectra) at different depths of the cortex (500-μm intervals).

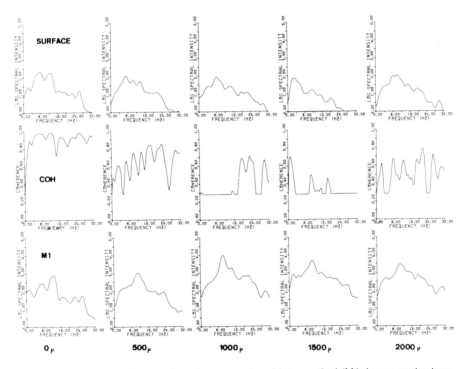

FIG. 1. Power spectra from surface (upper row) and intracortical (M1, lower row) microelectrode: periods of 4-sec seizure activity recorded simultaneously. The intracortical electrode was advanced at steps of 500 μm. (Middle row) Coherence estimates between surface and depth. Each of the five pillars of diagrams is from the first 4 sec of a fully developed seizure (topical application of penicillin). Abscissa, frequency range up to 32 Hz. Ordinate, log spectral intensity. Note the increase of power within the first millimeter of the cortex (M1) and the decrease of coherence between cortex and intracortical levels.

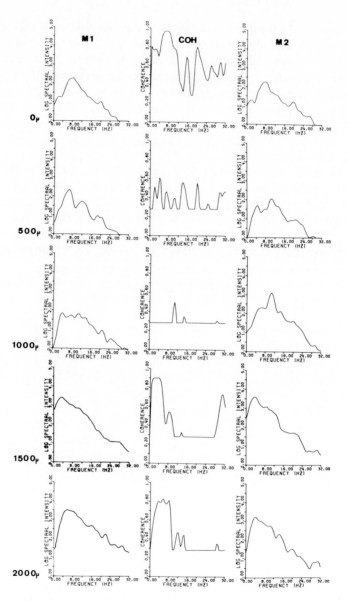

FIG. 2. Power spectra from adjacent microelectrodes (M1 and M2), 2 mm apart, and their corresponding coherence estimates, at steps of 500 μm. As in Fig. 1, the first 4 sec of a fully developed seizure were chosen for each analysis. The decrease of coherence with depth is also a prominent feature in the horizontal dimension. Increase of spectral intensity with depth as in Fig. 1. These findings suggest the "generator zones" to be smallest at about 1000 μm in this experiment. Below this zone the coherence of low frequencies increases again. (The horizontal lines in the coherence curves are the levels of significance below which no coherence was calculated.)

In between are drawn the coherence estimates between the corresponding power spectra. Each of these five analyses relates to a period of 4 sec at the begin of a seizure. The first column of diagrams was recorded at depth 0, i.e., the microelectrode recorded from the surface in the middle of the epicortical ring electrode. Two main observations may be made: (1) the power spectrum increases with increasing depth within the first millimeter of the cortex (logarithmic scale); (2) the coherence between surface and intracortical electrodes, being maximum at surface, decreases, attaining a minimum at 1,000 and 1,500 μm. Only coherences significantly different from zero were drawn (horizontal lines). One may conclude from this picture that epicortical and intracortical activities within a seizure are largely independent from a certain depth on. However, because of the finite length of the record the possibility of occasionally correlated transients between surface and depth cannot be excluded.

Figure 2 was chosen to demonstrate the electrical anisotropy of the cortex in the horizontal dimension. In this experiment, two surface electrodes, placed 2 mm apart, were used (power spectra and coherence function, upper row of diagrams). Two semimicroelectrodes were lowered through these electrodes; from these, recordings were made every 500 μm. In Fig. 2 each of the five subsequent rows of diagrams represents an analysis of the first 4 sec of seizures. This figure also demonstrates that the power spectrum increases with increasing depth and that the coherence function is lowest from a certain depth on. This means that at about 1,000 μm in this experiment, the activities recorded at 2-mm distances have no common source, whereas at still deeper levels, the low-frequency components of the seizures become coherent again. According to our above definition, the generator zones of potentials recorded at 500 μm and particularly at 1,000 μm have smaller horizontal extensions than those of the lowest layers. Because of this apparent complexity of generator zones it seemed worthwhile to study single and reproducible graphoelements.

In this context it should be remembered that single transients, i.e., the fast events called "spikes" in electroencephalography, were found to be correlated between surface and depth but phase-shifted, the deep electrode being the leading one (Petsche and Rappelsberger, 1973). Attempts at defining the range of the size of the generator zones for individual graphoelements were thought to help clarify the question of how constant these zones are and how they may be combined to produce surface transients of equal shape.

As one of the simplest models of ictal activity is the penicillin spike, an approach was designed to estimate the maximum size of their generator zones by comparing unipolar and bipolar records of paired microelectrodes at different depths.

Figure 3 shows a depth profile through the visual cortex during interictal penicillin spike activity. The surface electrode almost always shows a posi-

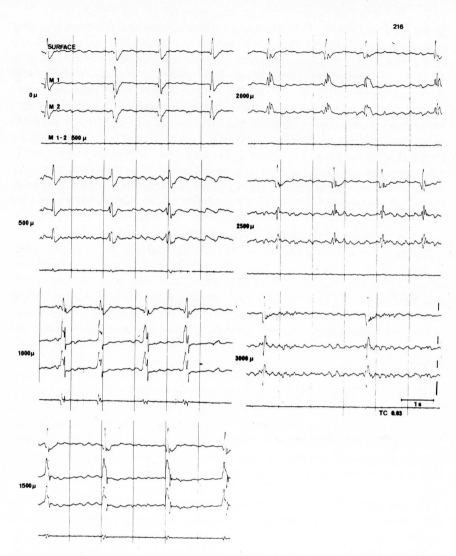

FIG. 3. Simultaneous recordings from a surface electrode and two adjacent semimicro-electrodes (M1 and M2) below, 500 μm apart, at steps of 500 μm. Unipolar and bipolar recordings. Penicillin spikes after topical application of Na-penicillin powder. Negativity upward. In these and the subsequent traces data on depth are related to agar surface. Note the lacking positive prepotential at 1,000 and 1,500 μm and the dissimilarity of the transients, most pronounced at these levels. This is best seen in the increasing voltage of the bipolar trace. These "spikes," therefore, are thought to be complex events and composed of different-sized and -shaped "generator zones" of diameters smaller than the electrode distance (500 μm) at 1,000 and 1,500 μm.

tive prepotential followed by a large negative spike. This is a common feature of penicillin spikes recorded briefly after topical application of the drug. This positive potential is only visible at the surface and within the upper cortical layers. It reappears below the pyramidal layer. Between these levels it is absent. Usually the interictal spikes appear, between 1,000 and 2,000 μm in Fig. 3, to be more complex than in the other layers, the amplitude being much larger than at the surface. In some cases potential gradients of up to 10 mV/mm in the vertical dimension were observed (Petsche et al., 1972). The position of the amplitude maxima indicates that the layer of the large pyramidal cells is involved with the origin of these potentials. The amplitudes at deeper cortical layers and in the white matter become even smaller than at the surface. Between 1,000 and 2,000 μm, the gross negative potentials appear to be composed of several components. The first large negativity appears at the same time as the surface positive prepotential and precedes the large negative potential at the surface (the so-called "penicillin spike"). The inverse time relationship holds true for deeper cortical layers and the white matter, as is clearly visible at 3,000 μm in Fig. 3.

The bipolar record where maximal activity is found in 1,000 and 1,500 μm deserves further attention. Because the amplitudes of the large transients are almost equal in both microelectrodes, it should be concluded that the bipolar activity is caused mainly by differences in the time domain. Because the bipolar derivation shows differences only at 1,000 and 1,500 μm, and disappears again with increasing depth, it may be concluded that in this case the horizontal diameter of the generator zone must be smaller than 500 μm, the electrode distance.

Another sample from a different experiment is demonstrated in Fig. 4. The distance of the microelectrodes is in this case 300 μm. This sample was chosen to demonstrate the variability of the time domain in this layer (1,000 μm). Again, no positive prepotential is found. Although the shape of the complex transients seems to be fairly equal in M1 and M2, the bipolar recording indicates the presence of several generators with different time relationships. As mentioned above the size of the generator zones is not stable.

This is also true for the graphoelements during seizures (Fig. 5). This seizure starts with a clonic pattern which is followed by 16 sec of tonic activity. From the bipolar trace it may be concluded that the spikes are events composed of several constituents with different time distribution whereby either M1 or M2 may lead. Attention should be focused on the tonic pattern, which consists roughly of three parts: in the first 4 sec the bipolar activity is low, indicating relatively large generator zones underlying these potentials; then comes a regular alternating pattern (5 sec), which is, bipolarly, characterized by only each second potential showing a phase difference; this means that the size of the generator zone also seems to

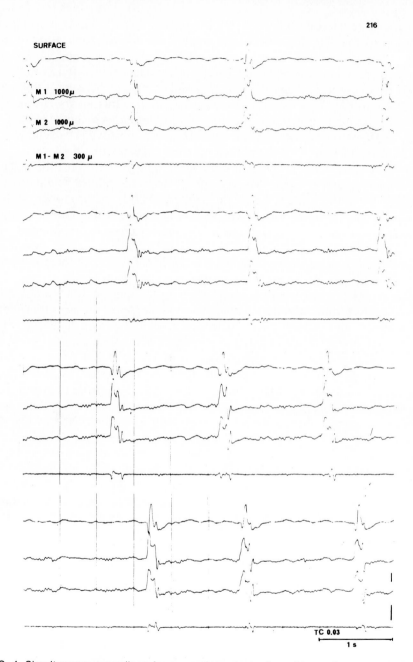

FIG. 4. Simultaneous recordings from a surface electrode and two adjacent semimicro-electrodes, 300 μm apart and 1,000 μm below. Penicillin spikes. The change of the time relationships of the different components of the transients may be concluded from the changing shape of the bipolar trace.

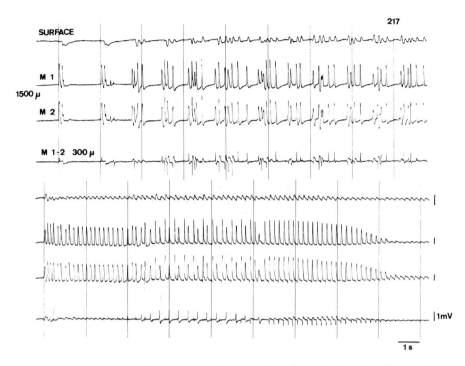

FIG. 5. Recordings as in Figs. 3 and 4. Clonic–tonic seizure. During the clonic pattern, the bipolar track, deviating toward negative and positive in an apparently random fashion, indicates that the groups of spikes that appear synchronously in the unipolar leads M1 and M2 are in fact composed of at least two electrical events arising shortly one after the other but with changing leadership. The tonic pattern consists of three parts: in the first 4 sec, the low bipolar activity indicates an almost synchronous activity at the two microelectrodes, i.e., relatively large generator zones; the next 5 sec are characterized by an alternating of a large and two small generator zones, and the last 5 sec demonstrate a constant sequence of at least two components forming each spike.

fluctuate. And finally, a rather stable generator zone appears to be present during the last 5 sec of the seizure.

In this context it is worth mentioning that the size of the generator zones of seizures may also be influenced by drugs. Benzodiazepines, for instance, which regularize seizure patterns and pronounce the limits of the electro-architectonic areas, give rise to a shortening of penicillin spikes and to an increase of the propagation speed along the cortex (*unpublished data*). Double microelectrode studies show that the bipolar record in the layer of apical dendrites significantly decreases in amplitude although the amplitude of the two unipolar records, as in Fig. 6, even increases. This means that the horizontal diameter of the generator zones underlying the seizure potentials becomes larger with the drug. Whether this effect is due to a better synchronization or to the decrease of the number of morphologic elements contributing to synchronization still has to be explored. However, it seems

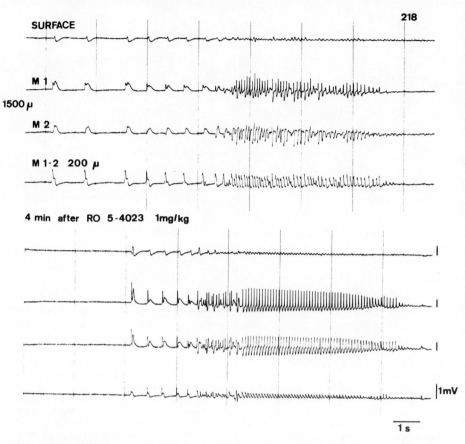

FIG. 6. Seizure patterns, recorded from the layer of apical dendrites by two microelectrodes, 200 μm apart, before and after the application of a benzodiazepine derivative. Note the regularization of the pattern and the decrease in amplitude of the bipolar track, whereas the unipolarly recorded activity increases. This means that the horizontal diameter of the generator zones underlying these potentials increases.

as if the latter, namely the gradual decrease of the number of active generators caused by the drug, may be the true explanation.

DISCUSSION

These results confirm our previous studies on the electrical anisotropy of the neocortex during seizures and may be briefly summarized as follows:

1. Seizure patterns recorded from adjacent surface electrodes have higher degrees of coherence than from electrodes at the same distance in deep cortical layers. The main differences were found in the region of pyramidal cells and in their apical dendrites.

2. A comparison of power spectra between surface and intracortical recordings resulted in the highest power to be found in a level that roughly corresponds to the deep pyramidal layer.

3. The power spectrum at this level contains more high-frequency components than at the surface.

4. The overall coherence between surface activity and deep layers is generally very low.

5. Single transients, however, propagated toward the surface (Petsche et al., 1972).

These findings underscore once more that even during such generalized and apparently uniform activities as seizure patterns, the electrical activity is quite complex and appears to be composed, even within the relatively small electrode distances of our experiments, of a quantity of more elementary electrical events. Therefore the question arose as to whether it might be possible to find the minimum volume of those cortical zones that are involved in the generation of the gross potentials of a seizure pattern. In other words, the problem was to define the possible size of that cortical volume within which equally shaped field potentials may be recorded. This zone was termed "generator zone." For their definition bipolar recordings from electrodes at different distances were used as explained above. When the unipolar records of two adjacent electrodes appeared to be identical and there was a zero bipolar trace, the two electrodes were concluded to be within a cortical zone that contributes uniformly to the production of this signal, i.e., to lie within one generator zone. We wish to emphasize that this term is merely descriptive and that it has been used as a functional concept, as a sort of working hypothesis. It neither implicates nor purports any information about the nature of underlying field potentials nor about current sources.

However, these studies resulted in several findings that are paralleled by some morphologic features of the cortex. Figure 7 is an attempt to summarize our findings in a hypothetical model. The generator zones, which up to now have been approached only in one dimension (by pairs of electrodes), are thought to be circular if the cortical architecture is uniform within this zone. This model, containing sharply limited generator zones, certainly gives some idea of their possible size and position. Nevertheless, a few features deserve mention: one is that generator zones of the uppermost and lowest cortical layers were found to be much larger than those within the layers of the large pyramids and apical dendrites (see also Figs. 1–6). From previous studies it is known that these zones may propagate in different directions horizontally. This is symbolized by vectors of different lengths. In contrast to these two layers the zone where the large pyramids and their apical dendrites are found behaves quite differently; here the generator zones may be much smaller (down to less than 120 μm diameter, the smallest

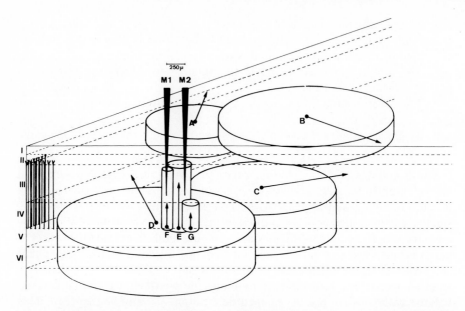

FIG. 7. Schematic presentation of the results. The "generator zones," i.e., cortical volumes with synchronous activity during a certain graphoelement, are characterized by the cylinders A–G. These volumes are small at approximately the layers of apical dendrites and relatively broad in the layers above and below. Besides, the small generator zones in the middle layers of the cortex (G,E,F) underlie the fast EEG components (e.g., penicillin spikes) and propagate in a corticopetal direction, whereas the large zones above and below (A–D), underlying the slow components in the EEG, propagate in different directions horizontally (indicated by the vectors) and are not necessarily linked to one another. The vertical lines on the left in III and IV represent dendritic bundles. M1 and M2: glass semimicroelectrodes.

electrode distance used in these experiments). They propagate too, but only in a corticopetal direction, and never horizontally.

These findings support the idea of a columnar structure in the electrogenesis of seizures. However, there is increasing evidence from morphologic findings that the apical dendrites of pyramidal cells are combined to bundles (Fleischhauer et al., 1972; Peters and Walsh, 1972; Massing and Fleischhauer, 1973; Fleischhauer, 1974; Feldman and Peters, 1974).

The concept of a columnar organization of the cerebral cortex is not new. Similar suggestions have been made by several authors. Lorente de Nó (1938), as one of the first, suggested from general anatomic considerations that the deeper layers of the cerebral cortex are organized in columns. The pillar-like formation of functionally linked nerve cells concluded from Hubel and Wiesel's (1962) experiments is another example of this concept. Especially organized zones of the cortex ("barrels") were described by Woolsey and van der Loos (1970) in the somatosensory cortex of mice. Therefore one may wonder whether our physiologic findings are related to dendritic bundles rather than to columnar cellular arrangements within the cortex.

Before this problem is approached, a short review of the possible mechanisms underlying the generation of "spikes" may be useful.

According to Creutzfeldt et al. (1966) who studied the relationships between cellular events and surface potentials, spiking activity on the surface consists of a biphasic positive–negative potential. They found that the positive surface potential is associated with intracellularly recorded excitatory postsynaptic potentials (EPSP's). The second phase, the negativity, was found to be associated with a postexcitatory silence of the cell under observation. This was found to be true for spiking activity after administration of pentylenetetrazol (Metrazol®) or strychnine or after local freezing, i.e., epileptogenic agents.

There is almost general agreement today that surface potentials are formed by a superposition of extracellular field potentials (for review, see Creutzfeldt, 1974). If EPSP's were located only near the soma, the apical dendrites would act as a source of current, and a positive surface potential would result. EPSP's arising somewhere in the middle of the apical dendrites would result in a smaller positive surface potential, and EPSP's arising close to the surface would produce a negative surface potential (see Fig. 28 in Creutzfeldt, 1974). Therefore an electrode invading the cortex along the dendritic tree "would record potentials of different polarity at different parts of the neuron, and a reversal of potentials near the active source or sink would be seen" (Creutzfeldt, 1974; see also Rall and Shepherd, 1968). According to these considerations one could interpret the positive prepotentials of surface spikes as being caused by EPSP's arising near the soma (Petsche et al., 1972). This is also evident from the work of other authors (see review by Ayala, Dichter, Gumnit, Matsumoto, and Spencer, 1973).

However, the mechanisms underlying the large negative surface potentials, the "spikes," seem to be different. Raabe and Lux (1972) and Humphrey (1968) suggested that electrotonic spreading of postsynaptic potentials (PSP's) from the soma along the apical dendrite was responsible for the surface potentials. But these conclusions were made on the basis of potentials evoked by antidromic pyramidal tract stimulation. It is questionable, however, if electrotonic transmission is sufficient to explain the findings of spike propagation through the cortex. If the length constant of the apical dendrites of pyramidal cells, which is on the order of 200 μm (Creutzfeldt, 1974), is taken into account, only about 5% of the voltage measured in the pyramidal layer should be found at the level where the apical dendrites ramify horizontally. However, with penicillin spikes the voltage gradient along the apical dendrites was shown to be much lower. Therefore at least several additional sources for the generation of penicillin spikes along the apical dendrites have to be assumed. As it is unlikely that these sources are caused by PSP's arising along the apical dendritic membrane in a strictly timed way, an active propagation along the dendritic membrane under the pathologic conditions of the interictal activity has to be considered.

According to a number of investigators, the concept of the dendritic membrane as a mere passive integration mechanism can no longer be maintained (for review see Purpura, 1971). There is general agreement today that under certain conditions dendrites begin to conduct like axons. This seems to be true particularly for seizures. One of the first observations supporting this assumption was made in 1960 on rabbit hippocampus by Green and Petsche who found that soon after the seizure had begun, the action potentials stopped and were replaced by very high and broad potentials, which could be followed with almost constant voltage down to the beginning of the stratum lacunosum. The authors concluded that these potentials may represent the "triggering of previously inactive membranes, presumably those of dendrites." For the present, what are presumably dendritic spikes have been recorded in cerebellum, hippocampus, spinal cord, neocortex, and in tissue cultures. Especially interesting are the observations by Purpura, Shofer, and Scarff (1965) who found no evidence for dendritic spikes in nonepileptic preparations of adult animals but succeeded in immature animals. As a result of their experiments, these authors thought that dendritic spike generation might be some kind of "atavistic feature" of membranes that are inexcitable under normal conditions. It seems not unlikely that epileptic seizures represent an occasion for remembering forgotten features.

Nevertheless, it is probable that dendritic membranes behave like axons also under certain physiologic conditions. Kwan and Murphy (1974a,b) were able to demonstrate by means of current-density analysis that active spike propagation occurs in Purkinje cell dendrites after activation of climbing fibers. An analogous report was given by Spear (1972) who found evidence for active propagation of potentials in ascending, vertically oriented, intracortical dendrites. Spear found the conduction velocity (0.1 to 50 cm/sec) to be slower in the more superficial layers of the cortex; this is the region in which the apical dendrites of the pyramids turn in an almost right angle to become merged in the fiber feltwork of the two uppermost cortical layers. We found that the electrical behavior does not change continuously, but changes fairly abruptly at about 200 μm below surface, a finding that roughly coincides with Spear's results.

With respect to these arguments and regarding the fact that distinct dendritic bundles are found in the neocortex one may wonder if this nonrandom distribution of apical dendrites is involved in the synchronization of fast EEG events.

The dendritic bundles of the neocortex are characterized by such a close packing that about 20% of the surface of every dendrite is common to adjacent dendrite surfaces, separated by the extracellular space only (Fleischhauer et al., 1972). If, according to the above considerations, the single dendrites become conductors during seizures, one may question the possibility of mutual electrotonic influences between the single dendrites within a bundle. Although distinct structures responsible for electrotonic transmission (dendrodendritic gap junctions) have been described in neocortex (Sloper, 1972), no gap junctions have been found in dendritic bundles up to now. There are, however, experimental findings that suggest a direct electrical interaction between closely arranged excitable membranes. Such "ephaptic" transmission was first reported by Arvanitaki on peripheral nerves (1942). Nelson (1966) who studied single motoneurons of the spinal cord, reported short-latency facilitation after antidromic stimulation of adjacent motoneurons, which implicates field effects. Terzuolo and Bullock (1956) were able to modify firing rates in the stretch receptor neuron of the crayfish even with such small voltage gradients as 1 mV/mm. The studies by Kaczmarek and Adey (1974) lend further support to this idea; they stimulated the neocortex with weak steady-current fields and found an increasing release of transmitter, which they concluded to be caused by increased nerve-cell activity caused by field effects.

Because the generator zones of the fast EEG events were found to be roughly in the layer of the apical dendrites with diameters of $< 120 \mu$m and to propagate exclusively in a corticopetal direction, it was postulated that one or several dendritic bundles may be the morphologic basis of these generator zones. This means that during EEG "spikes" the dendrites of a single bundle may discharge synchronously by electrotonic interaction. It is likely not only that single dendrites within one bundle discharge at the same time, but also that several bundles may be combined to form one generator zone and to discharge uniformly. The minimum size of these functional generator zones has not yet been determined in these experiments. Up to now it may only be claimed that these zones may be even less than 120μm, the smallest electrode distance used.

Synchronization phenomena underlying the generator of "slow" seizure potentials, which are mainly found in the uppermost and lowest cortical zones, are probably not connected to the interaction of dendritic bundles. Any hypothesis in this context would go beyond the scope of this chapter. Nevertheless, it may be mentioned that there seems to be some functional hierarchy in these three floors of generator zones insofar as the primary condition for the generation of seizure activity appears to be the formation of generator zones in the pyramidal cells and their apical dendrites by which the generators of the slow waves in the deep cortical layers are activated as aftereffects. Some tertiary effects seem to be the formation of generator zones in the uppermost cortical floor. The studies of Speckmann, Caspers, and Janzen (1972) explain the surface waves in seizures in a similar way. This assumption emerges also from experiments with vertical incisions into the cortex (Petsche and Rappelsberger, 1970), which clearly show that horizontal spreading of the waves (as indicated by the horizontal vectors in Fig. 7) is maintained in the highest and lowest layers of the cortex as long as the deepest cortical layers are not severed by the incision. Possible pathways for the maintenance of this synchronized slow activity in rabbit cortex were shown by Golgi studies (Tömböl, 1972) to exist in layers V and VI.

One may question the possible physiologic significance of dendrite bundles in general. Dendrite bundles were described in several regions of the nervous system: in the spinal cord of cat, frog, and monkeys, in the thalamus and formatio reticularis, and in the cerebral cortex (see Scheibel, Davis, Lindsay, and Scheibel, 1974). Pertinent to our findings may be the observation of the Scheibels (1974) that even the basilar dendrites of pyramidal cells of the neocortex are arranged in bundles. Matthews (1972) assumes that the close apposition of the single dendrites within a bundle probably supports the synchronization of those neurons that send their dendrites into the bundle by altering the threshold ephaptically. The Scheibels (1974) hypothesized that the bundling of dendrites creates subcenters for the motor output. They assert that a correlation between the formation of bundles and some types of behavior may be established.

At this moment, it is too early to draw such far-reaching conclusions from the available morphologic and neurophysiologic findings. Further research is needed to explain the functional significance of dendritic bundles. That the single dendritic tree of nerve cells can act rather independently has already been suggested (Rall and Shepherd, 1968; Llinás, 1974). But even if our findings are restricted to seizure activities, and therefore need not be valid under physiologic conditions, they suggest that dendritic bundles as a special geometric configuration of nerve-cell compartments may act as independent subunits.

ACKNOWLEDGMENTS

This work was supported by the Fonds zur Förderung der wissenschaftlichen Forschung (No. 1118 and 1402) and by the European Training Program in Brain and Behaviour Research. The computations were performed at the Interfakultäres Rechenzentrum der Universität Wien and at the Rechenzentrum der Medizinischen Fakultät, Wien.

REFERENCES

Arvanitaki, A. (1942): Effects evoked on an axon by the activity of a contiguous one. *J. Neurophysiol.,* 5:89–108.

Ayala, G. F., Dichter, M., Gumnit, R. J., Matsumoto, H., and Spencer, W. A. (1973): Genesis of epileptic interictal spikes. New knowledge of cortical feedback system suggests a neurophysiological explanation of brief paroxysms. *Brain Res.,* 52:1–17.

Creutzfeldt, O. D., Watanabe, S., and Lux, H. D. (1966): Relations between EEG-phenomena and potentials of single cortical cells. II. Spontaneous and convulsoid activity. *Electroencephalogr. Clin. Neurophysiol.,* 20:19–37.

Creutzfeldt, O. D. (1974): The neuronal generation of the EEG. In: *Handbook of Electroencephalography in Clinical Neurophysiology,* edited by A. Rémond, Vol. 2, Part C.

Feldman, M. L., and Peters, A. (1974): A study of barrels and pyramidal dendritic clusters in the cerebral cortex. *Brain Res., 77*:55–76.

Fleischhauer, K., Petsche, H., and Wittkowski, W. (1972): Vertical bundles of dendrites in the neocortex. *Z. Anat. Entwicklungsgesch., 136*:213–223.

Fleischhauer, K. (1974): On different patterns of dendritic bundling in the cerebral cortex of the cat. *Z. Anat. Entwicklungsgesch., 143*:115–126.

Green, J. D., and Petsche, H. (1961): Hippocampal electrical activity. IV. Unitary events and genesis of hippocampal seizures. *Electroencephalogr. Clin. Neurophysiol., 13*:868–879.

Hubel, D. H., and Wiesel, T. N. (1962): Receptive fields, binocular interaction and functional architecture in the cat's visual cortex. *J. Physiol., 160*:106–154.

Humphrey, D. R. (1968): Re-analysis of the antidromic cortical response. II. On the contribution of cell discharge and PSPs to the evoked potentials. *Electroencephalogr. Clin. Neurophysiol., 25*:421–442.

Kaczmarek, L. K., and Adey, W. R. (1974): Weak electric gradients change ionic and transmitter fluxes in cortex. *Brain Res., 66*:527–540.

Kwan, H. C., and Murphy, J. T. (1974a): A basis for extracellular current density analysis in cerebellar cortex. *J. Neurophysiol., 37*:170–180.

Kwan, H. C., and Murphy, J. T. (1974b): Extracellular current density analysis of responses in cerebellar cortex to climbing fiber activation. *J. Neurophysiol., 37*:333–345.

Llinás, R. (1975): Chapter 1, this volume.

Lorente de Nó, R. (1938): Architectonics and structure of the cerebral cortex. In: *Physiology of the Nervous System,* edited by J. F. Fulton. Oxford Univ. Press, London and New York.

Massing, W., and Fleischhauer, K. (1973): Further observations on vertical bundles of dendrites in the cerebral cortex of the rabbit. *Z. Anat. Entwicklungsgesch., 141*:115–123.

Matthews, M. A., Willis, W. D., and Williams, V. (1972): Dendrite bundles in lamina IX of cat spinal cord: A possible source for electrical interaction between motoneurons? *Anat. Rec., 171*:313–328.

Nelson, P. G. (1966): Interaction between spinal motoneurons of the cat. *J. Neurophysiol., 29*:275–287.

Peters, A., and Walsh, T. M. (1972): A study of the organization of apical dendrites in the somatic sensory cortex of the rat. *J. Comp. Neurol., 144*:253–268.

Petsche, H., and Rappelsberger, P. (1970): Influence of cortical incisions on synchronization pattern and travelling waves. *Electroencephalogr. Clin. Neurophysiol., 28*:592–600.

Petsche, H., and Rappelsberger, P. (1972): Spatio-temporal and laminar analysis of self-sustained cortical activity. *Riv. Patol. Nerv. Ment., 93*:16–44.

Petsche, H., and Rappelsberger, P. (1973): The problem of synchronization in the spread of epileptic discharges leading to seizures in man. In: *Epilepsy—Its Phenomena in Man,* edited by M. A. B. Brazier. Academic Press, New York and London.

Petsche, H., Rappelsberger, P., and Frey, Z. (1971): Intracorticale Mechanismen bei der Entstehung der Penicillin-Spitzen. *EEG-EMG, 2*:176–180.

Petsche, H., Rappelsberger, P., and Frey, Z. (1972): Intracortical aspects of the synchronization of self-sustained bioelectrical activities. In: *Synchronization of EEG Activity in Epilepsies,* edited by H. Petsche and M. A. B. Brazier. Springer-Verlag, Vienna.

Purpura, D. P., Shofer, R. J., and Scarff, T. (1965): Properties of synaptic activities and spike potentials in immature neocortex. *J. Neurophysiol., 28*:925–942.

Purpura, D. P. (1971): Dendrites: Heterogeneity in form and function. In: *Handbook of Electroencephalography in Clinical Neurophysiology,* edited by A. Rémond, Vol. 1, Part B, 1B3–1B17.

Raabe, W., and Lux, H. D. (1972): Studies on extracellular potentials generated by synaptic activity on single cat motor cortex neurons. In: *Synchronization of EEG Activity in Epilepsies,* edited by H. Petsche and M. A. B. Brazier. Springer-Verlag, Vienna.

Rall, W., and Shepherd, G. M. (1968): Theoretical reconstruction of field potentials and dendrodendritic synaptic interactions in olfactory bulb. *J. Neurophysiol., 31*:884–915.

Scheibel, M. E., Davies, T. L., Lindsay, R. D., and Scheibel, A. B. (1974): Basilar dendrite bundles of giant pyramidal cells. *Exp. Neurol., 42*:307–319.

Scheibel, M. E., and Scheibel, A. B. (1974): Dendrite bundles as sites for central programs. An hypothesis. *Int. J. Neurosci. (in press).*

Sloper, J. J. (1972): Gap junctions between dendrites in the primate neocortex. *Brain Res., 44*:641–646.

Spear, P. J. (1972): Evidence for spike propagation in cortical dendrites. *Exp. Neurol.*, 35: 111–121.

Speckmann, E.-J., Caspers, H., and Janzen, R. W. (1972): Relations between cortical DC shifts and membrane potential changes of cortical neurons associated with seizure activity. In: *Synchronization of EEG Activity in Epilepsies,* edited by H. Petsche and M. A. B. Brazier. Springer-Verlag, Vienna.

Terzuolo, C. A., and Bullock, T. H. (1956): Measurements of imposed voltage gradient adequate to modulate neuronal firing. *Proc. Natl. Acad. Sci. USA,* 42:687–694.

Tömböl, T. (1972): A Golgi analysis of the sensori-motor cortex in the rabbit. In: *Synchronization of EEG Activity in Epilepsies,* edited by H. Petsche and M. A. B. Brazier. Springer-Verlag, Vienna.

Woolsey, T. A., and van der Loos, H. (1970): The structural organization of layer IV in the somatosensory region (S1) of mouse cerebral cortex. *Brain Res.,* 17:205–242.

Advances in Neurology, Vol. 12, edited by
G. W. Kreutzberg, Raven Press, New York
© 1975.

Dendritic Bundling in the Cerebral Cortex

K. Fleischhauer and K. Detzer

Anatomical Institute, University of Bonn, Bonn, Germany

Golgi methods reveal the dendritic tree of only a small proportion of nerve cells present in any one section. In the literature, therefore, many figures showing dendrites in the cerebral cortex are, in fact, composite drawings in which well-impregnated cells from several sections are drawn as if being situated immediately adjacent to each other in one section. Such composite drawings seem to have been accepted unconsciously as depicting not only the structure of the dendritic arborizations, but also the true spatial relationship between the various elements shown in such a figure. Therefore it is perhaps not surprising that in most anatomic and electrophysiologic texts and considerations it has been tacitly assumed that in the mammalian cerebral cortex the apical dendrites of large layer V pyramids are distributed entirely at random.

However, this view was proved erroneous in 1972 when it was shown by two independent groups that in the somatosensory cortex of rat, rabbit, and cat apical dendrites of large layer V pyramids may approach each other to run in close association and to form vertical structures extending through layer IV. These structures were termed "clusters" by Peters and Walsh (1972) and "vertical bundles of dendrites" by Fleischhauer, Petsche, and Wittkowski (1972).

Close inspection, particularly of tangential sections, reconstruction of several bundles, and electron microscopy revealed that in this region of the rabbit brain the majority of dendrites take part in the formation of bundles; that one bundle contains about 15 dendrites; that the distance between two bundles is in the order of 50 μm; that within a bundle the individual dendrites lie very close to each other; and that there are stretches of direct contact between the plasmalemma of two adjacent dendrites (Fleischhauer et al., 1972; Massing and Fleischhauer, 1973).

These and other findings enabled us to propose the hypothesis that the vertical bundles of dendrites are the morphologic equivalent of a grid of homologous, densely packed, and vertically arranged functional units or generators. This had been postulated by Petsche, Rappelsberger, and Frey (1972) as a consequence of their electrophysiologic findings.

In order to test this hypothesis and to perform more specific experiments with respect to the electrophysiologic properties of dendritic bundles, it

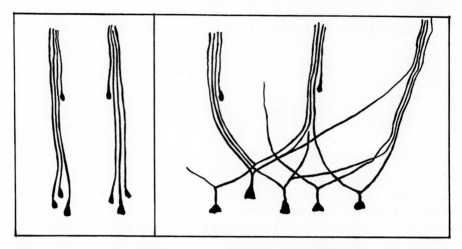

FIG. 1. Diagram illustrating the differences between the pattern of dendritic bundling in the visual (left) and in the sensorimotor cortex (right) of the cat. (From Fleischhauer, 1974.)

must be determined whether the composition and the morphology of the bundles differ in various regions of the cerebral cortex, and if so, whether these differences can be related to any known morphologic or electrophysiologic data.

Being most familiar with the cat brain and having a great number of serial sections at my disposal, I first investigated the cat (Fleischhauer, 1974) and studied the apical dendrites in two well-known regions that greatly differ in function as well as in cytoarchitectonic structure, i.e., the sensorimotor cortex in the superior sigmoid gyrus and the visual cortex in the splenial and suprasplenial gyri.

In the visual cortex [Fig. 1 (left)] a pattern was found that closely resembles that observed in the parietal cortex of rabbit and rat, i.e., apical dendrites of three or more layer V pyramids approach each other to form slender bundles that run straight through layer IV. Higher up, the bundles break up because the dendrites divide into obliquely running branches that become thinner and thinner and on entering layer II/I can no longer be traced with the ordinary methods.

In the second region, the sensorimotor cortex, however, an entirely different pattern of dendritic bundling was found [Fig. 1 (right)]. Here the large apical dendrites bifurcate immediately above layer V, and their secondary branches give rise to bundles that are joined by apical dendrites of what presumably are layer III pyramids. Initially, the bundles take an oblique course, but they then bend to become more perpendicular to the surface of the cortex.

The main result of comparing the two regions of cat brain was the conclusion, that there are, in fact, profound and characteristic regional differences of dendritic bundling, and that these can be related to the cytoarchitectonic picture. In the last few months this conclusion has been substantiated by additional studies of various regions in the cerebral cortex of the cat as well as of mouse and rabbit.

In the cat, another striking example for the existence of gross regional differences in the pattern of dendritic bundling is provided by a look at the gyrus genualis (area 32 of Winkler and Potter, 1914). In this region it is rather difficult to obtain a clear picture by studying frontal sections. But sections cut tangentially to the surface (for this particular region that means sagittal sections through the brain), reveal a prominent nonstatistical arrangement of the dendrites in very large bundles. In contrast to what is seen, for example, in the striate area where a bundle consists of 2 to 10 dendrites, the bundles in the gyrus genualis are much larger. As shown in Fig. 2 they may comprise 50 or more dendrites. The diameter of such bundles is, of course, considerably larger than the diameter of bundles in the visual cortex, and this explains why in the region of the gyrus genualis it is difficult to disentangle the picture in the comparatively thin frontal sections that are used for studying the dendritic pattern.

In the mouse, we have so far detected gross differences among the arrangements of apical dendrites in the barrel field of Woolsey and van der Loos (1970), in the adjacent region of the parietal cortex, and in the striate region. In the barrel field, the large apical dendrites of those layer V pyramids that are situated underneath a barrel take an oblique course; thus, they avoid the interior and enter the spaces between the barrels where bundles are formed, which can be traced into layer III. In the parietal region outside the barrel field, 8 to 10 apical dendrites of layer V pyramids form slender bundles, which ascend through layer IV. Here some additional small dendrites originating from cells situated in this layer and lying close to the respective bundles may be attached. In the striate cortex, similar bundles are found, but they usually consist of fewer dendrites than the bundles in the parietal region.

In the rabbit, our preliminary investigations have revealed differences between the pattern of dendritic bundling in the area parietalis, in the striate region, and in the retrosplenial region. Because the two last-mentioned regions are of particular interest with respect to electrophysiologic observations of Petsche and his co-workers, some of the differences found between these regions will be illustrated and described in more detail.

The striate region (i.e., area striata and peristriata) of the rabbit brain is comparatively thick. In Nissl sections there are easily discernible layers VI and V, a characteristically well-developed granular layer IV, and thick layers III and II. In contrast, the adjacent retrosplenial region is much thinner. Following a well-developed layer VI there is a broad layer V with large pyramids. This is bordered by a layer of extremely small, rounded cells passing into lamina II, making it difficult to differentiate between

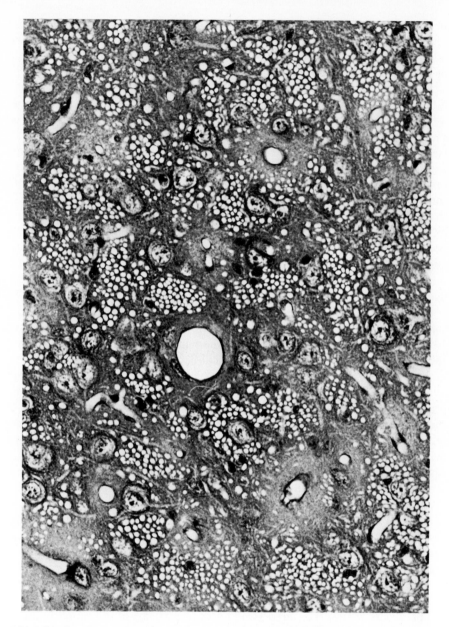

FIG. 2. Cat. Section tangential to the surface of the gyrus genualis showing cross sections of the particularly large dendritic bundles that are characteristic for this region. Bouin-fixed paraffin section stained with Klüver's Luxol fast blue followed by a periodic acid-Schiff reaction and counterstaining with hematoxylin. (~ x450.)

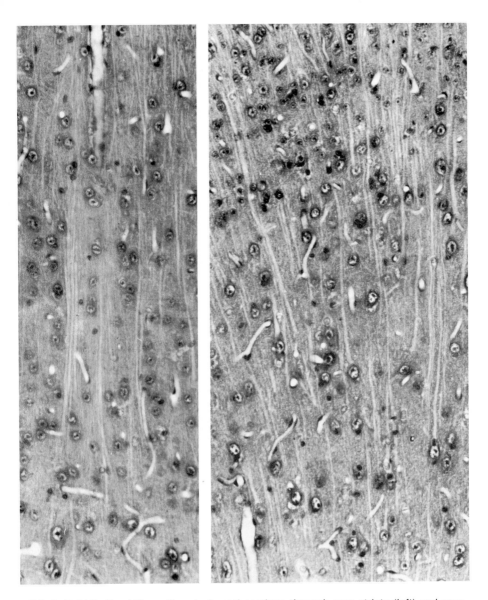

FIG. 3. Rabbit. Dendritic pattern in frontal sections through area striata (left) and area retrosplenialis granularis dorsalis (right). (Left) A small strip of layer V, the entire layer IV, and the beginning of layer III are seen. (Right) More than half of the picture is occupied by layer V, whereas the upper third shows the lower half of the layer comprising laminas IV to II. See text for details. Same technique as in Fig. 2. (~ x300.)

layers IV, III, and II. As described by Rose (1931), the layer comprising the laminas II to IV is comparatively broad and consists of an outer, more densely packed and an inner, less densely packed sublayer. The retrosplenial region of the rabbit is very extensive and can be subdivided into three different areas (equal to area 29a,b,c of Winkler and Potter, 1911; area retrosplenialis granularis ventralis-Rsgα-, dorsalis-Rsgβ- and infima-Rsgγ- of Rose, 1931).

According to our own observations, differences between the striate region on the one hand and the retrosplenial region on the other, as well as gradual changes between the three subdivisions of the retrosplenial region are also present with respect to the pattern of dendritic bundling. Figure 3 shows, at relatively low-power magnification, the dendritic pattern in the striate area and in the area retrosplenialis granularis dorsalis, i.e., in that part of area 29 that occupies the dorsomedial region of the hemisphere and is not yet buried in the interhemispheric sulcus. In the striate area [Fig. 3 (left)] several small bundles are seen. They originate in layer V and extend through

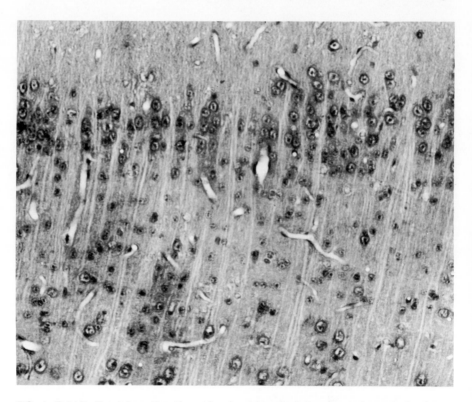

FIG. 4. Rabbit. Frontal section through area retrosplenialis granularis ventralis shows bundles of dendrites extending from layer V (lower rim) to the beginning of layer I. The upper half of the layer comprising laminas IV to II is divided by these bundles into vertically arranged packets or columns of cells. Same technique as in Fig. 2. (~ x260.)

layer IV. But on entering layer III and II most of the bundles can no longer be followed because many of the longer dendrites divide and give off small branches that take part in the formation of secondary bundles in the upper layers. In the retrosplenial area [Fig. 3 (right)], however, the picture is different. Here the large apical dendrites of layer V pyramids ascend undivided into the lower subdivisions of layers IV to II. Here they may be joined by smaller dendrites, some of which appear to originate in this layer, so that thick bundles are formed which pass through layer II and break up in layer I. These bundles, which become ever more prominent from the dorsomedial to the interhemispheric and lower parts of the retrosplenial area, actually appear to divide layer II into small, vertically arranged packets of cells. These vertical interruptions of layer II by easily discernible bundles of dendrites are so striking (Fig. 4) that they may be regarded as one of the most characteristic features of this particular part of the hemisphere.

Much further study is needed to obtain a clear picture of all the regional peculiarities and of how the pattern of dendritic bundling is related to the cytoarchitectonic structure. Although our investigations are still rudimentary and are hampered by many technical obstacles, which time prevents me from discussing, I think that even the preliminary findings show that we are dealing with a new and interesting structural feature of the mammalian cerebral cortex that may be of some physiologic significance and is therefore deserving of our attention.

ACKNOWLEDGMENT

This work was supported by grants from the Deutsche Forschungsgemeinschaft (F1 26/13) and by a Twinning Grant of the European Training Programme in Brain and Behavior Research.

REFERENCES

Fleischhauer, K. (1974): On different patterns of dendritic bundling in the cerebral cortex of the cat. *Z. Anat. Entwicklungsgesch.*, 143:115–126.

Fleischhauer, K., Petsche, H., and Wittkowski, W. (1972): Vertical bundles of dendrites in the neocortex. *Z. Anat. Entwicklungsgesch.*, 136:213–223.

Massing, W., and Fleischhauer, K. (1973): Further observations on vertical bundles of dendrites in the cerebral cortex of the rabbit. *Z. Anat. Entwicklungsgesch.*, 141:115–123.

Peters, A., and Walsh, T. M. (1972): A study of the organization of apical dendrites in the somatic sensory cortex of the rat. *J. Comp. Neurol.*, 144:253–268.

Petsche, H., Rappelsberger, P., and Frey, Z. (1972): Intracortical aspects of the synchronization of self-sustained bioelectrical activities. In: *Synchronization of EEG Activity in Epilepsies,* edited by H. Petsche and M. A. B. Brazier. Springer-Verlag, Vienna.

Rose, M. (1931): Cytoarchitektonischer Atlas der Grobhirnrinde des Kaninchens. *J. Psychol. Neurol.*, 43:353–440.

Winkler, C., and Potter, A. (1911): *An Anatomical Guide to Experimental Researches on the Rabbit's Brain.* Versluys, Amsterdam.

Winkler, C., and Potter, A. (1914): *An Anatomical Guide to Experimental Researches on the Cat's Brain.* Versluys, Amsterdam.

Woolsey, T. A., and van der Loos, H. (1970): The structural organization of layer IV in the somatosensory region (S1) of mouse cerebral cortex. *Brain Res.*, 17:205–242.

Advances in Neurology, Vol. 12, edited by
G. W. Kreutzberg, Raven Press, New York
© 1975.

Dendrodendritic Gap Junctions: A Developmental Approach

K. Møllgård and M. Møller

Anatomy Department A, University of Copenhagen, Universitetsparken 1, DK-2100
Copenhagen Ø, Denmark

Analysis of the ultrastructure of the mammalian central nervous system
(CNS) has shown that neighboring dendrites contact each other at various
sites. Four different types of dendrodendritic contacts have been recognized
(cf. Van der Loos, 1974): dendrodendritic membrane appositions often
with interdigitations, dendrodendritic puncta adherentia, dendrodendritic
synapses, and dendrodendritic gap junctions.

The purpose of the present study is to probe further into the nature of
dendrodendritic gap junctions. Gap junctions are now accepted as specialized areas of close membrane apposition, which permit the direct intercellular exchange of ions (electrical or ionic coupling) and low molecular
weight substances (metabolic coupling). For reviews and recent references
see, e.g., McNutt and Weinstein (1973), Satir and Gilula (1973), and Staehelin (1974).

The difficulties of finding and of clearly identifying dendrodendritic gap
junctions in thin sections of mammalian CNS are indicated by the fact that
only two reports have appeared in which these junctions are demonstrated
[between dendrites possibly of stellate cells in monkey neocortex (Sloper,
1972) and between basket-cell dendrites in rat cerebellum (Sotelo and
Llinás, 1972)]. To circumvent this problem, we have in the present study
used the freeze-cleave technique, which has the advantage over ultrathin
sectioning of both tremendously increasing the examinable membrane area
and of providing different criteria for the positive identification of true gap
junctions. In addition we have used Alcian blue as a marker substance to
facilitate the identification of gap junctions in thin sections because it per-
meates the gap and forms an electron-dense precipitate in the middle of the
junction. Because intercellular communication is one of the basic prerequi-
sites for the development of multicellular organisms, and because cell-to-
cell transfer of small substances may be of considerable importance for the
coordination and regulation of cellular activities both in development and
in mature tissues, it was considered of interest to investigate the presence
of dendrodendritic gap junctions also in fetal CNS.

MATERIALS AND METHODS

In order to apply the marker substance Alcian blue *in vivo* it is necessary to circumvent or avoid the blood-brain barrier (BBB). We therefore performed ventriculocisternal perfusions (Oldendorf and Davson, 1967) with Alcian blue in adult rabbits and intravenous injections in sheep fetuses at a stage at which the BBB is not developed.

In four adult rabbits the ventricular system was perfused for 1 hr with mock CSF containing Alcian blue (10 mg/100 ml) before the brains were fixed by perfusing a solution containing 2.5% glutaraldehyde in 0.1 M cacodylate buffer (pH 7.4) through an aortic catheter at a constant pressure of 150 mm Hg. After perfusion fixation the brains were removed and immersed for 6 hr in 2.5% glutaraldehyde fixative and from there were transferred to the buffer.

Four 60-day sheep fetuses (gestation period 150 days) were prepared in the following way. The ewes were anesthetized with i.v. thiopental (5% w/v in sterile water, 0.2 to 0.3 ml/kg body weight) followed by chloralose (1% w/v in 0.9% saline, up to 3 mg/kg body weight, supplemented at hourly intervals by 0.3 to 0.6 mg/kg). One horn of the uterus was exposed through an oblique lower midline abdominal incision in the anesthetized ewe. Cannulas were inserted into the umbilical vein and the umbilical artery was opened. One ml 0.5% Alcian blue in Locke's solution was injected into the placental cotyledon vein over 100 sec. Following that procedure, 1% Karnovsky fixative was injected over a period of 16 min; total amount of injected fixative, 40 ml. After perfusion fixation the brains were removed and immersed for 6 hr in 1% Karnovsky fixative, and from there were transferred to 0.1 M sodium cacodylate buffer.

After a thorough wash in buffer, tissue blocks were cut from the brainstem of the rabbits and from the visual cortex of the sheep fetuses. The blocks were postfixed in 2% OsO_4 in 0.1 M sodium cacodylate buffer, stained *en bloc* in 0.5% aq. uranyl acetate for 1 hr, dehydrated in increasing concentrations of ethanol, transferred to propylene oxide, and embedded in Epon.

The material examined with the freeze-etch technique comprises visual cortex from four human fetuses of 100 to 150 mm crown-rump length, which were removed by caesarian section in connection with legal abortion. Immediately following the operation the brain was taken out and immersed in ice-cold 2.5% glutaraldehyde in 0.1 M cacodylate buffer (pH 7.4). Small blocks of visual cortex were prepared after 1 hr of fixation and then kept for another 2 hr in the fixative. After 1 hr of infiltration with 30% buffered glycerol at room temperature, the specimens were mounted and oriented so that a transverse cleavage perpendicular to the cortical surface could be achieved. The specimens were then frozen in liquid Freon 22 cooled by liquid nitrogen. Freeze-fracturing followed by platinum–carbon shadowing was performed with a Balzer's apparatus (BAF 301) (Moor and Mühlethaler,

1963; Branton, 1966). Specimens were fractured at a stage temperature of $-115°C$. Replicas were cleaned in bleach.

RESULTS

Adult Rabbit Treated *In Vivo* with Alcian Blue by Ventriculocisternal Perfusion

Unstained thin sections of adult rabbit cut from the periaqueductal gray contain a material of high electron density that fills the extracellular space to a variable degree. Alcian blue has penetrated between the ependymal cells of the cerebral aqueduct to reach subependymal glial cell layers and underlying nervous tissue. All gap junctions present (e.g., between ependymal cells or between astrocytic endfeet) seem to be particularly well outlined by the marker substance Alcian blue. The width of the Alcian blue containing intermediate line in the gap junction is about 45 Å.

Many neighboring profiles in the periaqueductal gray identified as dendrites possess apposed plasma membranes that run strictly parallel to each other over large distances. The overall width of these appositions measured from cytoplasm to cytoplasm is about 170 Å, and the intercellular space is about 45 Å (Fig. 1). Therefore they are considered to be gap junctions. Cisternae of smooth endoplasmic reticulum are often found in the cytoplasm just below the junctional membrane.

Sheep Fetuses Treated *In Vivo* with Alcian Blue from the Blood Side

Alcian blue penetrates the vessels of neocortex in 60-day sheep fetuses (*unpublished observations*) and moves from the perivascular area into the clefts between the immature nervous processes. Numerous gap junctions (overall width, 170 Å; intercellular space, 45 Å) are found in the upper part of the cortical plate. In fortuitous sections it is possible to identify neighboring profiles as dendritic processes with certainty (e.g., an apical dendrite in continuity with its perikaryon and apposed to a dendrite with characteristically postsynaptic thickenings). Probably most of the numerous gap junctions identified in the present material are dendrodendritic gap junctions (Fig. 2A). Sometimes apposed dendrites enlarge the area of mutual apposition by interdigitation (cf. also Van der Loos, 1964). Dendrodendritic gap junctions can be observed in these interdigitations (Fig. 2B).

Freeze-Fracture Studies of Human Fetal Neocortex

The only replicas used for this study were those for which it was possible to distinguish clearly the cortical plate and the free surface of the cerebral wall.

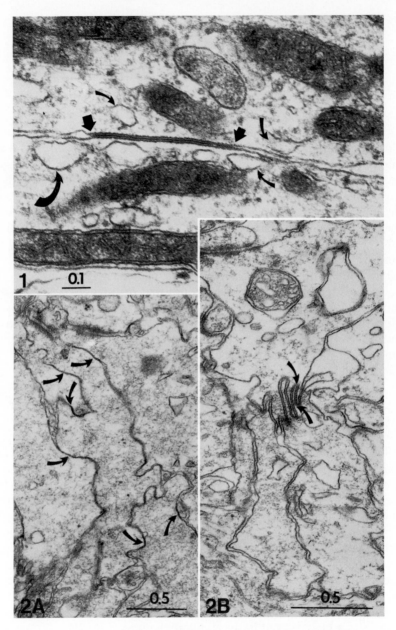

FIG. 1. Thin section of the periaqueductal gray (nucleus raphe dorsalis) from an adult rabbit subjected to ventriculocisternal perfusion with Alcian blue. A gap junction between two neighboring dendritic processes is seen between the two straight arrows. Curved arrows point to cisternae of endoplasmic reticulum. Bar indicates 0.1 μm.

FIG. 2. Typical dendritic profiles of the upper part of the cortical plate of 60-day sheep fetuses are demonstrated. Immature postsynaptic thickenings can be identified in the upper part of each picture. Gap junctions are indicated by arrows. Note the indentations in (B). Bars indicate 0.5 μm.

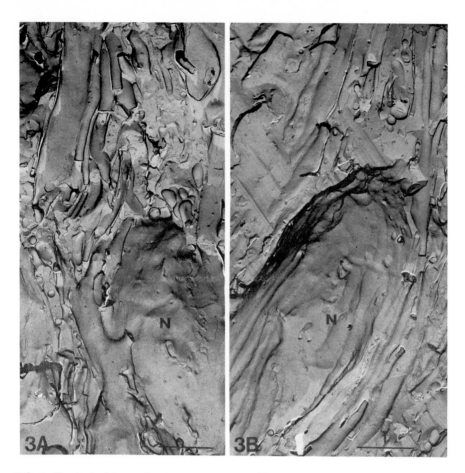

FIG. 3. The typical freeze-fracture appearance of immature nerve cell bodies (N) in the cortical plate. Note the surrounding long processes. Bars indicate 1 μm. Human fetal visual cortex.

Columnar groups of vertically oriented cells with long apical processes and surrounded by vertically oriented processes are characteristic of freeze-fracture replicas of the cortical plate (Figs. 3 and 4). Large apical processes can be followed a considerable distance from the cell bodies and can be seen to branch at various points. The intramembranous particles of the processes identified as dendrites have been analyzed.

Very small aggregates of membrane particles follow some longitudinal ridges or extensions that appear to be a characteristic freeze-fracture appearance of immature dendritic membranes. The large immature dendrites show some zones in the cell membrane where plaque-like differentiations are formed by aggregation of 80 to 90 Å particles (Figs. 5 to 7). A zone free of particles surrounds some of the larger aggregates. A packing of the

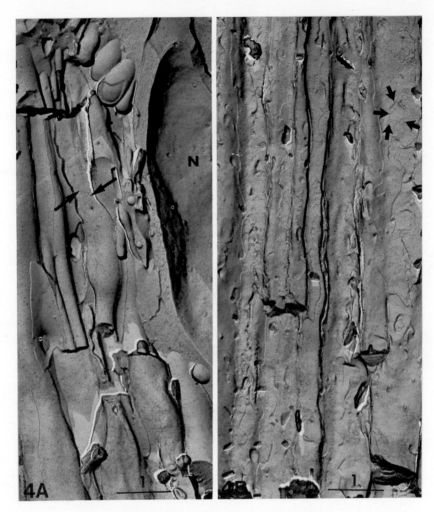

FIG. 4. Characteristic long processes extend from the middle of the cortical plate toward the free surface. A nucleus (N) with nuclear pores of an immature neuron is indicated in (A). Arrows point to small linear arrays of particles. (B) Arrows enclose an area that may contain tight junctional elements. Bars indicate 1 μm. Human fetal visual cortex.

particles into subcompartments separated by particle-free aisles can be found in these aggregates. Within the plaques many of the membrane particles are remarkably regular in both shape and dimensions. However, some larger particles are seen occasionally in the plaque between small linear arrangements of 80 to 90 Å particles (Fig. 7).

Very rarely small isolated ridges and furrows (tight junctional elements) have been observed associated with adjacent (probably dendritic) membranes. Small particles can be associated with either ridges or furrows (Fig. 8).

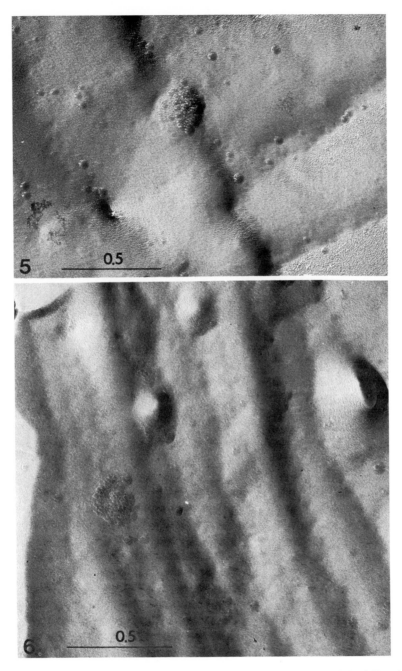

FIGS. 5 and 6. Plaque-like aggregates of small particles can be distinguished. Bars indicate 0.5 μm. Human fetal visual cortex.

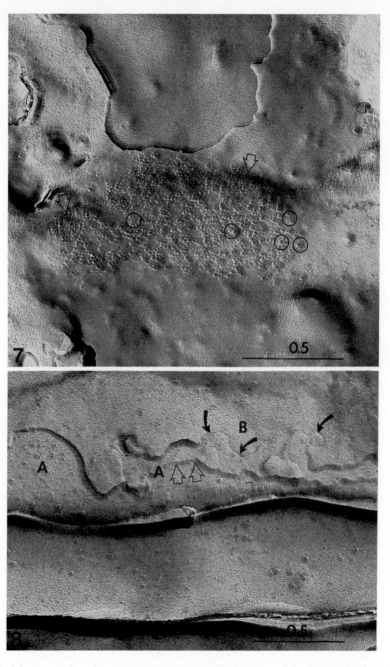

FIG. 7. A large gap junction is shown in a tangential fracture of the human fetal cortical plate. Note the variable packing of the junctional particles giving rise to particle-free zones between small patches of polygonally packed 85-Å particles. Regions of close packing are indicated by arrows. Some large particles (encircled) are also found in the junctional membrane. Bar indicates 0.5 μm.

FIG. 8. The upper part of the picture is occupied by a large dendrite. A particle-rich face (A) and the complementary face (B) can be distinguished. A small network of anastomosing grooves (curved arrows) is seen on the B face. A single array of particles (open arrows) extends from the region on the A face. Bar indicates 0.5 μm.

DISCUSSION

In this study we have positively identified gap junctions between dendritic processes. The identification of gap junctions is based on: (1) the overall thickness of the junction, which is about 170 Å measured from cytoplasm to cytoplasm; (2) a gap of about 45 Å revealed by Alcian blue impregnation of the zone of intercellular contact; and (3) freeze-fracture morphology typical of a gap junction.

The focal tight junctions, as well as the large particles found in association with the aggregates of 80 to 90 Å particles, might well represent stages in gap junction development (see Revel, Yip, and Chang, 1973; Decker and Friend, 1974).

The freeze-fracture appearance of dendrodendritic puncta adherentia of adult cerebellum (Landis and Reese, 1974; Palay and Chan-Palay, 1974) is different from most of the aggregates found in the present material.

The dendritic processes can be identified in freeze-fracture replicas of the human fetal neocortex (stage III–IV of Sidman and Rakic, 1974) because of their large size, irregular contours and branching, and their continuity with the characteristic young neurons in the cortical plate. Radial glial fibers are also present but their cell bodies lie in or near the subventricular zone (Sidman and Rakic, 1974).

The development of the neocortex in the 60-day fetal sheep corresponds to the neocortex of a 5-month human fetus (cf. Åström, 1967). Therefore the widespread occurrence of Alcian blue-containing dendrodendritic gap junctions in the sheep fetuses can be roughly correlated to the freeze-fracture findings in human fetuses. Abundant mature dendrodendritic gap junctions as demonstrated in the periaqueductal gray are also easily identified because of their affinity for Alcian blue. The precipitation of this dye probably indicates that the "gap substance" contains polyanionic substances (for a discussion of Alcian blue as a tracer molecule, see Møllgård and Sørensen, 1974).

The present study indicates that dendrodendritic gap junctions may be more widespread in the mammalian CNS than was previously supposed. They might well occur in association with the widespread type of dendrodendritic junctions analyzed in Golgi preparations of the cerebral neocortex by Van der Loos (1960). The spatial distribution of these junctions revealed a striking periodicity, and most of the contacts were between dendritic segments of the same branching order. The clusters of apical dendrites (Peters and Walsh, 1972) and the dendritic bundling (Fleischhauer, 1974) may represent columnar organizations of neurons electrotonically coupled by dendrodendritic gap junctions.

Dendrodendritic gap junctions (synchronizing synapses) allow more rapid transmission for mediation of short latency responses or highly synchronous activity; reciprocal action is also significant (see review by Bennett, 1973).

The dendrodendritic gap junctions found in the fetal material could also be necessary for the normal brain development, as it is supposed that normal tissue growth and differentiation depend on a flow of material from one cell interior to another through the junctional cell surfaces. Moreover, the gap junctions may serve a role in maintaining the differentiated state in adult tissues (see review by Loewenstein, 1973). However, the above-mentioned two functions of dendrodendritic gap junctions — electrotonic coupling and the role in morphogenesis — are, in fact, different manifestations of the same phenomenon, i.e., a low resistance to an intercellular flow of different types of ions and regulatory molecules.

SUMMARY

Dendrodendritic gap junctions have been identified in the periaqueductal gray substance of adult rabbits and in the visual cortex of sheep fetuses. The introduction of Alcian blue as a marker substance facilitated the positive identification of gap junctions. Dendrodendritic contacts in the human fetal neocortex have been examined in freeze-cleaved specimens. The contacts are identified as gap junctions by their freeze-fracture appearance. Features of the developing dendrodendritic gap junctions are described. The possible significance of these contacts is discussed, and it is suggested that they provide electrotonic coupling of neurons belonging to the same columnar organization. In addition it is suggested that the dendrodendritic gap junctions of fetal neocortex participate in cell differentiation and morphogenesis of the cerebral wall.

ACKNOWLEDGMENTS

The authors wish to thank Drs. N. Saunders, J. Reynolds, and M. Reynolds, Department of Physiology, University College, London, for providing the sheep material and Bjarne Lauritzen for his expert technical assistance in the freeze-fracture experiments.

REFERENCES

Åström, K. E. (1967): On the early development of the isocortex in fetal sheep. In: *Developmental Neurology*. Progress in Brain Research, edited by C. G. Bernhard and J. P. Schadé, Vol. 26, pp. 1–59. Elsevier, Amsterdam.

Bennett, M. V. L. (1973): Function of electrotonic junctions in embryonic and adult tissues. *Fed. Proc.,* 32:65–75.

Branton, D. (1966): Fracture faces of frozen membranes. *Proc. Natl. Acad. Sci. USA,* 55:1048–1056.

Decker, R. S., and Friend, D. S. (1974): Assembly of gap junctions during amphibian neurulation. *J. Cell Biol.,* 62:32–47.

Fleischhauer, K. (1974): On different patterns of dendritic bundling in the cerebral cortex of the cat. *Z. Anat. Entwicklungsgesch.,* 143:115–126.

Landis, D. M., and Reese, T. S. (1974): Differences in membrane structure between excitatory and inhibitory synapses in the cerebellar cortex. *J. Comp. Neurol.,* 155:93–126.

Loewenstein, W. R. (1973): Membrane junctions in growth and differentiation. *Fed. Proc.,* 32:60–64.

McNutt, N. S., and Weinstein, R. S. (1973): Membrane ultrastructure at mammalian intercellular junctions. *Prog. Biophys. Mol. Biol.,* 26:45–101.

Møllgård, K., and Sørensen, S. C. (1974): The permeability of cerebral capillaries to a tracer molecule, Alcian blue, with a molecular weight of 1390. In: *Pathology of Cerebral Microcirculation,* edited by J. Cervós-Navarro, pp. 228–232. de Gruyter, Berlin.

Moor, H., and Mühlethaler, K. (1963): Fine structure in frozen-etched yeast cells. *J. Cell Biol.,* 17:609–628.

Oldendorf, W. H., and Davson, H. (1967): Brain extracellular space and the sink action of cerebrospinal fluid. *Arch. Neurol.,* 17:196–205.

Palay, S. L., and Chan-Palay, V. (1974): *Cerebellar Cortex. Cytology and Organization.* Springer-Verlag, Berlin and Heidelberg.

Peters, A., and Walsh, T. M. (1972): A study of the organization of apical dendrites in the somatic sensory cortex of the rat. *J. Comp. Neurol.,* 144:253–268.

Revel, J.-P., Yip, P., and Chang, L. L. (1973): Cell junctions in the early chick embryo—A freeze etch study. *Dev. Biol.* 35:302–317.

Satir, P., and Gilula, N. B. (1973): The fine structure of membranes and intercellular communication in insects. *Annu. Rev. Entomol.,* 18:143–166.

Sidman, R. L., and Rakic, P. (1973): Neuronal migration, with special reference to developing human brain. A review. *Brain Res.,* 62:1–35.

Sloper, J. J. (1972): Gap junctions between dendrites in the primate neocortex. *Brain Res.,* 44:641–646.

Sotelo, C., and Llinás, R. (1972): Specialized membrane junctions between neurons in the vertebrate cerebellar cortex. *J. Cell Biol.,* 53:271–289.

Staehelin, L. A. (1974): Structure and function of intercellular junctions. *Int. Rev. Cytol.,* 39:191–283.

Van der Loos, H. (1960): On dendrodendritic junctions in the cerebral cortex. In: *Structure and Function of the Cerebral Cortex,* edited by D. B. Tower and J. P. Schadé, pp. 36–42. Elsevier, Amsterdam.

Van der Loos, H. (1964): Similarities and dissimilarities in submicroscopical morphology of interneuronal contact sites of presumably different functional character. *Prog. Brain Res.,* 6:43–58.

Van der Loos, H. (1974): Dendrodendritic junctions. *Neurosci. Res. Program Bull.,* 12:86–90.

Advances in Neurology, Vol. 12, edited by
G. W. Kreutzberg, Raven Press, New York
© 1975.

Dendritic Differentiation in Human Cerebral Cortex: Normal and Aberrant Developmental Patterns

Dominick P. Purpura

Department of Neuroscience and The Rose F. Kennedy Center for Research in Mental Retardation and Human Development, Albert Einstein College of Medicine, Bronx, New York 10461

The development of dendrites and the differentiation of dendritic spines are critical morphogenetic events in the development of neurons of the mammalian cerebral cortex (Cajal, 1911; Conel, 1939; Noback and Purpura, 1961; Poliakov, 1961; Rabinowicz, 1964; Scheibel and Scheibel, 1971; Marin-Padilla, 1970, 1971, 1972a). Dendrites provide the major proportion of membrane surface area for integration of synaptic inputs (Rall, 1962, 1967; Purpura, 1967; Rall and Rinzel, 1973), whereas dendritic spines are postsynaptic targets for a variety of afferent projections to cortical neurons (Berkley, 1897; Chang, 1952; Gray, 1959; Globus and Scheibel, 1967; Scheibel and Scheibel, 1968; Valverde, 1968; Colonnier and Rossignol, 1969; Jones and Powell, 1970; Garey and Powell, 1971; Szentagothai, 1973; Gruner, Hirsch, and Sotelo, 1974; Strick and Sterling, 1974). Hence, these morphogenetic events are also important determinants of the potential functional synaptic competency of the maturing brain. It follows from this that studies of dendritic development and dendritic spine differentiation may provide clues to the neural substrate underlying the ontogenesis of cortical functions. Attention to patterns of normal and abnormal development of dendritic systems and dendritic spines in the immature human brain may also shed light on the pathophysiologic basis of aberrant neurobehavioral development. Whereas these expectations may be currently unrealistic they are nevertheless worthy of serious pursuit. For if dendrites are as important for the elaboration of interneuronal transactions as is generally believed, then they are of sufficient importance to study in the context of normal and abnormal development of complex functions of the human brain, even at this primitive stage in the understanding of human developmental neurobiology.

Apart from the desirability of advancing knowledge concerning the structural organization of the brain there are several reasons why studies of dendritic development in the human cerebral cortex are useful, if not necessary, at this time. First, there is sufficient information available from descriptive and experimental studies of neurogenesis and dendritic differentiation in laboratory animals to permit reasonable interpretations of comparable descriptive studies of human brain development. Second, there is a need to provide data on the morphologic characteristics of neurons of the immature cerebral cortex in conditions that are known to place human infants at risk for neurobehavioral disorders. Obviously such an inquiry requires prior understanding of the range of normal variability of neuronal morphogenesis at different antenatal and postnatal epochs. The problem addressed in such studies is a central issue of developmental neurobiology, that is, the modifiability of neuronal development and synaptogenesis and its relationship to modifications of behavior (Purpura, 1973, 1975).

This chapter summarizes preliminary Golgi studies that bear upon several aspects of the general problem of dendritic morphogenesis in the immature human cerebral cortex. These include (1) consideration of the temporal and morphologic features of dendritic differentiation; (2) the nature of some abnormalities of dendritic development in the preterm infant; (3) the ontogenesis of dendritic spines; and (4) abnormalities of dendritic spine development.

GENERAL REMARKS

Observations summarized in this chapter are based on Golgi studies of the cerebral cortex (neocortex and hippocampus) from 60 brains removed at the time of postmortem examination in the Department of Pathology, Albert Einstein College of Medicine. Fetal brain specimens were obtained from spontaneously aborted, stillborn fetuses of 14 to 24 weeks gestational age (g.a.). Preterm infants (24 to 36 weeks g.a.) who survived a variable period in the Neonatal Intensive Care Unit, Department of Pediatrics, Albert Einstein College of Medicine, were also studied. Most of the preterm infants in this age group died as a result of massive intraventricular hemorrhages. All had "normal immature brains," as defined by routine gross and microscopic examinations. Older infants and children who succumbed were considered to have a "normal brain" if there was a negative neurologic history, normal neurobehavioral development, and a negative neuropathologic examination. Golgi studies were also carried out on a sample of cortical tissue obtained at the time of brain biopsy performed on a 10-month-old profoundly retarded child. The biopsy was primarily for biochemical, histochemical, and electron microscopic studies, and was initiated for diagnostic and family counseling purposes.

DENDRITIC DIFFERENTIATION IN IMMATURE HUMAN CEREBRAL CORTEX

The hippocampus is a particularly favorable cortical structure for examining the temporal and morphologic features of dendritic differentiation of pyramidal neurons. The youngest fetal brain studied with the rapid Golgi method in the present series of postmortem specimens was approximately 14 weeks g.a. At this stage apical dendrites are well differentiated, but basilar dendrites are barely detectable on most pyramidal neurons. From 18 to 22 weeks g.a. dendrites exhibit many of the growth characteristics described in detail in the subprimate mammalian brain most recently by Morest (1969, 1970). Examples of these growth processes in pyramidal neurons of the hippocampus from three fetal brains (spontaneous abortions) are shown in Fig. 1.

One of the features of dendritic growth is evident in Fig. 1A–C. This consists of the presence of marked irregularities in length and caliber of dendritic shafts. In most instances dendritic growth at a major bifurcation site proceeds equally in the two daughter branches (Fig. 1A). In some cells, however, only the most tentative outgrowth of a fine process with a prominent terminal head is evident at a major branch point (Fig. 1B). Dendritic branches may also exhibit relatively large expansions distal to their point of origin (Fig. 1C).

Preterminal and terminal growth cones with variable numbers of filopodia (Fig. 1D–G) are the most characteristic morphologic signs of rapid dendritic growth in pyramidal neurons of the fetal hippocampus (20 to 22 weeks g.a.). These growth cones may take the form of pleomorphic terminal expansions with multiple finger-like processes (Fig. 1E) or may consist of bulbous expansions with filopodia (Fig. 1F). Claw-like terminal enlargements with filopodia are also seen (Fig. 1G). Newly formed dendrites generally exhibit multiple varicosities with particularly large ones occurring at branch points (Fig. 1H). Filopodium-like fine processes are detectable on these developing dendrites. The characteristics of newly formed basilar dendrites of a hippocampal pyramidal neuron are in sharp contrast to the smooth and uniform caliber of the initial axonal segment of the neuron. Other developmental features of dendrites include the presence of lumpy enlargements, filopodia, and lacunae that are encountered in dendritic shafts undergoing rapid length increases. The lacunae appear to represent intradendritic organelles devoid of silver chromate precipitate. These and other features of differentiating dendrites have been described in laboratory animals (Morest, 1969, 1970).

On the basis of observations such as those illustrated in Fig. 1, it is evident that the maximal phase of dendritic growth and development of pyramidal neurons in the human hippocampus occupies a period between 18 to 24 weeks of gestation. Observations on motor cortex pyramidal neurons lead to a similar conclusion, but this is not the case for visual cortex neurons. Indeed, many pyramidal neurons of the visual cortex are just beginning to enter the maximal phase of dendritic differentiation toward the end of the sixth month of gestation. Visual cortex appears to lag behind hippocampus and motor cortex by at least 4 to 6 weeks during the antenatal period of dendritic development.

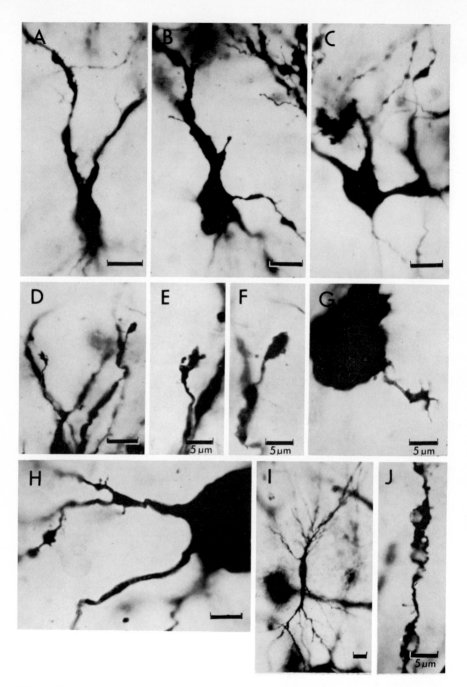

FIG. 1. Dendritic growth processes seen in rapid Golgi preparations of hippocampal neurons in 18 to 22-week-old human fetuses (natural abortions). (A) Pyramidal neurons of the regio inferior with bifid apical dendrites, both equally well developed. (B) Asymmetric development of dendritic branches from apical stem. (C) A cell with a lateral dendrite with a large distal expansion giving rise to several branches and branchlets. (D) Two forms of dendritic growth cones, seen at higher magnification in (E) and (F). Note multiple filopodia arising from these terminal processes. (G) Neuron with a small den-

Within the various subfields of the hippocampus, pyramidal neurons in the multilayered stratum pyramidale exhibit different degrees of dendritic differentiation at any one time. In the 18 to 20-week-old fetus deep pyramidal neurons of the regio superior (CA_1) have already acquired extensive apical dendrites that exhibit fine filopodium-like processes (Fig. 2A). In contrast, superficially located pyramids in the CA_1 area are poorly developed at this time (Fig. 2B). Although there is extensive dendritic differentiation in progress in "giant" pyramidal neurons of the regio inferior (CA_3) (Fig. 2C,D) overall apical dendritic growth is not as advanced as in (CA_1) large pyramids in the 18 to 20-week-old fetus.

The fascia dentata (FD) of the immature hippocampal formation provides the most striking example of regional variation in dendritic growth and differentiation of neurons of similar type at a particular phase of cortical development. Examples of immature neurons of the stratum granulosum are shown in Fig. 3A–F from an 18 to 20-week fetus. Neurons in the supra-pyramidal or lateral limb of the fascia dentata (adjacent to the entorhinal cortex) exhibit extensive dendritic growth processes and prominent dendrites that penetrate well into the molecular layer of the fascia dentata (Fig. 3A, B). Granule neurons in the infrapyramidal or medial limb (bordering the ventricle) (Fig. 3E, F), have poorly developed dendritic systems. Granule cells in the most distal segment of the infrapyramidal limb have cell bodies with a few small dendritic extensions. Between the supra- and infrapyramidal limbs a gradient of dendritic differentiation of granule cells is evident (Fig. 3C–E). An example of a multipolar pyramidal neuron in the hilus of the fascia dentata (CA_4 region) is shown in Fig. 3G. Its dendritic development is in synchrony with the large granule cells in superficial parts of the suprapyramidal limb of the stratum granulosum (Fig. 3A).

The striking gradient in dendritic development of granule neurons of the fascia dentata shown in Fig. 3 is evident from the earliest period of fetal development studied here (14 weeks) and persists throughout development. Indeed, the general pattern of regional variation in the fascia dentata observed at 33 weeks g.a. (Fig. 4) is not significantly different in the full-term newborn infant. Figure 4 shows the most prominent dendritic systems to be present in granule cells near the tip of the suprapyramidal limb (Fig. 4A), whereas the most primitively developed cells with neuroblast-like characteristics are located near the tip of the infrapyramidal limb (Fig. 4L–N). The developmental status of different pyramidal neurons in the hilus of the fascia dentata is noteworthy. Many of these cells are not

---

dritic process exhibits a preterminal expansion with multiple filopodia. (H) Basilar dendrite of pyramidal neuron exhibits multiple varicosities with spicules and filopodia. The initial axonal segment is smooth and of relatively uniform diameter. (I) Neuron of the regio inferior. (J) Magnification of dendrite of neuron in (I), to show dendritic lacunae and filopodia, which are morphologic features of rapid growth of dendritic shafts. Calibration: A–C, 15 μm; (D,H,I) 10 μm. B–H, from Purpura (1975).

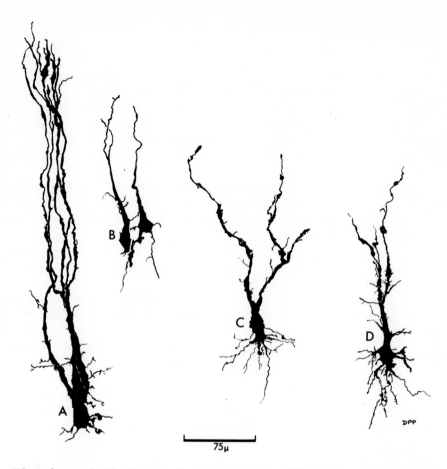

FIG. 2. Camera lucida drawings of pyramidal neurons of the hippocampus of an 18 to 20-week-old human fetus (natural abortion). (A) Cluster of pyramidal neurons of the regio superior (CA$_1$). Apical dendrites are well developed and exhibit a few fine filopodium-like spines and preterminal growth processes. Basilar dendrites are poorly represented. (B) Small pyramids in superficial layers of stratum pyramidale of CA$_1$. These exhibit few dendritic growth processes at this stage. (C) Pyramid of CA$_3$. (Photomicrograph of this cell is shown in Fig. 1A.) (D) Another pyramid of CA$_3$. Note the many growth processes on apical dendrites of these neurons.

significantly more advanced in dendritic development than the prominent granule cells of the suprapyramidal limb of the stratum granulosum. Obviously the fascia dentata and its most characteristic elements, the granule cells, is a complex cortical structure composed of a wide variety of cell types with uniquely different dendritic patterns (Cajal, 1911; Lorente de Nó, 1934). Details of these different patterns are shown in Fig. 5, the individual elements of which correspond to the locations noted in Fig. 4. The dendritic systems of granule cells of the fascia dentata in human surgical specimens have been studied by the Scheibels (1973) who have emphasized

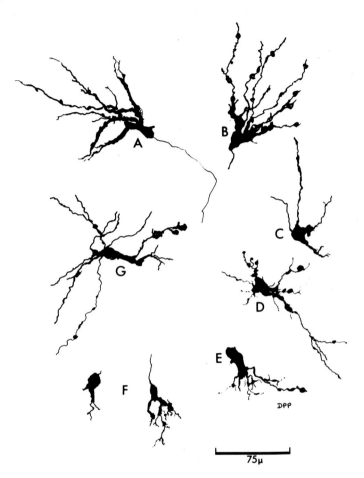

FIG. 3. Camera lucida drawings of cells of the fascia dentata (FD) in an 18 to 20-week fetus. (Hippocampal pyramidal neurons from this fetus are shown in Fig. 2.) Typical granule neurons are drawn as encountered in the stratum granulosum beginning in the supra-pyramidal (lateral) limb (A,B) and ending in the infrapyramidal (medial) limb (F). (G) Pyramidal neuron of the hilus of the FD. A gradient of dendritic differentiation is evident. Irregular shafts, varicosities, lumpy enlargements, and preterminal and terminal growth processes are seen to a variable degree in these elements. The most primitive and poorly differentiated granule cells occupy the tip of the infrapyramidal limb of the FD (F).

the extraordinary diversity of neuronal architecture in this structure in man. The present study demonstrates that this diversity is evident in the early fetal period of cortical development and is reflected in a gradient of dendritic differentiation that follows the curve of the stratum granulosum from suprapyramidal to infrapyramidal limbs.

Developmental studies in laboratory animals may provide important clues to the interpretation of the temporospatial patterns of dendritic differentiation of granule cells of the human fascia dentata. Autoradiographic

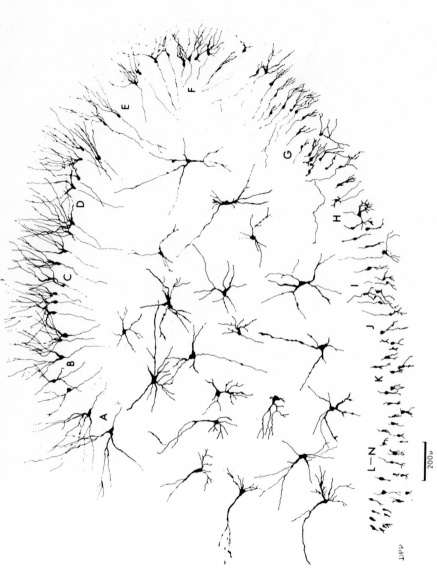

200μ

FIG. 4. Composite camera lucida drawings of cells of the fascia dentata in a 33-week-old preterm infant who survived 2 days. A gradient of dendritic differentiation from suprapyramidal (A–D) to infrapyramidal (H–N) limbs of the FD is demonstrated as in the 18 to 20-week fetus (Fig. 3). A number of different types of pyramidal neurons of the hilus of the FD in CA₄ are shown. The extraordinary variability in dendritic patterns of granule cells is noteworthy. Dendrites of some granule neurons (A) may be more extensive in development than those of CA₄ pyramids.

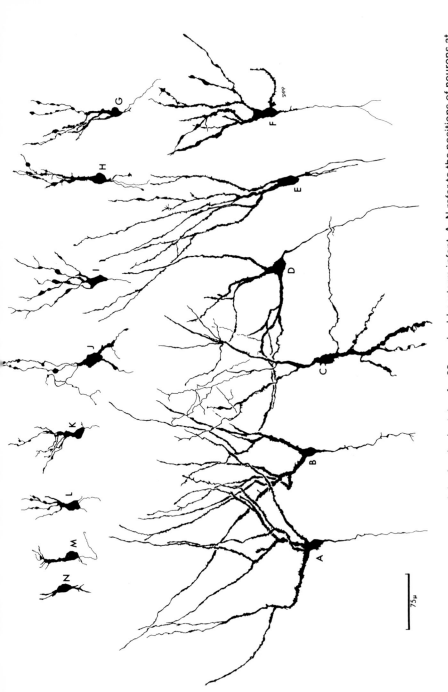

FIG. 5. Details of granule neurons of the fascia dentata of a 33-week-old preterm infant. A–N refer to the positions of neurons at approximate locations shown in Fig. 4. Neurons in the suprapyramidal limb of the stratum granulosum have extensive dendrites with many spines (A,B). At the curve of the FD, granule cell dendrites show lumpy enlargements and varicosities (F,G). Poorly developed granule cells are found near the tip of the infrapyramidal limb (L–N).

studies in the rodent indicate that the final position a cell attains in the stratum granulosum is dependent upon its time of origin (Angevine, 1965); Schlessinger, Cowan, and Gottlieb, 1975). Granule neurons of the supra-pyramidal limb of the fascia dentata in the mouse are generated on the 10th day of gestation, whereas neurons in the infrapyramidal limb are "born" as late as the 18th day of gestation. Extending these data from rodent to man it would seem that at least for the stratum granulosum of the fascia dentata there is a correspondence between time of origin of neurons and rate and extent of dendritic differentiation. Neurons generated early may not only develop dendrites early, but they may also have more extensive dendritic systems throughout the antenatal period. Other factors such as differences in the time of arrival of afferents to dendrites of fascia dentata granule cells (Gottlieb and Cowan, 1972) may also play a role in influencing the gradient of dendritic differentiation observed in the human fetal hip-pocampus.

SOME ABNORMALITIES OF DENDRITIC DEVELOPMENT IN THE PRETERM INFANT

It can be expected that with increasing attention to the morphologic char-acteristics of dendrites in the human immature brain a wide spectrum of unusual and perhaps abnormal patterns of dendritic growth will be found in association with different insults to the preterm infant while dendritic differentiation is in progress. These abnormalities of dendritic development may consist in generalized stunting of dendritic growth and reduction in number and distribution of dendritic spines. In view of the dependence of neuronal growth processes on the availability of appropriate metabolic machinery, it is not surprising that factors that compromise cellular bio-energetic operations will interfere with dendritic growth and development. Nevertheless, the possibility must also be entertained that abnormalities of dendritic growth may take the form of a "hypertrophy" or acceleration of dendritic growth involving certain classes of neurons and perhaps par-ticular dendritic systems. Examples of unusual dendritic growth patterns observed in two preterm infants in the present series serve to illustrate this point.

The first example is seen in the extraordinary long dendrites of some den-tate granule cells in a 33-week-old preterm infant who was born at 29 weeks g.a. and who survived for 4 weeks in a neonatal intensive care unit with the usual life-support systems. This infant had repeated bouts of cardiorespira-tory distress that necessitated prolonged assisted respiration. Death ensued after a number of transient cardiac arrests. In this infant examination of the hippocampus and neocortex revealed neurons in a relatively advanced state of morphogenesis (Purpura, 1975). Photomicrographs of some of the dentate granules observed in this subject are shown in Fig. 6. These cells

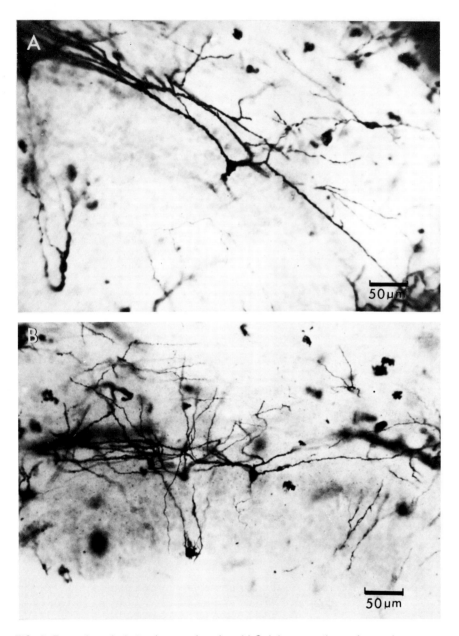

FIG. 6. Examples of photomicrographs of rapid Golgi preparations of granule neurons of the fascia dentata of a 33-week-old preterm infant who survived for 4 weeks. (A) Granule neuron in center of field has extensive dendrites that extend horizontally along the upper border of the stratum granulosum. (B) Granule neuron from another part of the fascia dentata also has massive dendritic development.

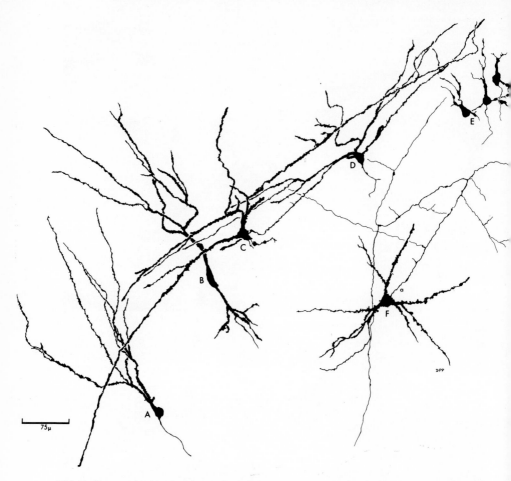

FIG. 7. Camera lucida drawings of granule neurons of the fascia dentata from the same preterm infant as in Fig. 6. Neurons (C) and (D) in this composite are shown in the photomicrographs of Fig. 6(A) and (B), respectively. Note that despite the massive development of dendrites of granule neurons in the suprapyramidal limb of the fascia dentata, (A–D), neurons in the infrapyramidal limb are poorly developed. The gradient of dendritic differentiation is maintained. (F) Pyramidal neuron of the CA_4 region has an axon (a) with collaterals that penetrate into the stratum granulosum.

together with others in the suprapyramidal and infrapyramidal limbs of the fascia dentata are illustrated in the composite camera lucida drawings of Fig. 7. The morphologic features of fascia dentata granule cells shown in Fig. 7 should be compared with those shown in Fig. 5, from a 33-week-old preterm infant who died within 2 days after birth. Suffice it to say that fascia dentata granule cells with such extensively developed dendrites, as shown in Figs. 6 and 7, have not been observed previously in the immature or mature monkey or human brain (Cajal, 1911; Lorente de Nó, 1934; Conel, 1939; Scheibel and Scheibel, 1973).

One comment may be made concerning these findings. It is obvious from the overt characteristics of the fascia dentata cells in Figs. 6 and 7 that survival of the preterm infant for 4 weeks in cardiorespiratory distress did not interrupt or compromise dendritic development. Rather it would seem

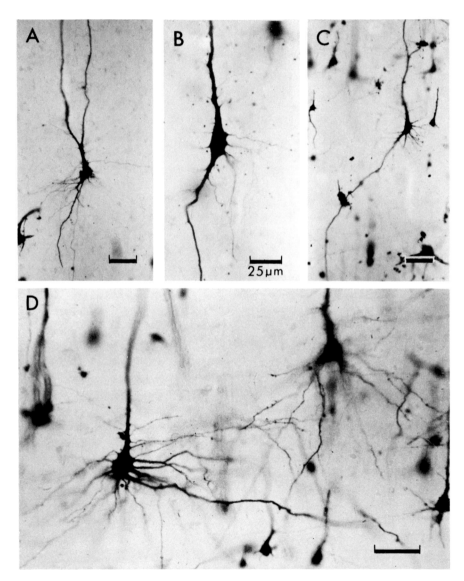

FIG. 8. Examples of Golgi–Cox preparations of pyramidal neurons of the motor cortex of a 36-week-old preterm infant, 2 days survival. (A–C) Unusual single basilar dendrites course downward. (D) Neuron lower left of center has a single large basilar dendrite (see text for further explanation). Calibration: 50 μm unless otherwise noted.

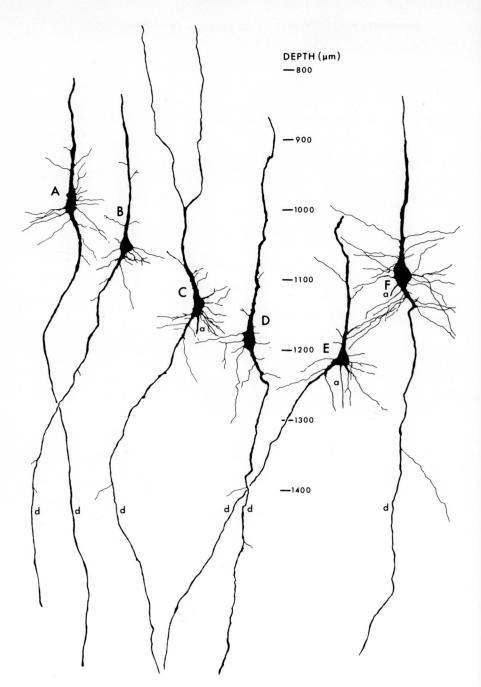

DEPTH (μm)
—800

—900

—1000

—1100

—1200

—1300

—1400

A
B
C
D
E
F
a
a
a

d   d   d   d d   d

FIG. 9. Composite camera lucida drawings of pyramidal neurons of the motor cortex of 36-week-old preterm infant as in Fig. 8. Cells (C) and (D) are (C) and (B) of Fig. 8, respectively. The single basilar dendrites (d) are shown extending downward into the depths of the cortex. Axon segments (a) are identified in some neurons. Note poor development of apical dendrites and thin, poorly developed basilar dendrites with exception of large branch (d). (Golgi–Cox preparation.)

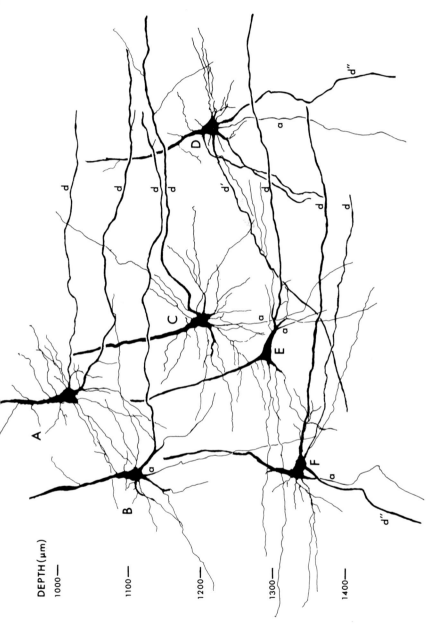

DEPTH (μm)

1000—

1100—

1200—

1300—

1400—

FIG. 10. Composite camera lucida drawings of pyramidal neurons of the motor cortex of a 36-week-old preterm infant as in Figs. 8 and 9. Some neurons (A,D,F) have two prominent basilar dendrites (d). Other neurons have basilar dendrites that curve downward (d″) as well as tangentially (d and d′). (Golgi–Cox preparations.)

that if any effect at all can be ascribed to the conditions that this preterm infant experienced, it was in the direction of stimulating or enhancing dendritic development. Additional pairs of age-related preterm infants, one of whom has survived one or more weeks with intensive care support systems, must be studied in a similar fashion to determine the validity of the notion that dendritic growth acceleration may occur in the young preterm infant.

The second example of an unusual dendritic growth pattern in cortical neurons comes from a 36-week-old preterm infant who survived for 2 days before death caused by intraventricular hemorrhage and respiratory distress syndrome. The mother of this infant had diabetes mellitus and preeclampsia. Routine neuropathologic examination revealed a normal immature brain with multiple acute subependymal hemorrhages.

Golgi–Cox preparations of the motor cortex of this preterm infant revealed neurons with generally poor dendritic development. For the most part basilar dendrites were thin and short with relatively few branches. A remarkable feature was the presence of one and occasionally several very prominent basilar dendrites on medium and large pyramidal neurons (Fig. 8). Two patterns of growth of these dendrites were discernible as illustrated in Figs. 9 and 10. One pattern consisted of "macrobundles" of basilar dendrites that extended downward into the cortical depths and even into the subcortical white matter (Fig. 9). The tendency was to replicate the upward pattern of apical dendritic growth in the opposite direction. The second pattern resulted in tangential asymmetric "macrobundles" of basilar dendrites of pyramidal neurons (Fig. 10). In some instances neurons contributed basilar dendrites to both radial and tangential arrays (Fig. 10D,F).

It has been suggested that dendritic bundling is a significant feature of the neuronal organization of the spinal cord (Scheibel and Scheibel, 1970a,b) and cerebral cortex (Fleischhauer, Petsche, and Wittkowski, 1972; Fleischhauer, 1974; Scheibel et al., 1974; cf. Fleischhauer, *this volume*). To the extent that the unusual growth of one or more basilar dendrites in the present example can be considered a regular finding in pyramidal neurons in this case, it follows that the resultant "macrobundles," as shown in Figs. 9 and 10, may produce significant distortions in neuronal operations subserved by normal patterns of dendritic bundles. Unfortunately, there are as yet no hard data on the functional significance of dendritic bundles in the cerebral cortex. Consequently it suffices only to indicate the potential importance of unusual patterns of dendritic growth in considerations of the pathophysiology of dendritic systems in the developing human cerebral cortex.

MORPHOGENESIS OF DENDRITIC SPINES OF CORTICAL PYRAMIDAL NEURONS

Peters and Kaiserman-Abramof (1970) have shown in a combined Golgi and electron microscopic study that dendritic spines are morphologically different in different parts of the dendritic systems of pyramidal neurons in the adult rat parietal cortex. They have broadly classified dendritic spines into three groups: thin, mushroom-shaped, and stubby. It is useful to apply this classification to the characteristics of fine processes observed in rapid Golgi preparations of apical dendritic shafts of motor cortex pyramidal neurons at different stages in the normal development of the human cerebral cortex. Preliminary observations relevant to this study are summarized in Fig. 11.

Apical dendritic shafts of proximal segments of motor cortex pyramidal neurons exhibit dramatic alterations in their associated fine processes during the latter half of gestation. In the 18-week-old human fetus a few long, thin filopodium-like processes with variable terminal expansions are detectable (Fig. 11,*1*). Dendritic shafts are highly irregular in contour, and occasionally mushroom-shaped elements are evident. By 26 weeks g.a. many more long, thin processes appear, some with multiple terminal heads (Fig.

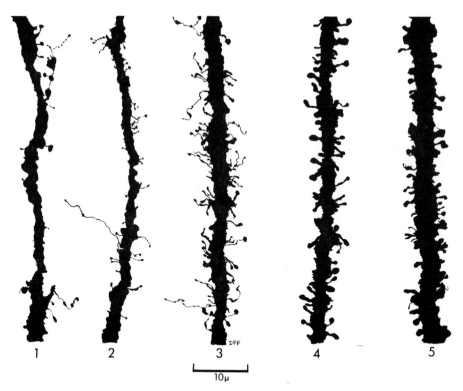

FIG. 11. Camera lucida drawings of proximal apical dendritic segments of motor cortex pyramidal neurons at different developmental stages. *1*, 18-week-old fetus; *2*, 26-week-old fetus; *3*, 33-week-old preterm infant; *4*, normal 6-month-old infant; *5*, normal 7-year-old child (accident case). Early phase of dendritic spine differentiation is associated with the development of long, thin filopodium-like spines and relatively few stubby and mushroom-shaped spines. The latter two types are prominent on proximal apical dendritic segments in the postnatal period and into early childhood. See text for further explanation.

11,2). Long, thin processes predominate at 33 weeks g.a. (Fig. 11,3) and are greatly increased in number. At this stage both mushroom-shaped and stubby spines are detectable but in small number.

During the early postnatal period there is a striking change in the characteristics of dendritic fine processes on proximal segments of pyramidal neuron apical dendrites of motor cortex (Marin-Padilla, 1972b). This is evident in the changing proportion of long-thin, short-thin and mushroom-shaped spines. Very thin, and long spine-like processes seen in the preterm infant (Fig. 11,3) are significantly reduced in the 6-month-old infant (Fig. 11,4). At the same time there is an increase in the number of mushroom-shaped and stubby spines, as well as short-thin spines. The trend toward a progressive increase in the number of stubby-necked spines with relatively large terminal heads is seen at least up to 7 years of age (Fig. 11,5). Although there is little change in the distribution of spines on proximal segments of apical dendrites of motor cortex neurons during early childhood, there appear to be more large-necked, short spines on proximal dendritic shafts in the 7-year-old child than in the 6-month-old infant.

It would be fatuous to assume that the foregoing brief description of what is obviously a complex sequence of overlapping developmental events satisfies present concerns for the problem of dendritic spine differentiation. Clearly quantitative analyses are required for spine characteristics, number, and distribution on different parts of the neuron and for different types of pyramidal neurons in different cortical layers. This will probably be forthcoming with computer-assisted techniques for automating data acquisition from Golgi preparations. In sum, dendritic spine typology has a developmental basis. The elaboration of short, thick-necked spines on proximal dendritic shafts proceeds through a fetal phase in which long–thin spines predominate (Marin-Padilla, 1972b). Whether long–thin spines seen in the latter half of gestation are progressively transformed into short, stubby spines or are replaced by the latter during continuing synaptogenesis is not known. It is also unclear whether a single class or different types of presynaptic inputs contact different types of spines. Apropos of these problems it is important to recall that different types of spines are distributed preferentially on different parts of the dendritic systems of pyramidal neurons (Peters and Kaiserman-Abramof, 1970).

ABNORMALITIES OF DENDRITIC SPINE DEVELOPMENT IN IMMATURE HUMAN CEREBRAL CORTEX

Marin-Padilla (1972b, 1974) was the first to apply the rapid Golgi method to the study of dendritic spine abnormalities in immature human cerebral cortex. He demonstrated that in infants with trisomic chromosomal aberrations known to be associated with mental retardation, dendritic spines were either very long, thin, and tortuous or short, thin, and barely detectable.

Variable spine loss and other degenerative processes were also encountered in his studies.

It is now clear from Golgi studies of dendritic spines in a series of children with unclassified mental retardation (normal karyotypes) (Purpura, 1974) that dendrites of cortical neurons may exhibit many of the abnormalities described in trisomic chromosomal disorders (Marin-Padilla, 1972*b*, 1974; Purpura, 1975). Examples of the morphologic features of dendritic spines in these cases are illustrated in the photomicrographs of Fig. 12B, C, $D_{3,4}$. Dendrites from a normal 6-month-old infant and a 7-year-old child (accidental death) are also shown for comparison. In an attempt to convey a better picture of the dendritic spine abnormalities seen in a 10-month-old infant with profound mental retardation, camera lucida drawings of different dendritic segments from the case illustrated in Fig. 12B are shown in Fig. 13B. Dendritic segments from the 6-month-old infant with a normal brain are shown in the photomicrographs of Fig. 12A; other segments from the same case are represented in Fig. 13A.

Description of the dendritic spines in the normal 6-month-old infant requires brief consideration of the relationship between spine type and location. In the camera lucida drawings of Fig. 13A dendritic segments *1* and *2* are proximal apical dendrites, whereas segment *3* is from a more distal location on an apical dendrite of a layer V pyramidal neuron. Segment *4* of Fig. 13A is from a basilar dendrite. In agreement with the findings of Peters and Kaiserman-Abramof (1970) it will be appreciated that thin spines are more prominent on distal apical dendritic segments and basilar dendrites of pyramidal neurons. All three types, thin (TH), mushroom-shaped (MS), and stubby (ST), are found on proximal segments of apical dendrites (Fig. 12A*1,2;* Fig. 13*1,2*), where long–thin spines are rarely encountered. These distribution differences are important in examination of the dendritic segments from the 10-month-old retarded infant (Figs. 12B and 13B) (cortical biopsy material). Several features characterize the dendritic spine abnormalities found on neurons from the retarded child – a reduction in mushroom-shaped and stubby spines on proximal segments and the presence of very long, thin, tortuous filopodium-like processes with single or multiple terminal heads. In some instances thin pedicles of these abnormally long spines appear to be in tangled arrays (Fig. 13B*3*). Although the tortuosity of abnormally long, thin spines has made it difficult to obtain complete thin sections of these elements for electron microscopy parallel, such studies have revealed normal axonal terminals in synaptic contact with thin dendritic spines in the 10-month-old retardate (K. Suzuki and D. P. Purpura, *unpublished findings*).

Additional examples of dendritic spine abnormalities from two other cases of profound mental retardation of unknown etiology are shown in Fig. 12C, 12D*3,4*. Proximal dendritic segments from a 3-year-old child with seizures and mental retardation show loss of spines and prominence

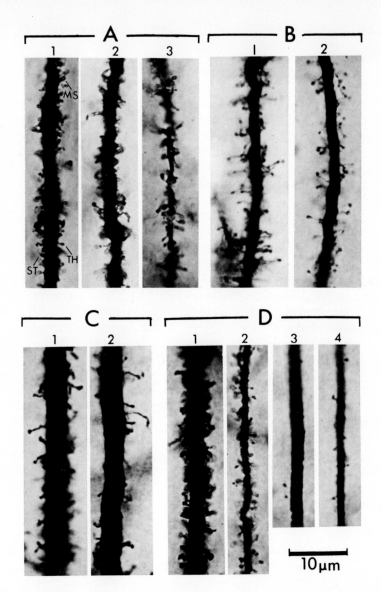

FIG. 12. Rapid Golgi preparations of dendrites of motor cortex neurons in normal and profoundly retarded subjects. (A) Normal 6-month-old infant with negative neurologic history, postoperative death. *1,2,* Proximal apical dendritic segments of medium sized layer V pyramidal neurons. Three basic types of dendritic spines are identified: thin (TH), stubby (ST), and mushroom-shaped (MS) spines. *3,* Basilar dendritic segment with a predominance of TH spines. B*1,2,* Proximal apical dendritic segments of medium sized pyramids in frontal cortex of a 10-month-old retardate. Brain biopsy case, infant currently alive. Abnormally long, thin spines predominate; many appear entangled. There is a marked reduction in MS and ST spines. (C)*1,2,* Proximal apical dendritic segments of medium pyramidal neurons in motor cortex of a 3-year-old retardate. Note variability in extent of spine loss and distribution of abnormally long, thin spines. (D)*1,2,* Proximal and distal segments of apical dendrites, from a normal 7-year-old child, accident case. *3,4,* Examples of apical dendritic segments from a 12-year-old profoundly retarded child. A few TH spines are seen, but otherwise there is almost complete absence of spines. (From Purpura, 1974.)

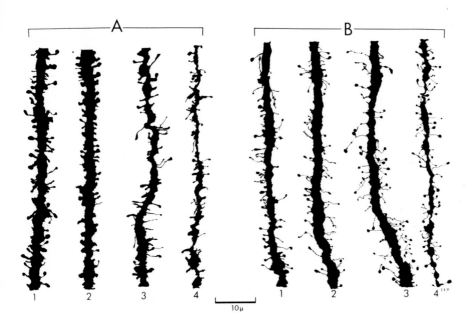

FIG. 13. Camera lucida drawings of dendritic segments of motor cortex neurons, rapid Golgi preparations. (A) Normal 6-month-old infant. *1,2,* Proximal apical dendritic segments with a predominance of stubby and mushroom-shaped spines; *3,* Distal apical dendritic segment and *4,* basilar dendritic segment have many more thin spines. (B) From a 10-month-old retarded child. *1,2,3,* Proximal apical dendritic segments. Note presence of many very long, thin spines with large terminal heads. *4,* Basilar dendritic segment. See text for further explanation.

of long, thin-necked spines with large terminal heads (Fig. 12C). Dendritic segments of cortical neurons from a 12-year-old profoundly retarded child (with a "developmental age" of about 1 year) are shown in Fig. 12D*3,4.* Only a few very thin-necked, short spines remain on these segments. Dendritic segments of motor cortex neurons from a normal 7-year-old child are shown in Fig. 12D*1,2,* by way of contrast.

A few comments are appropriate concerning the observations on dendritic spine abnormalities in infants and children with unclassified mental retardation (Purpura, 1974). It should be pointed out that the proportion of well-impregnated pyramidal neurons exhibiting a particular type of spine abnormality (e.g., spine loss, or long–thin spines) varied from case to case. Variations were also observed in any one case depending upon the cortical area examined. Not infrequently did two adjacent pyramidal neurons with similar dendritic branching patterns and apical dendrites in the same plane show different degrees of spine loss and spine abnormality. This remarkable finding is illustrated in the case of a profoundly retarded 8-month-old infant who also had negative chromosomal studies (Fig. 14).

Neurons exhibiting spine loss or spine abnormalities showed variable

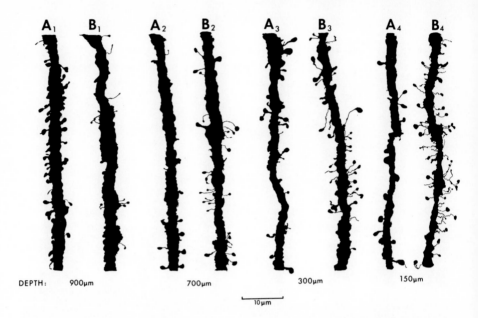

FIG. 14. Camera lucida drawings of dendritic segments from two closely adjacent medium sized pyramidal neurons of the motor cortex in an 8-month-old profoundly retarded child. The apical dendrites of these neurons were no more than 50 to 75 μm apart throughout the entire extent of their passage through the upper half of cortex. Depths at which parallel segments are illustrated are shown below. Dendrite of neuron A (A_1–A_4) exhibits more normal appearing short, stubby and mushroom-shaped spines in proximal segment (A_1) than dendrite of neuron B (B_1). In superficial regions of cortex neuron B exhibits many more long, thin and tangled spines (B_3,B_4), whereas dendritic segments of neuron A (A_2,A_3,A_4) are relatively depleted of all types of spines. The large-necked spines and thick lumpy protuberances on the superficial dendritic segments of neuron A are noteworthy. (Rapid Golgi preparations.) This composite drawing illustrates the marked variability in dendritic spine abnormalities observed in two closely adjacent pyramidal neurons.

changes in dendrites. In general no obvious relationship existed between the degree of dendritic spine abnormality in these elements and dendritic length or branching patterns. Indeed dendritic spine abnormalities appear to be more closely correlated with the severity of retardation and age of the subject than were changes in basic dendritic geometry. Huttenlocher (1974) has recently reported that dendritic branching in frontal cortex neurons is significantly reduced in young but not older retardates.

The fact that dendritic spine abnormalities similar to those described in infants with chromosomal aberrations are also found in retarded infants and in children with normal karyotypes indicates that abnormalities of dendritic spine generation are common to a variety of developmental disorders that are beyond current methods of identification. However different the etio-pathologic factors may be in the cases considered here and by Marin-Padilla (1972*b*, 1974) it is reasonable to suspect that these factors converge upon and interfere with processes regulating dendritic spine genesis and differentiation.

The morphologic similarity of the abnormally long, thin spines shown in Figs. 11 and 12 and the long, thin spines observed in the normal preterm infant of 26 to 33 weeks g.a. (Fig. 10*2,3*) is especially noteworthy. Marin-Padilla (1972*b,* 1974) first pointed out the similarity of bizarre long, thin cortical dendritic spines in a stillborn infant with D_1 (13–15) trisomy and developing spines of primitive neurons. This suggestion has considerable merit. Its significance would be to commit to hypothesis the concept of "maturational arrest" as the basis for the appearance of abnormally long, thin spines in cases of profound mental retardation. To the extent that this concept accounts for the spine abnormalities noted in this study, it follows that the absence of small, stubby spines in retardates may reflect failure of spine generation rather than loss of spines in the postnatal period. Alternatively it may be argued that there is failure of transformation of fetal long–thin spines into mature stubby and mushroom-shaped spines during spine differentiation. In the final analysis these may be trivial distinctions as the end effect is probably the same, i.e., dendrites relatively devoid of spines. From the standpoint of "synaptic competency," spine loss may be equated with loss of axospinodendritic synapses, whereas the presence of long–thin spines can be expected to provide less effective elements for injecting postsynaptic currents into dendrites (Llinás and Hillman, 1969). Rall (1974) recently examined the theoretical consequences of changes in the relationship between spine-neck resistance and dendritic branch resistance for different types of spines. From these considerations it seems reasonable to infer, especially for large dendritic shafts, that absence of normal small thick-necked spines and predominance of long, thin-necked spines as occurs in the cases illustrated above may significantly modify the efficacy of integrative operations of dendritic systems. Additional work along these lines may validate these speculations with respect to functional activities of normal and abnormal dendritic spine synapses. In the meantime the particular emphasis here on dendritic spine dysgenesis as a common feature of the microstructural pathology of profound mental retardation may be viewed as an affirmation of the central importance of axodendritic synaptic dysfunction in a wide range of developmental disorders of infancy and childhood (Marin-Padilla, 1972, 1974*b;* Purpura 1973, 1974, 1975).

RECAPITULATION AND CONCLUSION

Many of the morphologic features that characterize dendritic growth processes in laboratory animals are detectable in neurons of the immature human cerebral cortex at mid-gestation (18 to 22 weeks). These morphogenetic features, indicative of a phase of maximal dendritic development, are evident at different times in different cortical neuronal organizations.

One of the most striking illustrations of the differential rate of maturation of dendritic systems of cortical neurons is seen in the gradient of dendritic development in neurons of the stratum granulosum of the fascia dentata. Observations on such differences emphasize the interplay of genetic and local "environmental" factors in the regulation of neuronal morphogenesis.

Dendritic development is susceptible to many perturbations that place the human infant at risk. Although such insults are likely to produce generalized nonspecific stunting of dendritic growth, in some circumstances dendritic growth may be accelerated. Several examples of neural patterns of dendritic development are considered in this context.

Dendritic spine differentiation in cortical pyramidal neurons commences at mid-gestation and continues throughout early childhood. During this prolonged period of dendritic spine morphogenesis sequential changes in spine morphology and distribution are evident.

Infants and young children with unclassified profound mental subnormality show significant alterations in dendritic spines of cortical pyramidal neurons. For the most part these consist of a variable loss or absence of thick, short spines and prominence of abnormally long, thin spines. It is inferred that such microstructural alterations may influence the functional competency of axospinodendritic synapses sufficiently to compromise the integrative operations of cortical dendritic systems.

Routine neuropathologic studies generally provide no direct information on the morphologic status of dendrites. Yet, as shown in the foregoing survey, extraordinary changes in dendrites and dendritic spines may occur in the immature human brain despite negative findings in routine histologic studies. It is hoped that the present studies will encourage analysis of the normal and pathologic features of dendrites in the continuing search for the morphologic substrate of developmental disorders of higher nervous activities.

ACKNOWLEDGMENTS

The expert technical assistance of Mrs. M. Buschke in the preparation of the histologic material, and S. Brown for the preparation of photographic material is greatly appreciated. I also wish to thank my colleagues Drs. D. Ghetti, J. Powers, I. Rapin, K. Suzuki, M. Valsamis, and D. Wolfe for facilitating the acquisition of human brain tissue for this study. This work was supported in part by the National Institute of Neurological Diseases and Stroke (NS 07512), the National Institute of Child Health and Human Development (HD 01799), and the Alfred P. Sloan Foundation.

REFERENCES

Angevine, J. B. (1965): Time of neuron origin in the hippocampal region. *Exp. Neurol. (Suppl.),* 2:1–70.

Berkley, H. J. (1897): The intracerebral nerve-fibre terminal apparatus and modes of transmission of nervous impulses. *Johns Hopkins Hosp. Rep.,* 6:89–93.

Cajal, S. Ramon y (1911): *Histologie du système nerveaux de l'homme et des vertébrés.* Maloine, Paris.

Chang, H. T. (1952): Cortical neurons with particular reference to the spical dendrites. *Cold Spring Harbor Symp. Quant. Biol.,* 17:189–202.

Colonnier, M., and Rossignol, S. (1969): Heterogeneity of the cerebral cortex. In: *Basic Mechanisms of the Epilepsies,* edited by H. H. Jasper, A. A. Ward, and A. Pope, pp. 29–40. Little, Brown, Boston, Massachusetts.

Conel, J. L. (1939): *Postnatal Development of the Human Cerebral Cortex.* Harvard Univ. Press, Cambridge, Mass.

Fleischhauer, K., Petsche, H., and Wittkowski, W. (1972): Vertical bundles of dendrites in the neocortex. *Z. Anat. Entwicklungsgesch.,* 136:213–223.

Fleischhauer, K. (1974): On different patterns of dendritic bundling in the cerebral cortex of the cat. *Z. Anat. Entwicklungsgesch.,* 143:115–126.

Garey, L. J., and Powell, T. P. S. (1971): An experimental study of the termination of the lateral geniculo-cortical pathway in the cat and monkey. *Proc. R. Soc. Lond. (B),* 179:41–63.

Globus, A., and Scheibel, A. B. (1967): Synaptic loci on visual cortical neurons of the rabbit: The specific afferent radiation. *Exp. Neurol.,* 18:116–131.

Gottlieb, D. I., and Cowan, W. M. (1972): Evidence for a temporal factor in the occupation of available synaptic sites during the development of the dentate gyrus. *Brain Res.,* 41:452–456.

Gray, E. G. (1959): Axo-somatic and axo-dendritic synapses of the cerebral cortex: An electron microscope study. *J. Anat.,* 93:420–434.

Gruner, J. E., Hirsch, J. C., and Sotelo, C. (1974): Ultrastructural features of the isolated suprasylvian gyrus in the cat. *J. Comp. Neurol.,* 154:1–28.

Huttenlocher, P. R. (1974): Dendritic development in neocortex of children with mental defect and infantile spasms. *Neurology,* 24:203–210.

Jones, E. G., and Powell, T. P. S. (1970): An electron microscopic study of the laminar pattern and mode of termination of afferent fiber pathways in the somatic sensory cortex of the cat. *Philos. Trans. R. Soc. Lond. (Biol. Sci.),* 257:45–62.

Llinás, R., and Hillman, D. E. (1969): Physiological and morphological organization of the cerebellar circuits in various vertebrates. In: *Neurobiology of Cerebellar Evolution and Development,* edited by R. Llinás, pp. 43–73. American Medical Association, Chicago, Illinois.

Lorente de Nó, R. (1934): Studies on the structure of the cerebral cortex. I. Continuation of the study of the Ammonic system. *J. Psychol. Neurol. (Lpz),* 46:113–177.

Marin-Padilla, M. (1970): Prenatal and early postnatal ontogenesis of the human motor cortex: A Golgi study. 1. The sequential development of the cortical layers. *Brain Res.,* 23:167–183.

Marin-Padilla, M. (1971): Early prenatal ontogenesis of the cerebral cortex (neocortex) of the cat (*Felis domestica*). A Golgi study. *Z. Anat. Entwicklungsgesch.,* 134:117–145.

Marin-Padilla, M. (1972*a*): Prenatal ontogenetic history of the principal neurons of the neocortex of the cat (*Felis domestica*). A Golgi study. *Z. Anat. Entwicklungsgesch.,* 136:125–142.

Marin-Padilla, M. (1972*b*): Structural abnormalities of the cerebral cortex in human chromosomal aberrations. A Golgi study. *Brain Res.,* 44:625–629.

Marin-Padilla, M. (1974): Structural organization of the cerebral cortex (motor area) in human chromosomal aberrations. A Golgi study. 1. D_1 (13–15) trisomy, Patau syndrome. *Brain Res.,* 66:373–391.

Morest, K. (1969): The differentiation of cerebral dendrites. A study of the post-migratory neuroblast in the medial nucleus of the trapezoid body. *Z. Anat. Entwicklungsgesch.,* 128:271–289.

Morest, D. K. (1970): A study of neurogenesis in the forebrain of opossum pouch young. *Z. Anat. Entwicklungsgesch.,* 130:265–305.

Noback, C. R., and Purpura, D. P. (1961): Postnatal ontogenesis of neurons in cat neocortex. *J. Comp. Neurol.,* 117:291–308.

Peters, A., and Kaiserman-Abramof, I. R. (1970): The small pyramidal neuron of the rat cerebral cortex. The perikaryon, dendrites and spines. *Am. J. Anat.,* 127:321–356.

Poliakov, G. I. (1961): Some results of research into the development of the neuronal structure of the cortical ends of the analysers in man. *J. Comp. Neurol.,* 117:197–212.

Purpura, D. P. (1967): Comparative physiology of dendrites. In: *The Neurosciences: A Study Program,* edited by G. C. Quarton, T. Melnechuck, and F. O. Schmitt, pp. 372–393. Rockefeller Univ. Press, New York.

Purpura, D. P. (1973): Analysis of morphophysiological developmental processes in mammalian brain. In: *Biological and Environmental Determinants of Early Development. Res. Publ. Ass. Nerv. Ment. Dis.,* 51:79–110.

Purpura, D. P. (1974): Dendritic spine "dysgenesis" and mental retardation. *Science,* 186: 1126–1128.

Purpura, D. P. (1975): Normal and aberrant neuronal development in the cerebral cortex of human fetus and young infant. In: *Brain Mechanisms in Mental Retardation,* UCLA Forum in Medical Sciences. Academic Press, New York.

Rabinowicz, T. H. (1964): The cerebral cortex of the premature infant of the 8th month. In: *Growth and Maturation of the Brain. Prog. Brain Res.,* edited by D. P. Purpura and J. D. Schadé, 4:39–92.

Rall, W. (1962): Electrophysiology of a dendritic neuron model. *Biophys. J.,* 2:145–167.

Rall, W. (1967): Distinguishing theoretical synaptic potentials computed for different soma-dendritic distributions of synaptic input. *J. Neurophysiol.,* 30:1138–1168.

Rall, W. (1974): Dendritic spines, synaptic potency and neuronal plasticity. In: *Cellular Mechanisms Subserving Changes in Neuronal Activity,* edited by C. D. Woody, K. A. Brown, T. J. Crow, and J. D. Knispel, pp. 13–21. Brain Inf. Service, UCLA, Los Angeles.

Rall, W., and Rinzel, J. (1973): Branch input resistance and steady attenuation for input to one branch of a dendritic neuron model. *Biophys. J.,* 13:648–688.

Scheibel, M. E., and Scheibel, A. B. (1968): On the nature of dendritic spines – Report of a workshop. *Comm. Behav. Biol. A,* 1:231–265.

Scheibel, M. E., and Scheibel, A. B. (1970a): Organization of spinal motoneuron dendrites in bundles. *Exp. Neurol.,* 28:106–112.

Scheibel, M. E., and Scheibel, A. B. (1970b): Developmental relationship between spinal motoneuron dendrite bundles and patterned activity in the hind limb of cats. *Exp. Neurol.,* 20:321–355.

Scheibel, M. E., and Scheibel, A. B. (1971): Selected structural–functional correlations in postnatal brain. In: *Brain Development and Behavior,* edited by M. B. Sterman, D. J. McGunty, and A. M. Adinolphi, pp. 1–21. Academic Press, New York.

Scheibel, M. E., and Scheibel, A. B. (1973): Hippocampal pathology in temporal lobe epilepsy. A Golgi survey. In: *Epilepsy,* edited by M. A. B. Brazier, pp. 311–337. UCLA Forum in Medical Sciences, Academic Press, New York.

Scheibel, M. E., Davies, T. L., Lindsay, R. D., and Scheibel, A. B. (1974): Basilar dendrite bundles of giant pyramidal cells. *Exp. Neurol.,* 42:307–319.

Schlessinger, A. R., Cowan, W. M., and Gottlieb, D. I. (1975): An autoradiographic study of the time of origin and the pattern of granule cell migration in the dentate gyrus of the rat. *J. Comp. Neurol.,* 159:149–176.

Strick, P. L., and Sterling, P. (1974): Synaptic termination of afferents from the ventrolateral nucleus of the thalamus in the cat motor cortex. A light and electron microscope study. *J. Comp. Neurol.,* 153:77–106.

Szentagothai, J. (1973): Synaptology of the visual cortex. In: *Handbook of Sensory Physiology, Vol. VIII/3: Central Visual Information B,* edited by R. Jung, pp. 269–324. Springer-Verlag, New York.

Valverde, F. (1968): Structural changes in the area striata of the mouse after enucleation. *Exp. Brain Res.,* 5:274–292.

Advances in Neurology, Vol. 12, edited by
G. W. Kreutzberg, Raven Press, New York
© 1975.

Role of Cell Interaction in Development
of Dendritic Patterns

Pasko Rakic

*Department of Neuropathology, Harvard Medical School and Department of Neuro-
science, Children's Hospital Medical Center, Boston, Massachusetts 02115*

Growth of the neuronal dendritic arborization and establishment of its size and pattern are major developmental processes that occur both pre- and postnatally in mammals. Specific cell populations become arranged in a precisely organized fashion in relation to each other and to the afferent input; cytoplasmic processes grow in an ordered, sequential manner, ultimately resulting in characteristic neuronal morphology essential to the function of a mature brain (Rakic, 1975). Numerous morphologic observations dating back to Ramón y Cajal (1896, 1911) indicate that the formation of dendrites may depend on interactions with the processes of other cells. The most explicit examples are in brain structures in which processes are arranged in a clear geometric fashion (Fig. 1). Developmental analyses have shown that the ingrowth and elaboration of afferents coincides with the development of dendrites, which suggests that the growth and differentiation of dendrites may be both instigated and shaped by a contact with their specific axonal input (Ramón y Cajal, 1896; Terrazas, 1897; Barron, 1944; Morest, 1969; Mugnaini, 1969; Skoff and Hamburger, 1974; Vaughn, Henrikson, and Griesharber, 1974). The hypothesis that dendritic development depends on afferent axons has been supported by experiments in which axonal input was severed early in development (e.g., Levi-Montalcini, 1949; Kelly and Cowan, 1972; Berry and Hollingworth, 1973; Peusner, 1974). On the basis of such studies it has been suggested that the shape and size of the dendritic arborization of a given neuron is controlled partially by intrinsic factors that depend on the active part of individual cell genome, but also by extrinsic factors through interaction with neighboring cells (Rakic, 1974). The extrinsic factors may be basically structural (e.g., mechanical, adhesive, or repulsive forces), or they may be exercised through the presence or absence of function (functional validation, to use the term favored by Jacobson, 1970). However, because there is a temporal overlap and a close interdependence of structural and functional factors, the distinction between them is not at all clear.

Although it is difficult to argue with the validity of the generalization that both intra- and extracellular factors control the genesis of dendrites, it is

117

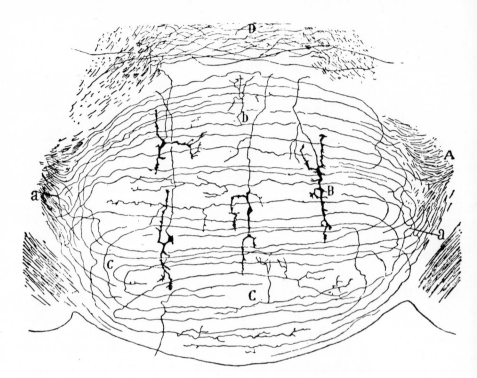

FIG. 1. A transverse section through the interpenduncular nucleus of the 4-day-old mouse (from Ramón y Cajal, 1911). In this nucleus, as in many other examples in the CNS, the dendrites of neurons are predominantly oriented in a plane lying 90° to the main orientation of axons. Such a perpendicular orientation of dendrites can provide a maximal number of possible contacts with fibers from the habenulointerpeduncular tract (fasciculus retroflexus of Meynert), many of which are in addition folded several times as if to increase such a possibility. However, the existence or the degree of interdependence of dendrites and axons in this example cannot be resolved because the developmental sequences, the time of axonal arrival, the time of neuron origin, and the time and mode of dendritic elaboration are not known.

not easy to sort out which dendritic properties are determined intrinsically and which are established by forces outside the cell. One approach to this problem is through the morphologic analysis of normal dendritic development in a highly geometric structure, such as the cerebellar cortex, and then to compare the results with dendritic development when the extrinsic conditions are changed. This chapter is limited to a consideration of the Purkinje cells and interneurons of the molecular layer (the latter term includes both the "stellate" and "basket" cells), that is, to those cerebellar neurons the dendrites of which are confined to a well-defined milieu consisting mainly of an array of parallel fiber axons oriented at a right angle to those dendrites.

The magnificent, fan-shaped dendritic tree of Purkinje cells is perhaps the most frequently used example of a cell region shaped by the precise geometry of its major axonal input. Yet the extent of this dependence, i.e., which features and details of Purkinje cell morphology are intrinsic and which are shaped by extrinsic influences, is not completely understood. I will not dwell here on a detailed description of the morphogenesis of Purkinje cell dendrites, which can be found in the works of Ramón y Cajal (1911), Addison (1905), Dadoune (1966) and others; instead I will mention several more recent studies that have relevance for a discussion of the role of cell interactions in the formation of dendritic arborizations.

In the last decade numerous experiments involving destruction of granule cell populations by X-ray irradiation (e.g., Shofer, Pappas, and Purpura, 1964; Altman and Anderson, 1972), by viruses (Herndon, Margolis, and Kilham, 1971; Llinás, Hillman, and Precht, 1972), by toxins (Hirano, Dembitzer, and Jones, 1972), or by genetic compromise (Sidman, 1968; Rakic and Sidman, 1973a,b), indicate that despite the absence or severe reduction of parallel fibers, Purkinje cells develop surprisingly well. This point is well illustrated in the cerebellar cortex of the neurologic mutant weaver mouse (gene *wv*), in which, despite a virtual absence of granule cells (and thus parallel fibers) in a homozygous animal, an extensive outgrowth of Purkinje cell dendrites occurs at the normal time during the second postnatal week (Rakic and Sidman, 1973b). The Purkinje cell dendrites form relatively large primary and secondary dendrites studded by numerous dendritic spines. However, it should be emphasized that the dendritic arbor does not assume the typical sagittally oriented, espalier shape, and generally lacks third and fourth order branches (Fig. 2).

The development of Purkinje cell dendritic arborization and the geometry of its orientation may also be studied under different circumstances in another neurologic mutant mouse, reeler (gene *rl*), which exhibits profound changes in the arrangement of cerebellar cells (Sidman, 1968; Rakic and Sidman, 1972). In homozygous affected animals Purkinje cell bodies are distributed throughout the cerebellum (Fig. 3A). Most granule cell bodies occupy a broad band beneath an attenuated molecular layer, but this band is external to Purkinje cell bodies rather than internal to them as it is in normal animals. Those Purkinje cells that remain close to the ventricular surface do not come into contact with granule cell axons, but their dendrites form typical primary stems and some secondary branches that are covered with numerous spines (Rakic, 1974). As in the weaver, tertiary branches are poorly developed and the orientation of the dendritic arbor appears to be completely random (Fig. 3B). A Golgi analysis of the Purkinje cells situated close to the external cerebellar surface discloses that normally oriented dendrites with extensive tertiary dendritic branching are present only in areas of the molecular layer in which parallel fibers are abundant and relatively normal in their orientation (Fig. 3C). Occasionally one encounters a Purkinje cell with one primary dendritic stem that is displaced away from the molecular layer and that possesses only misoriented branches, whereas another primary stem projects among bundles of parallel fibers

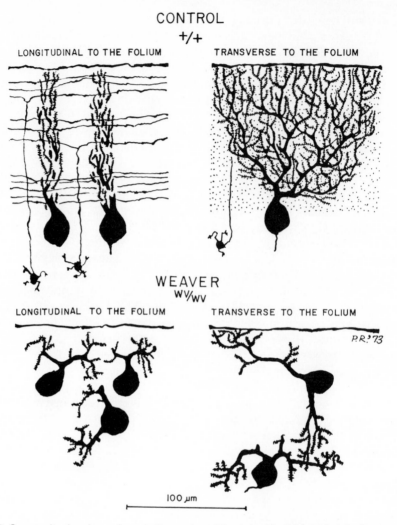

FIG. 2. Composite drawings of cerebellar cortex of 3-week-old wild-type (+/+) mice (upper row) and their homozygous weaver (C57BL/6J, *wv/wv*) littermates (lower row). Sections at the left are made longitudinal to the folium (coronal) and at the right transverse to the folium (sagittal). Note a precise orientation of dendritic sphere 90° to the parallel fibers in control animals. Although Purkinje cells in weaver mice develop an easily recognizable dendritic arborization studded with spines, the dendritic arbor is reduced in size and the orientation of dendrites is apparently random.

and has more elaborate secondary and tertiary dendritic branches oriented in a normal fashion (arrow, Fig. 3C). Such examples clearly indicate that initiation and growth of Purkinje cell dendrites as well as development of their spines appears to proceed relatively uninfluenced by parallel fiber input, but that the site and final detailed orientation of the dendritic arbor does depend on the parallel fibers.

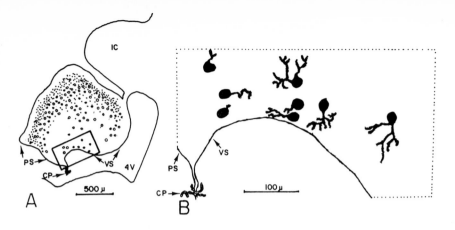

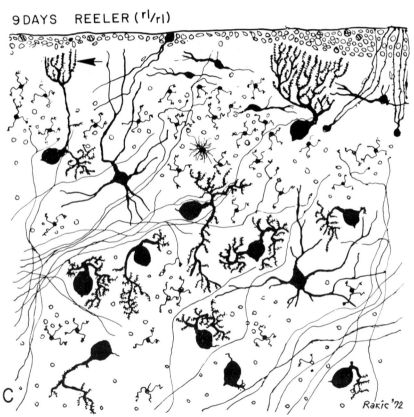

9 DAYS REELER (rl/rl)

Rakic '72

FIG. 3. (A) Midsagittal outline of the cerebellum in 19-day-old reeler mouse (C57BL/6J, *rl/rl*). Open circles represent Purkinje cells and dots indicate position of granule cells. Both cell types are abnormally placed: Purkinje cells are distributed throughout the cerebellum and granule cells occupy a broad band beneath a shallow molecular layer. (B) The Golgi-impregnated cells in the area of the cerebellum within quadrangle A, drawn at higher magnification, to show the dendritic morphology of Purkinje cells which remain in proximity of ventricular surface. Note the typical primary dendritic stems, with branches covered with spines that develop on displaced Purkinje cells in spite of the absence of any granule cells in the vicinity. (C) Composite drawing of Golgi-impregnated cerebellum of a 9-day-old reeler. Position of granule cells and still active external granular layer is made from toluidine blue counterstained sections. *Abbreviations:* CP, choroid plexus; IC, inferior colliculus; PS, pial surface; VS, ventricular surface; 4V, fourth ventricle. Drawing from a rapid Golgi preparation.

Similar observations have been made in rat cerebellum in which the orientation of parallel fibers in the superficial strata of the molecular layer has been altered by X-ray irradiation during development (Altman, 1973). In a given Purkinje cell of such animals the orientation of segments of the dendritic arbor at different depths of the molecular layer may vary so as to be consistently at a right angle to corresponding sheaves of parallel fibers.

The observation that dendritic spines of Purkinje cells can develop independently of the parallel fibers with which they normally have synaptic contacts is worth special emphasis. This has been observed in the mutant mice reeler (Rakic and Sidman, 1972) and weaver (Hirano and Dembitzer, 1973; Rakic and Sidman, 1973b; Sotelo, 1973) and in the virus, X-irradiation and drug experiments mentioned above. Homozygous weaver mice on a hybrid genetic background often have a normal life expectancy, and in them the Purkinje dendritic spines not only develop initially but then persist indefinitely despite the absence of synaptic input by parallel fibers (Rakic and Sidman, 1973b).

A further observation relevant to the issues discussed in this volume is that even in the absence of contact with axonal input, Purkinje dendritic spines can maintain a "postsynaptic" thickening in granuloprival cerebellar cortex (Herndon, 1968; Herndon, Margolis, and Kilham, 1971; Altman and Anderson, 1972; Hirano, Dembitzer, and Jones, 1972; Hirano and Dembitzer, 1973; Llinás, Hillman, and Precht, 1973; Rakic and Sidman, 1973b). Perhaps it is erroneous to assume an analogy between membrane thickenings in normal and experimental animals in the absence of precise chemical characterizations; however, the dimensions, electrodensity, and location of the membrane thickening on the naked spines resembles those of the normal postsynaptic web (Fig. 4). As a working hypothesis, the membrane specializations are interpreted as an abortive attempt by the cell to form a postsynaptic thickening. If this indeed proves to be the case, it appears that Purkinje cells not only form dendritic spines independently of parallel fibers, but also have the information that these spines would under normal circumstances establish asymmetric (excitatory?) synapses. In anticipation of such contact they form some sort of postsynaptic thickening, even though they have not actually come into contact with their prospective presynaptic partner at any point in time.

The nonsynaptic spines, which form on the normal schedule during the second postnatal week in weaver mouse, eventually become enveloped by a thick astroglial coating (Fig. 4). However, it seems unlikely that the thickening of the membrane is either induced or maintained in any specific way by the contact with glial cells, as it is frequently present also on the segment of membrane attached directly to other spines (arrow in Fig. 4C), and because the glial enveloping occurs after the thickening has formed.

The formation and maintenance of spines with postsynaptic thickenings but with no presynaptic element may be taken as an indication that the

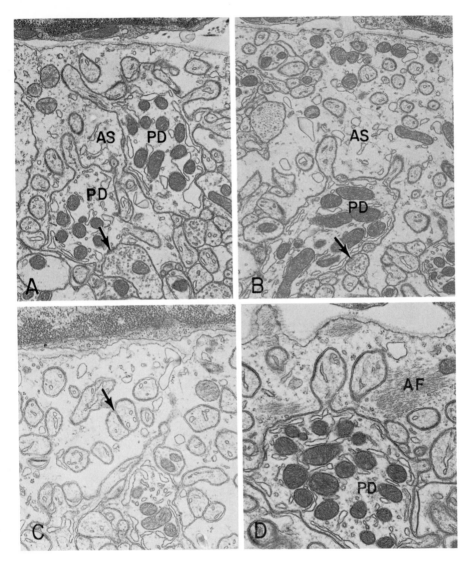

FIG. 4. Electron micrographs of the cerebellar cortex close to pial surface in a 13-month-old noninbred weaver mouse (*wv/wv*). Sections are made in the vermis close to the midline. Numerous spines with "postsynaptic thickening" are enveloped by astroglial cytoplasm. *Abbreviations:* AF, astroglial fibrils; AS, astrocyte; PD, Purkinje dendrites. See text for further explanation.

mosaicism of the dendritic surface membrane is programmed intrinsically or under the influence of other extrinsic factors than the parallel fiber. This mosaicism is well illustrated in the weaver mouse, in which axons of the interneurons of the molecular layers (stellate cells) form symmetric synapses with the smooth surface of Purkinje cell dendritic shafts, as they do in normal animals, although numerous bare spines are present in the immediate vicinity (arrows in Fig. 4A,B). Similarly, in most instances climbing fiber terminals in the weaver mouse form appropriate synapses with elongated spines on the primary dendrites as they do normally, rather than with the small spines on secondary dendrites which would normally form junctions with parallel fibers (Rakic and Sidman, 1973b). Although some unusual synaptic formations are observed in weaver mice (Rakic and Sidman, 1973b; Sotelo, 1973) the striking feature is that the basic normal pattern is retained in both weaver and reeler mice. In such cases, where both normal and abnormal synaptic arrangements are encountered, it is essential to make at least some rough quantitative estimates. We have the impression that in both weaver and reeler mice, normal synaptic connections are surprisingly well preserved and significantly outnumber "unusual" types. It should be underscored that even in normal animals certain numbers of synapses are encountered that are also bizarre and difficult to classify.

The presence of Purkinje cell dendritic spines and their membrane thickenings in granuloprival cerebella, however, does not prove that these features develop completely independently, governed by intrinsic cell forces alone, because other exogenous agents may have acted earlier in development. For example, the climbing fiber input of Purkinje cells might act as an extrinsic determinant of Purkinje cell dendritic morphology and as a trigger to spine development. These cerebellar axons form the earliest afferent contacts with Purkinje cells, initially on the tips of the basal somatic spines, then on apical spines, and finally they transfer to the primary stems of growing dendrites (Ramón y Cajal, 1911; Larramendi, 1969; Mugnaini, 1969; Kornguth and Scott, 1972). It should be emphasized that climbing fibers themselves do not make direct synaptic contact with the small type of dendritic spines on which parallel fibers normally synapse (e.g., see Mugnaini, 1972; Palay and Chan-Palay, 1973). Recent experiments in which climbing fibers have been surgically severed indicate that these afferents may have a profound influence on spine maintenance in the rat (Hámori, 1973a). Because typical climbing fiber terminals are present on the dendrites of Purkinje cells in both weaver (Rakic and Sidman, 1973b) and reeler (Rakic and Sidman, 1972) mice, they cannot be excluded as a possible inducer of dendritic differentiation in granuloprival mice.

Another type of cerebellar afferent that also forms relatively early arises in the nucleus locus coeruleus. These adrenergic fibers seem to be already intermingled with Purkinje cells at the premigratory stage, as has been elegantly shown by fluorescence histochemistry in human embryos (Olson, Boreus, and Seiger, 1973). It has been suggested that the monoamines present early in these axons might have a morphogenetic role during development before they assume a synaptic impulse-transmitting function (Olson and Seiger, 1972; Seiger and Olson, 1973). The fibers from the locus coeruleus are present in both weaver and reeler mice even on the ectopic and misoriented Purkinje cells and their dendrites (Landis and Bloom, 1974).

If climbing fibers or axons from the locus coeruleus do indeed have an influence on spine formation they probably act at early stages, as numerous spines develop in Purkinje cells in cerebellar tissue cultures explanted at the first postnatal day (Privat, 1975). However, the formation of spines in such experiments does not rule out the possibility that climbing fibers might induce spines, as suggested by Hámori (1973a,b) because their influence may be mediated prenatally before morphologically detectable synaptic contact is established. The presence of some unidentified axosomatic synapses in rat cerebellum at birth (del Cerro and Snider, 1972) should also be taken into account. The issue is even further complicated by the observation that terminal boutons, with ultrastructural characteristics of climbing fibers, may originate from deep cerebellar nuclei which are usually present in this type or organotypic cultures (Hendelman, 1973). It should be emphasized that even if climbing fibers or axons from the locus coeruleus do influence Purkinje cell differentiation, they probably serve as a trigger for the growth only of primary and secondary dendrites or the formation of spines or both, because, as described above, the development of tertiary branches and dendritic orientation seems to be modulated significantly by the presence and organization of parallel fibers.

The other class of cerebellar neurons that develop their dendrites exclusively within the milieu of parallel fibers are the interneurons of the molecular layer (i.e., the "basket" and "stellate" cells). These cells represent a typical example of local circuit neurons (Rakic, 1975). The analysis of their development in rhesus monkey cerebellum has indicated possible effects of extrinsic influences on the shapes of these neurons and on their assembly into local neuronal circuits (Rakic, 1972, 1973, 1974). The combination of Golgi, autoradiographic, and electron microscopic methods employed to study genesis of dendrites of the interneurons of the cerebellar molecular layer has shown that the pattern and volume of their dendritic distribution depends both on the time of interneuron origin and on the orientation and rate of maturation of adjacent parallel fibers.

Figures 5–7 summarize diagrammatically the evidence that indicates that these interneurons form a single class of cells by developmental criteria and that the precise shape of their dendrites is attained under the direct influence of the local cellular environment (Rakic, 1972, 1974). The major synaptically relevant components of their local environment are parallel fibers. In considering the development of those fibers, one should keep in mind the morphogenetic transformation that leads to their T-shaped axon as described originally by Ramón y Cajal (1911) and recently reconstructed in three dimensions from electron micrographs in the fetal monkey cerebellum (Rakic, 1971, 1973). It is important to note that the earliest granule cell neurons have been generated and have formed their parallel fiber axons be-

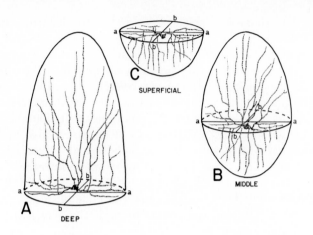

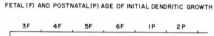

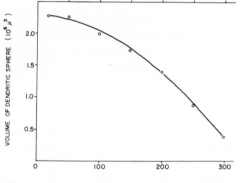

FIG. 5. Summary of the shapes and volumes of dendritic arborization of interneurons in the cerebellar molecular layer (stellate and basket cells) in adult rhesus monkey. (A) Diagrammatic representation of the space occupied by the dendritic arbors of typical deep, middle, and superficial interneurons. (B) Graphic representation of the progressively decreasing volumes occupied by interneuron dendrite arborization (expressed in $10^6 \mu^3$ on the vertical scale) as a function of the distance of interneuron somas from the bottom of the molecular layer (lower horizontal scale) and of the age at which dendrites begin to grow (upper horizontal scale in fetal, F, and postnatal, P, months). (From Rakic, 1972.)

fore the first interneurons are generated (Fig. 7A), and continue to be produced for a relatively long time after the last interneuron has appeared (Rakic, 1973). Those interneurons that in the adult lie deepest in the molecular layer (basket cells) are generated earliest, and the progressively more superficial interneurons (stellate cells) arise at progressively later times (Fig. 7).

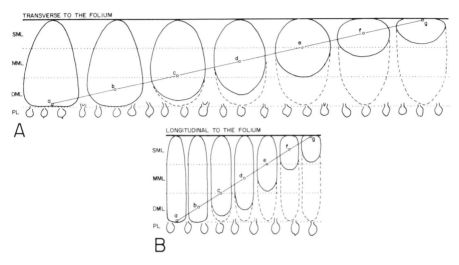

FIG. 6. Diagrammatic representation of the average areas occupied by dendritic arborizations of interneurons situated at different levels of the molecular layer as seen in plane transverse (upper row) and longitudinal (lower row) to the folium. The molecular layer is arbitrarily divided into 100-μ-wide deep (DML), middle (MML), and superficial (SML) zones. Note the systematic change in the shape and size of actual dendritic distributions (outlined by solid line) from the deepest-lying cell (a) to the most superficial cell (g). (From Rakic, 1972.)

Let us see how the volumes and shapes of dendritic domains of the mature interneurons are correlated systematically with their position in the molecular layer in the rhesus monkey. The earliest interneurons begin to generate their processes while they lie close to the Purkinje cell somas on a shallow bed of previously generated parallel fibers (Fig. 7). Subsequently, more parallel fibers are laid down externally and at right angles to them, so that the somas of these interneurons become permanently fixed in position; their growing dendrites, however, can lengthen freely by growing externally as additional strata of parallel fibers are added. Thus the earliest formed interneurons lie deepest in the molecular layer and acquire the largest volumes of dendritic spheres (Figs. 5 and 6). An interneuron that begins to generate dendrites when about half the parallel fibers have been laid down will become fixed in position in the middle of the molecular layer. Its dendrites can grow internally into the parallel fiber territory occupied in part by dendrites of earlier-generated interneurons and, along with the dendrites of the earlier-generated interneurons, also grow externally as new parallel fibers are laid down (Fig. 7C). However, these interneurons will have smaller volumes than the earlier-generated cells, because their dendrites do not generally extend all the way to the bottom of the molecular layer. Finally, an interneuron that forms its dendrites late will have a soma fixed in the external

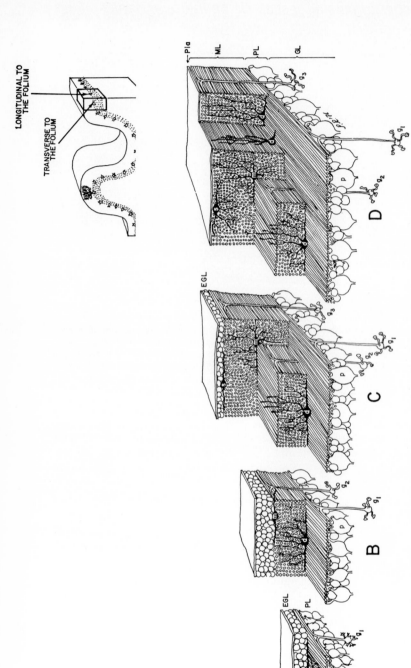

FIG. 7. Three-dimensional reconstruction of histogenetic events in the molecular layer with emphasis on the relationship between the development of interneuron dendritic pattern and the sequence of genesis of parallel fibers. The diameters of cell processes, particularly of parallel fibers, are exaggerated to make the reconstruction more explicit. (A–C) Correspond roughly to the early, middle and late developmental stages described in the text. (D) Reconstruction of the adult cortex. For orientation the planes transverse and longitudinal to the folium are indicated on the sketch in the right upper corner. *Abbreviations:* d, deep interneurons; EGL, external granular layer; g_{1-3}, granule cells; GL, granular layer; m, middle interneuron; ML, molecular layer; p, Purkinje cell; PL, Purkinje cell layer; s, superficial interneuron. (From Rakic, 1972.)

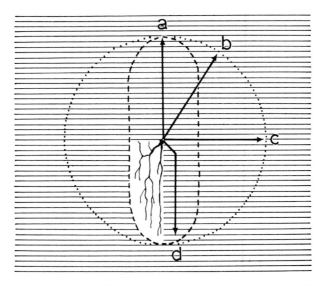

FIG. 8. An idealized model to illustrate the relationship between dendritic growth and orientation of parallel fibers in the plane parallel to pia. For the same extent of growth dendrites a, b, and c would achieve 100%, 80%, and 0% of the possible interactions with parallel fibers (horizontal lines). In actual specimens most of the dendrites grow close to the axis which maximizes the number of interactions; growth in direction c has not been encountered in electron micrographs. However, after an initial growth at a sharp angle, many fibers may curve in the direction that could account for the observed dendritic distribution within the area of a flattened ellipse (broken line). The actual pattern of the dendritic arborization as seen from above in the plane parallel to pia is inscribed on the left lower portion of the ellipse. (From Rakic, 1972.)

stratum of the molecular layer and its dendrites directed inward (Fig. 7D); its volume will be even smaller compared to earlier interneurons (Figs. 5 and 6).

On the basis of such data, it is reasonable to speculate that adult interneurons, the somas of which are situated at various levels of the molecular layer, may be identical cells with respect to their intrinsic gene expression, but that their dendritic pattern is extrinsically determined, presumably on the basis of surface membrane-mediated signals, to respond in a particular way to parallel fibers, i.e., to establish a maximal number of interactions with parallel fibers for a given length of growth, as graphically illustrated in Fig. 8 (Rakic, 1972). However, the molecular nature of membrane specificities in developing cell processes, their time of appearance, quantitative distribution and turnover are less understood than in other less complex tissues (e.g., Bennett, Boyse, and Old, 1972; Lowenstein, 1973).

From such analysis it appears that the dendritic branching patterns and the volume of dendritic sphere are exclusively dependent on the orientation of the adjacent parallel fibers. Not only do the dendrites grow predominantly in the plane transverse to the orientation of the folium, but the individual growing branchlets appear to realign quickly to that same orientation, as though obeying the principle of maximizing the number of parallel fiber contacts per unit length of interneuron dendrite (Fig. 8). The systematic decrease in volume of dendritic sphere reflects the progressive decrease in territory available for dendritic growth as successive waves of interneurons are generated (Rakic, 1972). The paucity and misorientation of dendritic arborization on otherwise normally differentiated interneurons in the weaver mouse supports the hypothesis that their dendritic growth and orientation depends on the presence of parallel fibers (Rakic and Sidman, 1973*b*). Although a similarly detailed developmental analysis has not been made for any other neuron class that grows predominantly in the plane perpendicular to their major axonal input (e.g., Fig. 1), it is tempting to speculate that some other systems might obey the same principle.

If the pattern and size of dendritic ramifications depend, with virtually mathematical precision, on the status of the ever-changing local milieu encountered at the time a given neuron class begins to differentiate, this allows for a significant morphologic diversity among them on the basis of local extrinsic influences without the need to invoke further subspecialization in gene expression. However, we should be careful not to lapse into the erroneous overemphasis of external influences. For example, the basic difference between neuron classes, such as the 90° difference in orientation of bipolar phase of granule cell compared with bipolar phase of interneurons (Fig. 7) probably reflects a fundamental difference in intrinsic gene expression that determines what type of response a cell makes to its milieu (Rakic, 1974). These basic differences are probably already specified in the proliferative tissue of the external granular layer where prospective interneurons and granule cells behave differently with respect to kinetics of their proliferation and have possibly already formed separate cell lines (Rakic, 1973).

Another aspect of genesis of dendrites concerns the signal that terminates the latent period between the time of interneuron genesis and the time that cell begins to generate dendrites. Our results in monkey fetuses show that this latent period lengthens progressively during development. Deep interneurons make dendrites relatively soon after the cell itself is generated, but cells destined for superficial strata of the molecular layer apparently are in a latent stage for a period of 2 months before they begin to generate dendrites (Rakic, 1973). These cells actually arise long in advance of the appropriate sheaves of parallel fibers and sprouts of climbing fiber terminals that will constitute most of their synaptic contacts. Therefore they appear to wait, presumably as round, undifferentiated cells on the thickening bed of parallel fibers, until they become completely enveloped by the newly-formed processes of other cells that constitute their proper local environment. Among these processes in addition to parallel fibers and climbing fibers, we have been able to identify axons of previously generated interneurons and Purkinje dendrites (Rakic, 1973). It is not possible to discern which particular class of processes or combination of classes in the local environment induces the genesis of dendrites by those interneurons.

Both examples of neuronal differentiation, that of Purkinje cells and of interneurons of the cerebellar molecular layer reviewed in this chapter show that a given neuron may be considered partly as an autonomous and active individual unit and partly as a passive element subordinate to forces that lie outside its boundary. There appears to be a balance of intrinsic and extrinsic factors (Rakic, 1972, 1974). In different neuron classes, however, one or the other influence may prevail (e.g., Van der Loos, 1965; Hamori, 1973*b*). Cell interaction during neurogenesis probably occurs in various ways, and recent investigations not only have begun to disclose the immense complexity of the problems, but they have also opened an exciting new approach for distinguishing among intrinsic and extrinsic factors. Future research, however, clearly should not be carried out in the spirit of a renaissance of the old philosophic dialogue of epigenesis versus preformation, but rather as an exact scientific inquiry into minute details of neuronal development.

The development of dendrites in other brain regions has not been analyzed in comparable detail, probably because the geometric organization of neuropil in most brain structures is not as obvious as it is in the cerebellar cortex. This problem might be overcome, however, through the use of recently developed computer-aided analytic systems for the rapid and accurate measurement of different dendritic parameters as visualized by impregnation according to the Golgi method (Glaser and Van der Loos, 1965; Garvey, Young, Coleman, and Simon, 1973; Wann, Woolsey, Dierker, and Cowan, 1973; Hilman, Chujo, and Llinás, 1974; Marin-Padilla and Stibitz, 1974). These systems can be used to view three-dimensional shapes of dendritic arborizations, and they also have the capability to rotate the entire neuron and to provide quantitative data on the total dendritic length, number of branchings, number of spines, etc.

For some specific questions such as analysis of specific synaptic input on dendrites, another promising approach is the computer-aided neuron reconstruction from serial electron microscopic sections (Levinthal and Ware, 1972; Macagno, Lopresti, and Levinthal, 1973; Rakic, Stansaas, Sayre, and Sidman, 1974). This method is based on the use of an uninterrupted sequence of ultrathin serial sections through the neural structure of interest. From each section or from alternate sections (depending on the specific objectives of the study) overlapping fields are photographed with the electron microscope, and photomontages are prepared. A set of planar profiles of selected cells are digitized and then reassembled into three-dimensional solids in space by a computer. In addition to visual display and printouts of neuron contours and synaptic input, it is possible to measure total surface areas, fractional surface areas (e.g., areas occupied by morphologically definable synaptic junctions, by glial coatings, or by dendritic spines), and volumes of cells and their parts. In a pilot study we have demonstrated the feasibility of obtaining such measurements on relatively simple immature neurons in the developing cerebral cortex (Rakic et al., 1974). The reconstruction of the dendritic tree of a more complex, mature neuron and particularly the quantitative plotting and measurement of synaptic inputs is going to be a much more formidable task, but technically it is within reach. This methodology will probably become an indispensible tool for neurobiologists in the near future. For example, the problem of ✓ modifiability and plasticity of dendritic morphology might be determined quantitatively by objective analysis rather than by subjective inspection of sections. To be reliable, pertinent measurements must be done on a large sample. Quantitative and qualitative data of this type, presently not available, are likely to promote understanding of the modes of dendritic genesis and possibly will provide more reliable evidence on the possible modifiability of dendritic morphology in the adult and on possible changes in their synaptic relations under different experimental conditions.

REFERENCES

Addison, W. H. F. (1911): The development of the Purkinje cells and of the cortical layers in the cerebellum of the albino rat. *J. Comp. Neurol.*, 21:459–487.

Altman, J. (1973): Experimental reorganization of the cerebellar cortex. IV. Parallel fiber reorientation following regeneration of the external germinal layer. *J. Comp. Neurol.*, 149:181–192.

Altman, J., and Anderson, W. J. (1972): Experimental reorganization of the cerebellar cortex. I. Morphological effects of elimination of all microneurons with prolonged X-irradiation started at birth. *J. Comp. Neurol.*, 146:355–406.

Barron, D. H. (1944): The early development of the sensory and internucleal cells in the spinal cord of the sheep. *J. Comp. Neurol.*, 81:193–225.

Bennett, D., Boyse, E. A., and Old, L. J. (1972): Cell surface immunogenetics in the study of morphogenesis. In: *Cell Interactions. Proceedings of the Third Lepetit Colloquium*, edited by L. G. Silvestri. North-Holland, Amsterdam.

Berry, M., and Hollingworth, T. (1973): Development of isolated neocortex. *Experientia*, 29:204–207.

del Cerro, M. P., and Snider, R. S. (1972): Axo-somatic and axo-dendritic synapses in the cerebellum of the newborn rat. *Brain Res.*, 43:581–586.

Dadoune, J. P. (1966): Contribution à l'étude de la différentiation de la cellule de Purkinje et du cortex cérébelleux chez le rat blanc. *Arch. Anat. Hist. Embryol.*, 49:383–393.

Garvey, C. F., Young, J. H., Coleman, P. D., and Simon, W. (1973): Automated three-dimensional dendrite tracking system. *Electroencephalography*, 35:199–204.

Glaser, E. M., and Van der Loos, H. (1965): A semi-automatic computer-microscope for the analysis of neuronal morphology. *IEEE Trans. Biomed. Engl.*, 12:22–31.

Hámori, J. (1973a): The inductive role of presynaptic axons in the development of postsynaptic spines. *Brain Res.*, 62:337–344.

Hámori, J. (1973b): Developmental morphology of dendritic postsynaptic specializations. In: *Results in Neuroanatomy, Neuroendocrinology, Neurophysiology and Behavior*, edited by K. Lissák. Akadémia Kiadó, Budapest.

Hendelman, W. J. (1973): The synaptology of cerebellar cultures of the vermis. *Anat. Rec.*, 172:327–328.

Herndon, R. M. (1968): Thiophen-induced granule cell necrosis in the rat cerebellum. An electron microscope study. *Exp. Brain Res.*, 6:49–68.

Herndon, R. M., Margolis, G., and Kilham, L. (1971): The synaptic organization of the malformed cerebellum induced by prenatal infection with the feline leukopenia virus. *J. Neuropathol. Exp. Neurol.*, 30:557–570.

Hillman, D. E., Chujo, M., and Llinás, R. (1974): Quantitative computer analysis of the morphology of cerebellar neurons. I. Granule cells. *Anat. Rec.*, 178:375–376.

Hirano, A., and Dembitzer, H. (1973): Cerebellar alteration in the weaver mouse. *J. Cell Biol.*, 56:478–486.

Hirano, A., Dembitzer, H. M., and Jones, M. (1972): An electron microscopic study of cycasin-induced cerebellar alteration. *J. Neuropathol. Exp. Neurol.*, 31:113–125.

Jacobson, M. (1970): Development, specification, and diversification of neuronal connections. In: *The Neurosciences, Second Study Program*, edited by F. O. Schmitt. Rockefeller Univ. Press, New York.

Kelly, J. P., and Cowan, W. M.. (1972): Studies on the development of the chick optic tectum. III. Effects of early eye removal. *Brain Res.*, 42:263–288.

Kornguth, S. E., and Scott, G. (1972): The role of climbing fibers in the formation of Purkinje cell dendrites. *J. Comp. Neurol.*, 146:61–82.

Landis, S. C., and Bloom, F. E. (1974): Fluorescence and electron microscopic analysis of catecholamine-containing fibers in mutant mouse cerebellum. *Anat. Rec.*, 178:398.

Larramendi, L. M. H. (1969): Analysis of synaptogenesis in the cerebellum of the mouse. In: *Neurobiology of Cerebellar Evolution and Development*, edited by R. Llinás. American Medical Association Education and Research Foundation, Chicago, Illinois.

Levi-Montalcini, R. (1949): The development of the acoustico-vestibular centers in the chick embryo in the absence of the afferent root fibers and of descending fiber tracts. *J. Comp. Neurol.*, 91:209–241.

Levinthal, C., and Ware, R. (1972): Three dimensional reconstruction from serial sections. *Nature*, 236:207–210.

Llinás, R., Hillman, D. E., and Precht, W. (1973): Neuronal circuit reorganization in mammalian agranular cerebellar cortex. *J. Neurobiol.*, 4:69–94.

Lowenstein, W. R. (1973): Membrane junctions in growth and differentiation. *Fed. Proc.*, 32:60–64.

Macagno, E. R., Lopresti, V., and Levinthal, C. (1973): Structure and development of neuronal connections in isogenic organisms: variations and similarities in the optic system of *Daphnia magna*. *Proc. Natl. Acad. Sci. USA*, 70:57–61.

Marin-Padilla, M., and Stibitz, G. R. (1974): Three-dimensional reconstruction of the basket cell of the human motor cortex. *Brain Res.*, 70:511–514.

Morest, D. K. (1969): The differentiation of cerebral dendrites: a study of post-migratory neuroblast in the medial nucleus of the trapezoid body. *Z. Anat. Entwicklungsgesch.*, 128:271–289.

Mugnaini, E. (1969): Ultrastructural studies on the cerebellar histogenesis. II. Maturation of the nerve cell populations and establishment of synaptic connections in the cerebellar cortex of the chick. In: *Neurobiology of Cerebellar Evolution and Development*, edited by R. Llinás. American Medical Association and Research Foundation, Chicago, Illinois.

Mugnaini, E. (1972): The histology and cytology of the cerebellar cortex. In: *The Comparative Anatomy and Histology of the Cerebellum. Vol. III. The Human Cerebellum, Cerebellar Connections and Cerebellar Cortex*, edited by O. Larsell and J. Jansen. The Univ. of Minnesota Press, Minneapolis, Minnesota.

Olson, L., Boreus, L. O., and Seiger, A. (1973): Histochemical demonstration and mapping of 5-hydroxytryptamine- and catecholamine-containing neuron systems in the human fetal brain. *Z. Anat. Entwicklungsgesch.*, 139:259–282.

Olson, L., and Seiger, A. (1972): Early prenatal ontogeny of central monoamine neurons in the rat: fluorescence histochemical observations. *Z. Anat. Entwicklungsgesch.*, 137:301–316.

Palay, S. L., and Chan-Palay, V. (1973): *Cerebellar Cortex: Cytology and Organization*. Springer-Verlag, New York.

Peusner, K. D. (1974): Neurogenesis in chick tangential nucleus and the effect on otocyst removal. *Anat. Rec.*, 178:438.

Privat, A. (1975): this volume.

Rakic, P. (1971): Neuron-glia relationship during granule cell migration in developing cerebellar cortex. A Golgi and electronmicroscopic study in Macacus rhesus. *J. Comp. Neurol.*, 141:283–312.

Rakic, P. (1972): Extrinsic cytological determinants of basket and stellate cell dendritic pattern in the cerebellar molecular layer. *J. Comp. Neurol.*, 146:335–364.

Rakic, P. (1973): Kinetics of proliferation and latency between final division and onset of differentiation of the cerebellar stellate and basket neurons. *J. Comp. Neurol.*, 147:523–546.

Rakic, P. (1974): Intrinsic and extrinsic factors influencing the shape of neurons and their assembly into neuronal circuits. In: *Frontiers in Neurology and Neuroscience Research,* edited by P. Seeman and G. M. Brown. The Univ. of Toronto Press, Toronto.

Rakic, P. (1975): Local neuronal circuits. A report based on NRP work session. *Neurosci. Res. Program Bull. (in press.)*

Rakic, P., and Sidman, R. L. (1972): Synaptic organization of displaced and disoriented cerebellar cortical neurons in reeler mice. *J. Neuropathol. Exp. Neurol.,* 31:192.

Rakic, P., and Sidman, R. L. (1973a): Sequence of developmental abnormalities leading to granule cell deficit in cerebellar cortex of weaver mutant mice. *J. Comp. Neurol.,* 152:103–132.

Rakic, P., and Sidman, R. L. (1973b): Organization of cerebellar cortex secondary to deficit of granule cells in weaver mutant mice. *J. Comp. Neurol.,* 152:133–162.

Rakic, P., Stensaas, L. J., Sayre, E. P., and Sidman, R. L. (1974): Computer aided three-dimensional reconstruction and quantitative analysis of cells from serial electron microscopic montages of fetal monkey brain. *Nature,* 250:31–34.

Ramón y Cajal, S. (1896): Les épines collaterales des cellules du cerveau colorée au bleu de méthyléne. *Rev. Trim. Microgr.,* 1:5–19.

Ramón y Cajal, S. (1911): *Histologie du Système Nerveux de l'Homme et des Vertébrés.* Maloine, Paris. (Reprinted by Consejo Superior de Investigaciones Cientificas, Madrid, 1955.)

Seiger, A., and Olson, L. (1973): Late prenatal ontogeny of central monoamine neurons in the rat: fluorescence histochemical observations. *Z. Anat. Entwicklungsgesch.,* 140:281–318.

Shofer, R. J., Pappas, G. D., and Purpura, D. P. (1964): Radiation-induced changes in morphological and physiological properties of immature cerebellar cortex. In: *Response to Ionizing Radiation. Second International Symposium,* edited by T. J. Haley and R. S. Snider. Little, Brown, Boston, Massachusetts.

Sidman, R. L. (1968): Development of interneuronal connections in brains of mutant mice. In: *Physiological and Biochemical Aspects of Nervous Integration,* edited by F. D. Carlson. Prentice-Hall, Englewood Cliffs, New Jersey.

Skoff, R. P., and Hamburger, V. (1974): Fine structure of dendritic and axonal growth cones in embryonic chick spinal cord. *J. Comp. Neurol.,* 153:107–148.

Sotelo, C. (1973): Permanence and fate of paramembranous synaptic specializations in "mutants" and experimental animals. *Brain Res.,* 62:345–351.

Terrazas, R. (1897): Notas sobie la neuroglía del cerebelo y el crecimiento de los elementos nerviosos. *Rev. Trim. Microgr.,* 2:4a–65.

Van der Loos, H. (1965): The "improperly" oriented pyramidal cell in the cerebral cortex and its possible bearing on problems of neuronal growth and cell orientation. *Bull. Johns Hopkins Hosp.,* 117:228–250.

Vaughn, J. E., Henrikson, C. K., Grieshaber, J. A. (1974): A quantitative study of synapses on motor neuron dendritic growth cones in developing mouse spinal cord. *J. Cell Biol.,* 60:664–672.

Wann, D. F., Woolsey, T. A., Dierker, M. L., and Cowan, W. M. (1973): An on-line digital-computer system for the semiautomatic analysis of Golgi-impregnated neurons. *IEEE Trans. Biomed. Eng.,* 20:233–247.

Advances in Neurology, Vol. 12, edited by
G. W. Kreutzberg, Raven Press, New York
© 1975.

Can Dendrites Be Presynaptic?

E. Ramon-Moliner

Department of Anatomy, School of Medicine, Sherbrooke University, Sherbrooke, Quebec, Canada

According to the classic conception, functional junctions between neurons in the vertebrate nervous system are represented by axosomatic and axo-dendritic synapses. The neuron theory (Ramón y Cajal, 1909, 1934) did not explicitly state that these two types of synapses offered the only polarity of conduction observed in higher vertebrates, but it was implied that, in most neuronal circuits, nervous signals were conveyed by axons to dendrites or perikarya, and that in turn these signals traveled from dendrites and peri-karya to the efferent axon. This simple conception is still used in models of the nervous system in which individual neurons are regarded as operational modules, each provided with multiple inputs and one single output. We now know that this notion can be proposed only as a first approximation and that, without ruling out the neuron theory, the past two decades have contributed a number of data that appear to be incompatible with the assignment of a pure receptor role to dendrites and perikarya.

Even before the impact of electron microscopy, a few disconcerting facts were known. The internal granule cells of the olfactory bulb had consistently failed to show an axon, and the same applied to the amacrine cells of the retina. In addition, the myelinated distal process of sensory ganglion cells provided the example of an axon-like structure which conveys signals, if not toward the perikaryon, at least away from its distal ramifications.

With the progressive refinement of electron microscopy and its application to the study of every region of the nervous tissue it soon became evident that the conventional notion of synapses converging upon dendrites and perikarya constitutes only a particular case of a number of complex possibilities. Unfortunately, the present evidence points to the insufficiencies of the classic theory without substituting a new one for it. Perhaps the only legitimate conclusion that one can now propose is that the terms dendrite, axon, presynaptic, and postsynaptic, are no longer easy to apply.

MATERIALS AND METHODS

Guinea pigs, rats, and young cats were anesthetized with Nembutal and perfused by intracardiac injection of a solution of 0.08 M sodium cacodilate buffered at pH 7.3 containing 1% formaldehyde and 1.25% glutaraldehyde.

Once signs of fixation began to appear, the perfusing solution was replaced by one with the same cacodilate concentration and pH, but with 4% formaldehyde and 5% glutaraldehyde. If the brain is to be impregnated with the formaldehyde variants of the Golgi method, no glutaraldehyde is added to the second solution. Direct electron microscopy of Golgi-stained structures was carried out after lead chromate substitution (Ramon-Moliner and Ferrari, 1972) according to a modified technique. The tissue was impregnated with the Golgi-Kopsch variant and was sectioned by hand. Those regions in which the reaction was successful were then processed as follows: (1) osmication in a 1% solution of osmium tetroxide in 2% silver nitrate; (2) partial lead chromate substitution in a 6% solution of lead nitrate buffered at pH 5.5 with 1% sodium cacodilate and lactic acid; (3) acetones of ascending concentration; (4) one night in a saturated solution of potassium ferricyanide and potassium phosphate in 70% acetone; (5) 3 hr in a 3% solution of potassium thiocyanate in 80% acetone; and (6) dehydration followed by embedding in an epoxy resin according to standard procedures. The polymerized blocks were studied under incident light to select the structures of interest and trimmed for ultramicrotomy.

OBSERVATIONS AND DISCUSSION

Characterization of Typical Axons and Dendrites

According to classic criteria (Ramon-Moliner, 1968; Peters et al., 1970), a typical axon is characterized by its even thickness, absence of tapering with progressive distance from its origin, and by a ramification pattern that usually bears no relationship to the location of the perikaryon. In addition, it may often be surrounded by myelin. In electron micrographs, it is characterized by the scarcity or absence of ribosomes, the tendency of microtubules to arrange themselves in parallel clusters, the submembranous accumulation of a layer of dense material in the axon hillock and the initial segment, and by the presence of synaptic vesicles in the terminal boutons and preterminal ramifications. Typical dendrites, by contrast, are relatively short, taper out as they diverge from the perikaryon, and ramify in such a way that the resulting branches course, as a rule, away from the latter. In electron micrographs, they show evenly spaced microtubules which funnel into their initial portion, clusters of ribosomes, and relatively abundant cisternae of endoplasmic reticulum. It is interesting that typical dendrites never show a myelin sheath or enveloping Schwann cells.

In typical vertebrate synapses, the selective accumulation of synaptic vesicles in the neighborhood of the presynaptic membrane, and the presence of the postsynaptic, or subsynaptic web constitute about the only features that have so far survived as a clue to determine polarity.

It is generally accepted that most vertebrate neurons have multiple dendrites but never more than one axon. For some unknown reason, all the signals reaching a neuron must converge toward one single process. This is an intriguing circumstance, particularly if one bears in mind that many axons ramify or give collaterals immediately after leaving the perikaryon. Admittedly, it is not completely proven that neurons never have more than one axon. The horizontal cells of the outermost layer of the neocortex may constitute one exception and the same applies to the Golgi II neurons of the cerebellum (Fox et al., 1967). In any case, the rule whereby there is only one axon per neuron seems to hold for most of the vertebrate nervous system and must, therefore, have a physiologic explanation. This point is particularly important in view of recent claims that, in some exceptional cases, perikarya could be presynaptic to the structures that contact them (Setalo and Szekely, 1967; Wong, 1970; Peute, 1971; Lieberman, 1973; Ramon-Moliner, 1973). Why should a perikaryon generate impulses in two different ways: by means of a typical axon and by means of somatofugal synapses? This question was formulated in a previous communication (Ramon-Moliner, 1973) in view of the polarity that had to be attributed to mitral somatic synapses if the current electron microscopic criteria are accepted. Should their somatofugal polarity be confirmed, it will become necessary to clarify why Nature has not used, instead, a multiplicity of axons.

Atypical Processes and Synapses

The past decade has witnessed a progressive erosion of the criteria that could be used to differentiate the two known types of neural processes and to establish synaptic polarity. Hirata (1964) and Andres (1965) were probably the first authors who pointed out the existence of reciprocal synapses in the olfactory bulb. This finding was subsequently used (Rall et al., 1966) to propose a model of the electrical activity of the olfactory bulb on the basis of dendrodendritic interaction. In this neural territory, the presence of junctions between processes containing synaptic vesicles is now a well-documented fact (Pinching, 1970; Price and Powell, 1970; and many others). One could account for these atypical synapses as an indication of the "primitive nature" of the olfactory bulb. In this regard, there are reports of similar reciprocal synapses in other regions of the central nervous system of lower vertebrates (Setalo and Szekely, 1967; Peute, 1971; and others). However, atypical synapses between vesicle-containing processes have also been demonstrated in various regions of the central nervous system of higher vertebrates, i.e., the lateral geniculate nucleus (Gray, 1969; Guillery, 1969; Szentagothai, 1970; Wong, 1970; Lieberman and Webster, 1972; Lieberman, 1973; and others), the medial geniculate nucleus (Morest, 1971), and other thalamic nuclei (Harding, 1971; Ralston, 1971). Therefore there is a possibility that somatofugal signals could be propagated along dendrites and along somatic synapses even in phylogenetically recent nerve centers.

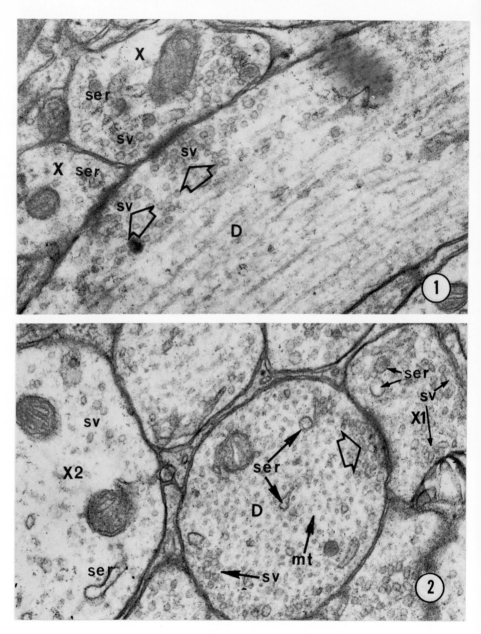

FIG. 1. A mitral dendrite, D, synapses with two boutons, X, that probably belong to internal granule cell dendrites. The latter appear to be postsynaptic to the mitral dendrite. There are transitional forms between the smooth endoplasmic reticulum, ser, and the synaptic vesicles (sv) of the boutons. (×54,500.)

FIG. 2. A tranversely cut mitral dendrite, D, synapses with one bouton, X1. Process X2 probably is a transversely cut dendrite of an internal granule cell. Microtubules, mt, are abundant in the mitral dendrite but not in the granule cell dendrite. (×54,500.)

When first discovered, these contacts between processes that contained synaptic vesicles were interpreted as axoaxonic (Gray, 1962), and were regarded as a morphologic substrate for presynaptic inhibition (Eccles et al., 1961). But if, as recently claimed by Morest (1971), some of these vesicle-filled processes must be classified as dendrites, the picture becomes so complex that a radical revision of current theories regarding neuronal interaction will become necessary. An attitude of cautious reserve may be justified at present, because the assignment of dendritic or axonal parentage to the profiles seen in electron micrographs is not an easy task. Whenever two processes containing synaptic vesicles are seen synapsing with each other, discrepancies of interpretation become inevitable. Current literature abounds in examples.

In the case of the olfactory glomerulus, at least six types of processes can be expected to be intimately intermingled: the dendritic arborizations of mitral cells; the processes, axonal or dendritic, of the external granule cells; the dendritic arborizations of tufted cells; the axons of olfactory neuroepithelial cells, the axons of the external granule cells; and the axons of the periglomerular neurons. In our opinion, there is, as yet, no reliable way to identify every one of these processes in electron micrographs of the glomerulus. Certain criteria that have been proposed should be viewed with caution. The olfactory axons are the only structures that can possibly be identified with some degree of confidence but not with absolute certainty.

In regions outside the glomerulus, large and rectilinear dendrites (Figs. 1 and 2) could possibly belong to mitral cells. But the processes with which they make contact may well belong to several categories, all of which may contain synaptic vesicles—axons or dendrites of periglomerular cells and tufted cells; axons of external granule cells; and possibly other processes of neuronal types as yet unidentified with light microscopy.

If classic criteria are accepted, the polarity that should be attributed to the synapses illustrated in Figs. 1 and 2 is dendrifugal. Rall et al. (1966) have shown examples of adjacent paired synapses with opposite polarities. Such reciprocal arrangements are so rarely observed that we are inclined to think that their theoretical importance has been overrated.

In our material, large dendrites displayed mostly the apparently dendrifugal type of synapse illustrated in Figs. 1 and 2, both in the external plexiform layer and in the interglomerular regions. Many of these processes must be mitral dendrites. Therefore it would appear that mitral cells are presynaptic to most of their surrounding neuropil, at least in the extraglomerular regions. This appears so unlikely that one may be inclined to question the dendrifugal nature of the synapses illustrated in Figs. 1 and 2. But this is also difficult to accept, unless it can be proven that the axons of the olfactory neuroepithelial cells also have synapses comparable to those of processes labeled with X in Figs. 1 and 2. Indeed, if this were the case, one would have to reject the only criteria that so far have survived in deter-

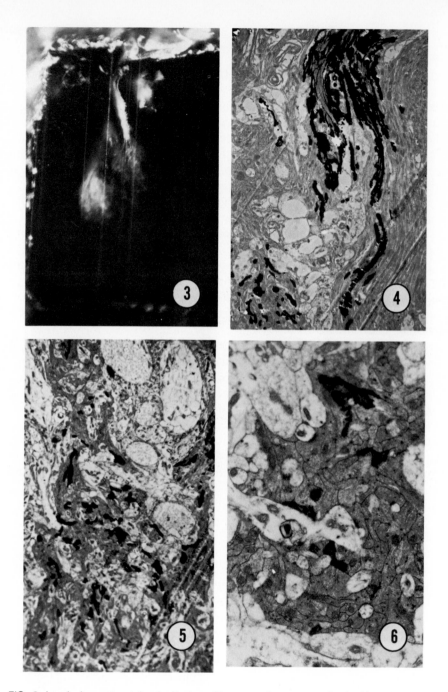

FIG. 3. Lead chromate-stained olfactory fibers can be seen under incident light in the araldite-embedded block. (×210.)

FIG. 4. One bundle of lead chromate-stained fibers coursing in the superficial layers of the olfactory bulb. (×3,200.)

FIG. 5. The terminal olfactory ramifications within the glomerulus. It can be seen that the lead chromate-stained fibers are confined to the polypoid formations and do not reach the light areas. (×3,200.)

FIG. 6. The olfactory polypoid formations made out of compact aggregates of olfactory fibers. The lead chromate-stained fibers are confined to these formations. (×12,540.)

mining polarity. In view of this, it becomes desirable (1) to establish beyond doubt that no aberrant olfactory fibers are found in the extraglomerular neuropil, and (2) to identify these olfactory fibers and their synapses within the glomeruli. This can be achieved by carrying out direct electron microscopy of Golgi-stained olfactory axons (Figs. 3–6). The sequence of chemical insults to the tissue has resulted in a rather poorly preserved ultrastructure. Nevertheless, the material permits unambiguous identification of the olfactory fibers. These appear as densely stained profiles within certain polypoid formations made out of the aggregation of many olfactory axons. It can be seen that, contrary to what one could have expected, the latter do not terminate in the form of freely ramifying branchlets scattered between the dendritic ramifications of the remaining components of the glomerulus, and that they are confined to the polypoid formations. If one studies the surface of these formations in material prepared according to standard electronmicroscopic technology, it is a relief to find that the classic criteria for synaptic polarity still hold (Figs. 7 and 8). However, large extraglomerular dendrites display synapses comparable to those of Figs. 9 and 10, and it would appear that mitral cells are presynaptic to most of their surrounding neuropil, with the exception of the olfactory fibers. Within the glomerulus, only on two occasions profiles that looked like olfactory fibers appeared to show synapses with a reversed arrangement of vesicle clusters and subsynaptic web (Figs. 9 and 10). Hopefully, these were not real synapses with olfactory fibers. They are shown here because the possibility, however remote, cannot be excluded.

At least four different types of processes containing synaptic vesicles have been described in the lateral geniculate nucleus (Guillery, 1969). The central process XI in Fig. 11 is probably of retinal origin; it synapses with another vesicle-containing process, in X2, and with others possibly devoid of vesicles. According to the criteria put forth, among others, by Guillery (1969) and Szentagothai (1970), the process in X2 should be regarded as the axon of a Golgi II cell, whereas the work of Morest (1971) and Lieberman (1973) opens the possibility that it should be a dendritic appendage of a Golgi II cell. To make matters more complicated, the synapse indicated by an open arrow displays a synaptic web on the side of the process which should be regarded as an extrinsic axon. The latter, in turn, appears to be presynaptic to processes X3 and X4, which do not contain evident synaptic vesicles and which could represent dendritic spines. Figure 12 shows a large bouton that surrounds a spine, in X2, with which it synapses. It appears likely that profile X1 in Fig. 11 resulted from the tangential section of a bouton comparable to that of Fig. 12. If, as seems likely, process X1, in Fig. 11, is an extrinsic afferent axon, one must conclude that synaptic polarity has nothing to do with the side on which the synaptic web is located. One may then wonder about the value that can be attributed to similar webs to determine synaptic polarity in other regions of the nervous system.

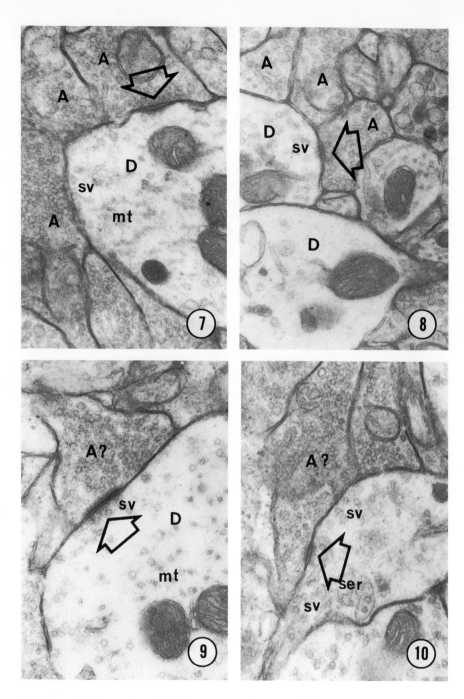

FIGS. 7 and 8. Aggregates of olfactory axons, A, surround dendrites, D, within the olfactory glomerulus. Most, if not all, of the synapses on the olfactory fibers (open arrows) display a subsynaptic web on the dendritic side. (×37,000.)

FIGS. 9 and 10. Two synapses (open arrows) within the olfactory glomerulus. In view of their apparent polarity, the axonal nature of the boutons (A?) can be questioned. Otherwise, the latter resemble olfactory fibers. (×37,000.)

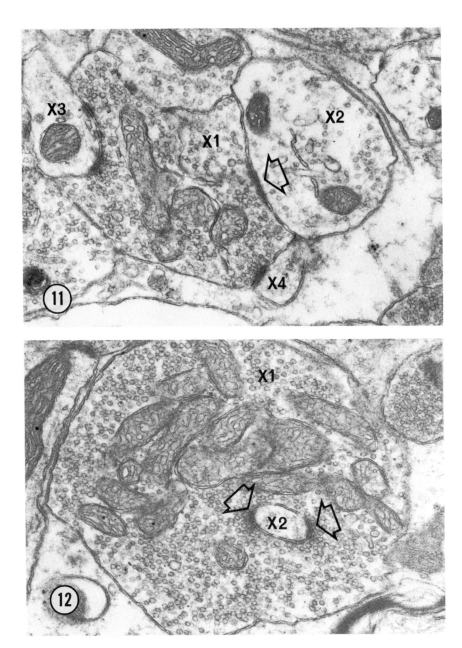

FIG. 11. Dorsolateral geniculate nucleus of rat. The central process (X1) could be an axon of retinal origin. It synapses (open arrow) with one vesicle containing bouton, as well as with other processes (X3 and X4). The polarity of the synapse indicated by an open arrow has probably no relation to the location of the synaptic web. (×31,500.)

FIG. 12. Dorsolateral geniculate nucleus of rat. A large spherical bouton (X1) within which a dendritic spine is invaginated. (×31,500.)

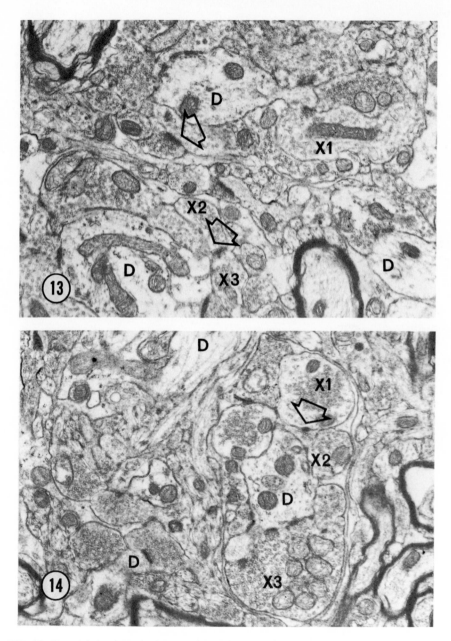

FIG. 13. Dorsal lateral geniculate nucleus of rat. In the neuropil of this center, typical synapses between vesicle-filled axons (as for example, in X1), and dendrites, D, are considerably more abundant than between vesicle-filled processes (open arrows). This is a general feature of the LGN neuropil. (×21,000.)

FIG. 14. Dorsolateral geniculate nucleus of rat. Note the rarity of synapses between processes containing synaptic vesicles. The only possible one is indicated by an open arrow. (×22,000.)

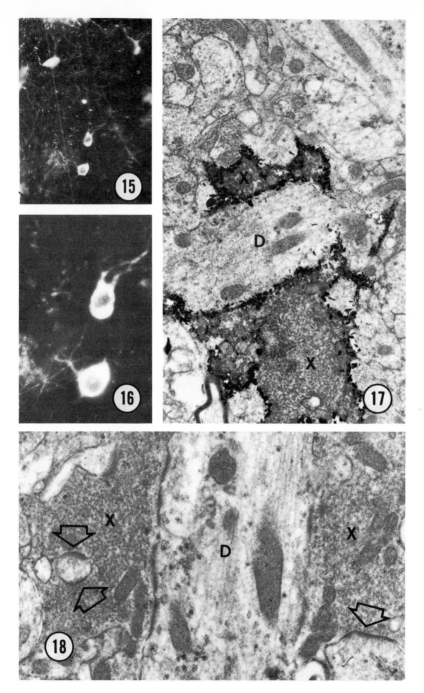

FIGS. 15 and 16. Neurons of VA nucleus of thalamus of rat, stained with lead chromate, embedded in araldite, and illuminated with incident light.

FIG. 17. Electron micrograph of the material shown in Figs. 15 and 16. A dendrite, D, is enveloped by a lead chromate-stained structure, X, within which a granular material is present. The latter could be made out of synaptic vesicles distorted by the Golgi impregnation. (×21,000.)

FIG. 18. A field from the same section illustrated in Fig. 17, showing a large enveloping profile, X, filled with synaptic vesicles and probably synapsing at the points indicated by open arrows. (×21,000.)

Although synapses between vesicle-containing processes are well documented in the lateral geniculate nucleus (LGN), it may be worthwhile to mention that they are far from numerous. Figures 13 and 14 illustrate representative regions of the LGN neuropil. It can be seen that there are numerous synapses but that only a few — those indicated with open arrows — are established between vesicle-containing processes. Moreover, the open arrow in Fig. 14 could point to a desmosome-like junction and not to a proper synapse.

The combined approach of experimental degeneration and electron microscopy can be useful in the identification of extrinsic axonal endings. But differentiating between local short axons and dendrites, when both are reported to contain synaptic vesicles, cannot be accomplished easily. One possible approach to this challenge could be the direct electron microscopic study of Golgi-stained material. The lead chromate substitution technique (Ramon-Moliner and Ferrari, 1972) used to obtain the material illustrated in Figs. 3–6 can show a depleted impregnation without fading of the borderlines under certain circumstances. In such cases it is possible to see that the cytoplasm of the impregnated structures contains occasionally relatively well-preserved organelles. As yet, we have failed to obtain convincing images of synaptic vesicles within previously identified processes. Figures 15–18 illustrate this attempt. Under incident light, neurons and dendrites of the nucleus ventralis anterior of the thalamus of rat are seen in Figs. 15 and 16 in Golgi-stained material treated for lead chromate substitution and embedded in araldite. Electron microscopy of this material showed occasional profiles with a granular texture that could be synaptic vesicles crushed by the silver chromate impregnation (Fig. 17). This possibility appears to be endorsed by the vesicular appearance of the cytoplasm of adjacent structures in the same block of tissue (Fig. 18). It goes without saying that the technique will require considerable improvement in order to provide intelligible and useful images.

ACKNOWLEDGMENT

This work was supported by grant MA-4183 of the Medical Research Council of Canada.

REFERENCES

Andres, K. H. (1965): Der Feinbau des Bulbus olfactorius der Ratte. *Z. Zellforsch. Mikrosk. Anat.,* 65:530–561.

Eccles, J. C., Eccles, R. M., and Magni, F. (1961): Central inhibitory action attributable to presynaptic depolarization. *J. Physiol.,* 159:147–166.

Famiglietti, E. V., Jr. (1970): Dendro-dendritic synapses in the lateral geniculate nucleus of the cat. *Brain Res.,* 20:181–191.

Fox, C. A., Hillman, D. E., Siegesmund, K. A., and Dutta, C. R. (1967): The primate cerebellum: A Golgi and electron microscopic study. In: *The Cerebellum,* edited by C. A. Fox and R. S. Snider. Elsevier, Amsterdam.

Gray, E. G. (1962): A morphological basis for presynaptic inhibition? *Nature*, 193:82–83.

Guillery, R. W. (1969): The organization of synaptic interconnections in the laminae of the dorsal lateral geniculate nucleus of the cat. *Z. Zellforsch. Mikrosk. Anat.*, 96:1–38.

Harding, B. N. (1971): Dendro-dendritic synapses, including reciprocal synapses, in the ventrolateral nucleus of the monkey thalamus. *Brain Res.*, 34:181–185.

Hirata, Y. (1964): Some observations on the fine structure of the synapses in the olfactory bulb with particular reference to the atypical synaptic configurations. *Arch. Histol. Jap.*, 24:293–302.

Lieberman, A. R., and Webster, K. E. (1972): Presynaptic dendrites and a distinctive class of synaptic vesicle. *Brain Res.*, 42:196–200.

Lieberman, A. R. (1973): Neurons with presynaptic perikaria and presynaptic dendrites in the lateral geniculate nucleus. *Brain Res.*, 59:35–59.

Morest, D. K. (1971): Dendrodendritic synapses of cells that have axons: The fine structure of the Golgi type II cell in the medial geniculate body of the cat. *Z. Anat. Entwicklungsgesch.*, 133:216–246.

Peters, A. (1968): The morphology of axons of the central nervous system. In: *The Structure and Function of Nervous Tissue*, edited by G. F. Bourne. Academic Press, New York.

Peters, A., Palay, S. L., and Webster, H. F. (1970): *The Fine Structure of the Nervous System.* Harper, New York.

Peute, J. (1971): Somato-dendritic synapses in the paraventricular organ of two anuran species. *Z. Zellforsch. Mikrosk. Anat.*, 112:31–41.

Pinching, A. J. (1970): Synaptic connexions in the glomerular layer of the olfactory bulb. *J. Physiol.*, 210:14–15.

Price, J. L., and Powell, T. P. S. (1970): The synaptology of the granule cells of the olfactory bulb. *J. Cell Sci.*, 7:125–155.

Rall, W., Shepherd, G., Reese, T. S., and Brightman, M. W. (1966): Dendro-dendritic synaptic pathway for inhibition in the olfactory bulb. *Exp. Neurol.*, 14:44–56.

Ralston, H. J. (1971): Evidence for presynaptic dendrites and a proposal for their mechanism of action. *Nature*, 230:585–587.

Ramón y Cajal, S. (1909): Histologie du système nerveux. Malouin, Paris.

Ramón y Cajal, S. (1934): Les preuves objectives de l'unité anatomique des cellules nerveuses. *Trav. Lab. Invest. Biol.*, 29:1–137.

Ramon-Moliner, E. (1968): The morphology of dendrites. In: *Structure and Function of the Nervous Tissue*, edited by G. F. Bourne. Academic Press, New York.

Ramon-Moliner, E. (1973): Presynaptic perikaria in olfactory bulb of guinea pig. *Brain Res.*, 63:351–356.

Ramon-Moliner, E., and Ferrari, J. (1972): Electron microscopy of previously identified cells and processes within the central nervous system. *J. Neurocytol*, 1:85–100.

Scheibel, M. E., Davies, T. L., and Scheibel, A. B. (1972): An unusual axonless cell in the thalamus of the adult cat. *Exp. Neurol.*, 36:512–518.

Setalo, G., and Szekely, G. (1967): Somatodendritic synaptic junctions in the optic tectum of the frog. *Exp. Brain Res.*, 4:237–242.

Sloper, J. J. (1971): Dendro-dendritic synapses in the primate motor cortex. *Brain Res.*, 34:186–192.

Szentagothai, J. (1970): Glomerular synapses, complex synaptic arrangements, and their operational significance. In: *The Neurosciences: Second Study Program*, edited by F. O. Schmitt. Rockefeller Univ. Press, New York.

Wong, M. T. T. (1970): Somato-dendritic and dendro-dendritic synapses in the squirrel monkey lateral geniculate nucleus. *Brain Res.*, 20:135–139.

Zelena, J. (1970): Ribosome-like particles in myelinated axons of the rat. *Brain Res.*, 24:359–363.

Advances in Neurology, Vol. 12, edited by
G. W. Kreutzberg, Raven Press, New York
© 1975.

Postnatal Differentiation of "Presynaptic Dendrites" in the Lateral Geniculate Nucleus of the Rhesus Monkey

Jozsef Hámori,* Pedro Pasik, and Tauba Pasik

First Department of Anatomy, Semmelweis University Medical School, Budapest, Hungary
and Department of Neurology, Mount Sinai School of Medicine, New York, New York
10029

The recognition of dendritic profiles containing synaptic vesicles in the ventrobasal thalamus of the cat (Ralston and Herman, 1969) has been followed by increasingly frequent observations of these elements in other thalamic relay nuclei of various mammalian species (Famiglietti, 1970; Wong, 1970; Morest, 1971; Le Vay, 1971; Lieberman and Webster, 1972). The occurrence of these "presynaptic dendrites" is usually paralleled by the presence of "presynaptic perikarya" (Wong, 1970; Le Vay, 1971; Pasik, Pasik, Hámori, and Szentágothai, 1973; Lieberman, 1973). Serial reconstructions (Lieberman, 1973; Famiglietti and Peters, 1972) and experimental studies (Pasik et al., 1973) in the pars dorsalis of the lateral geniculate nucleus (LGN) suggest that such unorthodox elements belong to Golgi type II interneurons exhibiting both presynaptic and postsynaptic sites distributed along their membrane.

The position of presynaptic dendrites in the LGN neuronal circuitry has been clarified more recently. They contribute to the formation of a triadic unit (Famiglietti and Peters, 1972; Hámori, Pasik, Pasik, and Szentágothai, 1974), which is the most characteristic synaptic arrangement in this nucleus appearing both within the synaptic glomerulus as well as in the extraglomerular neuropil (Hámori et al., 1974). The "triad" comprises three elements: (1) a retinal terminal, which is presynaptic to (2) a principal cell dendrite (or soma), and to (3) an interneuron dendrite (or soma), the latter being in turn presynaptic to the same principal cell profile.

Despite a few opinions to the contrary (Le Vay, 1971; Scheibel, Davies, and Scheibel, 1972), there is ample evidence that LGN interneurons have axons (Guillery, 1966; Szentágothai, Hámori, and Tömböl, 1966; Famiglietti and Peters, 1972; Pasik et al., 1973). The possible role of these axons as well as that of the presynaptic dendrites has been discussed in a recent publication (Hámori et al., 1974). In order to gain more understanding of the relative contribution of these elements in the synaptic circuitry, an ultrastructural developmental approach was selected for the present study, both at the qualitative and quantitative levels.

MATERIALS AND METHODS

Seven normal monkeys (*Macaca mulatta*) were perfused under deep barbiturate narcosis through the abdominal aorta after ligating the two axillary arteries and the descending aorta distal to the introduction of the cannula. Drainage was secured by cutting the inferior vena cava. Details of composition and amount of the buffered 1% paraformaldehyde–1% glutaraldehyde perfusate were given elsewhere (Pasik et al., 1973; Hámori et al., 1974). The ages of the monkeys as per their known birth dates were: newborn, 1, 2 (two animals), 4, and 8 weeks. The seventh monkey was an adolescent of approximately 100 weeks as estimated by the dental formula. Blocks of LGN were dissected, washed in buffer, postfixed in buffered 2% osmium tetroxide, and embedded in Epon 812. Ultrathin sections were contrasted with uranyl acetate and lead citrate and examined with a Hitachi 12A electron microscope.

Quantitative assessment was made on randomly taken electron micrographs of optimally fixed neuropil obtained at a magnification of 10,000 and further enlarged to 25,000. Five samples from each age were analyzed covering a mean area of 200 μm^2 (SD = 3). An electronic graphic calculator (Numonics Corp., North Wales, Pa.) was used to compute the areas and to measure the total membrane length (surface) of identified interneuron dendrites and axons as well as the length of presynaptic and postsynaptic sites exhibited by these elements.

RESULTS

Identification of Interneuron Profiles

The criteria for recognition of perikarya, dendrites, and axons of interneurons in the monkey LGN have been described elsewhere (Famiglietti and Peters, 1972). Briefly, both perikaryon (Fig. 1) and proximal dendrites (Fig. 2) have a light matrix, small and dense mitochondria, a few scattered strands of rough endoplasmic reticulum, ribosomes, and, most characteristically, groups of small, pleomorphic synaptic vesicles, which at some locations are opposed to presynaptic membrane specializations. In the latter instance the postsynaptic element may belong to a principal cell dendrite or to another interneuron profile. Axon terminals can frequently be seen ending on interneuron somata or dendrites or both.

More distally, the dendrites become devoid of rough endoplasmic reticulum and ribosomes, and have only a few smooth endoplasmic cisterns and scattered synaptic vesicles (Fig. 3). In agreement with light microscopic

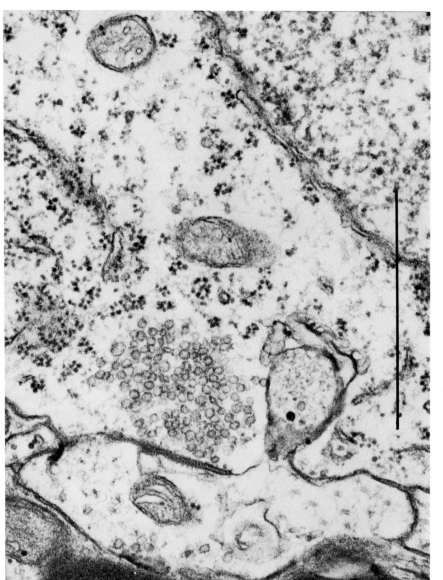

FIG. 1. Part of an interneuron soma that is presynaptic to a dendrite containing synaptic vesicles from 100-week-old monkey LGN (lateral geniculate nucleus). (Scale: 1μm.)

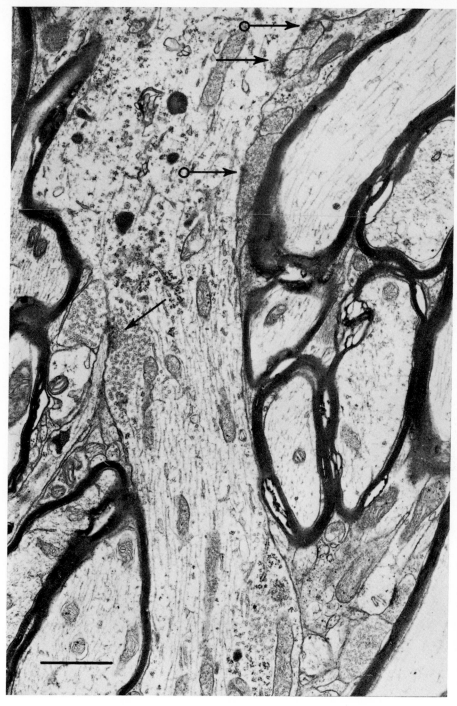

FIG. 2. Proximal part of an interneuron dendrite with presynaptic (arrows) and post-synaptic sites (ringed arrows) from 100-week-old monkey LGN. (Scale: 1 μm.)

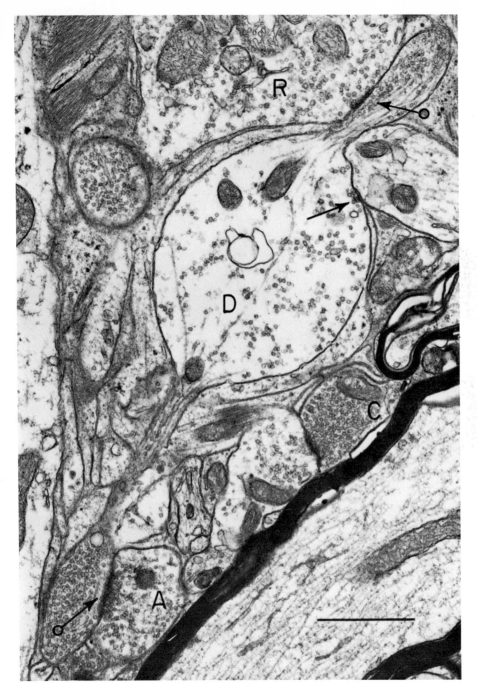

FIG. 3. Distal portion of an interneuron dendrite, D, with presynaptic (arrow) and post-synaptic (ringed arrow) sites from 100-week-old monkey LGN. Note that thin axon-like portions are exclusively postsynaptic. R, Retinal ending; A, interneuron axon; C, cortical terminal. (Scale: 1 μm.)

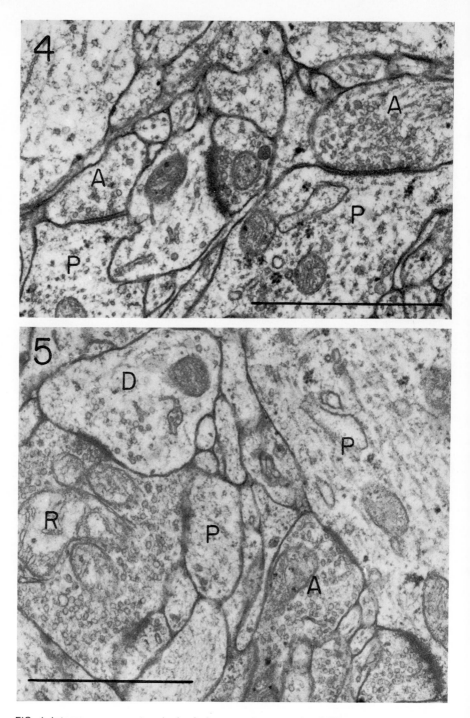

FIG. 4. Interneuron axon terminals, A, from newborn monkey LGN, presynaptic to principal cell dendrites, P. Note the long synaptic contact and poorly developed postsynaptic density. (Scale: 1 μm.)

FIG. 5. Interneuron axon terminal, A, from 1-week-old monkey LGN presynaptic to a principal cell dendrite, P. The retinal ending, R, is presynaptic to both principal cell dendrite, P, and interneuron dendrite, D. (Scale: 1 μm.)

observations of Golgi-impregnated interneurons (Pasik et al., 1973), the dendrites can show varicosities and thinner portions. The latter are usually packed with synaptic vesicles but are always in a postsynaptic position. As depicted in Fig. 3 the dendrite shows its additional presynaptic character in the enlarged portion, which can be either a varicosity or a dendritic appendage.

The axon profiles are more difficult to identify particularly in their distal endings (Hámori et al., 1974). However, they can be recognized because they have the same type of small, pleomorphic vesicles as present in the dendrites and/or somata of interneurons, although the vesicle population density is higher and the distribution is more uniform. The axon profiles are less than 1 μm in size and are exclusively presynaptic. The synaptic membrane specialization is always considerably longer than that of the presynaptic dendrite, as can be seen by comparing Fig. 3 with Figs. 4 and 5. Interneuron axons can be distinguished from other small axonic endings, such as those of cortical origin, because the latter contain a homogeneous and very dense population of small round vesicles (Hámori et al., 1974).

Developmental Aspects

Qualitative Observations

The synaptic glomeruli (Szentágothai, 1963) are already present in the LGN of the newborn monkey (Fig. 6). The retinal afferent is surrounded by both principal cell and interneuron dendrites with which it establishes synaptic contacts. Some of these synapses are mature at this stage. Although the interneuron dendrites contain synaptic vesicles, they exhibit only postsynaptic ties (Fig. 7). Presynaptic membrane specializations and contacts are conspicuously absent. Conversely, numerous axon terminals, presumably belonging to interneurons, are seen making the characteristic long synaptic contact with both principal cell dendrites (Figs. 4 and 5) and presynaptic dendrites. These general characteristics are maintained in the LGN of the 1-week-old monkey except that interneuron profiles, both dendritic and axonic, appear to be more abundant.

The first observed presynaptic dendritic specializations are seen in the 2-week-old specimen (Fig. 8). Therefore the first triadic units are formed at this age (Fig. 9) and are similar to those found in the fully mature monkey (Fig. 10). The frequency of occurrence of presynaptic dendrites increases in the LGN of older monkeys, whereas the number of axonal profiles and concomitant axonal presynaptic sites decreases with age.

Quantitative Measurements

Table 1 gives some of the results of the quantitative analysis of electron micrographic data in terms of mean percentage of the total membrane length

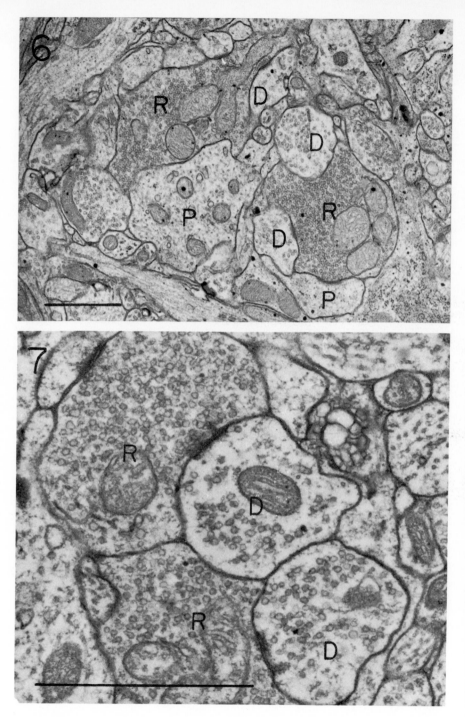

FIG. 6. Low-power electron micrograph of developing synaptic glomerulus from the new-born monkey LGN. The retinal terminals, R, are surrounded by principal cell dendrites, P, and also by interneuron dendritic profiles, D, containing synaptic vesicles and having only postsynaptic sites. (Scale: 1 μm.)

FIG. 7. High-power electron micrograph to show detail of the developing glomerulus from the newborn monkey LGN. The retinal terminals, R, are presynaptic to two interneuron dendrites, D, containing synaptic vesicles but exhibiting only postsynaptic specializations. (Scale: 1 μm.)

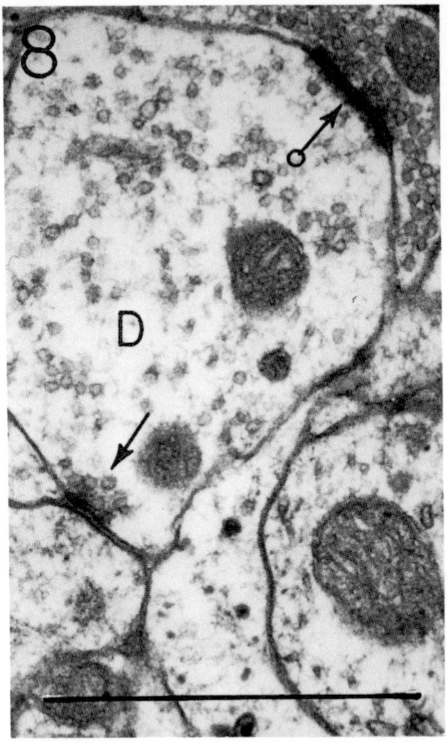

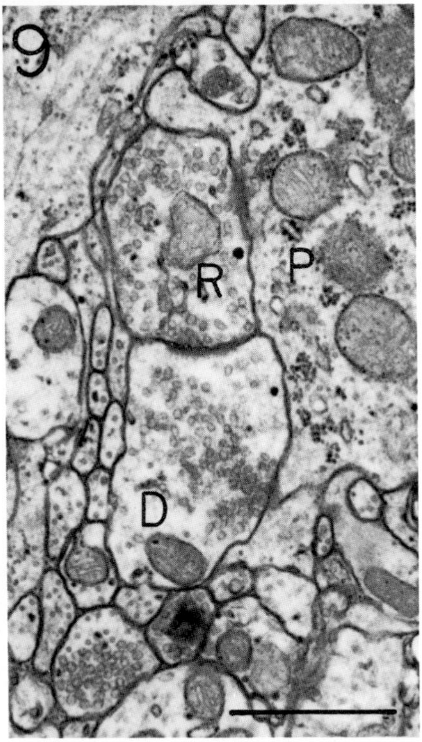

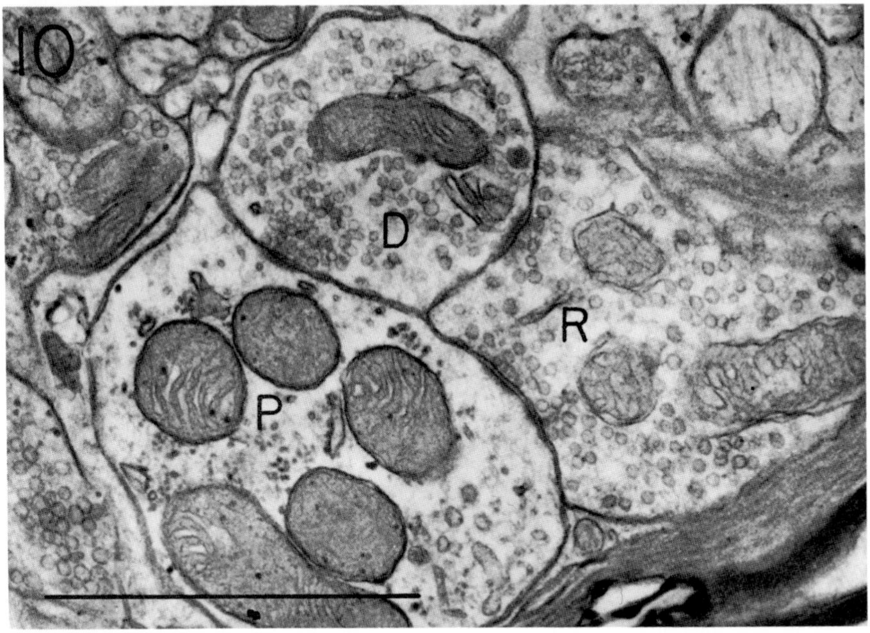

FIG. 8. Presynaptic dendrite, D, from a 2-week-old monkey LGN showing both presynaptic (arrow) and postsynaptic (ringed arrow) sites. (Scale: 1 μm.)

FIG. 9. Maturing synaptic triad from 2-week-old monkey LGN. Retinal terminal, R, principal cell dendrite, P, interneuron presynaptic dendrite, D. (Scale: 1 μm.)

FIG. 10. Synaptic triad from the 100-week-old monkey LGN. The retinal terminal, R, is presynaptic to principal cell dendrite, P, and to interneuron dendrite, D, the latter being presynaptic to the same principal cell profile. (Scale: 1 μm.)

TABLE 1. *Mean percentage of interneuron membranes exhibiting presynaptic and post-synaptic sites in 200 μm² of LGN neuropil (n = 5)*

Type of contact[a]	Age (weeks)					
	0	1	2	4	8	100
Presynaptic	2.71 [0.72]	2.71 [0.52]	2.54 [0.87]	2.28 [0.42]	2.64 [0.73]	2.63 [0.40]
Postsynaptic	1.86 [0.94]	2.73 [0.64]	3.06 [0.73]	2.40 [0.87]	3.52 [1.69]	2.60 [0.72]

[a] Presynaptic data: Percentage of dendritic plus axonal surfaces. Postsynaptic data: Percentage of dendritic surfaces only. Numbers in brackets are standard deviations.

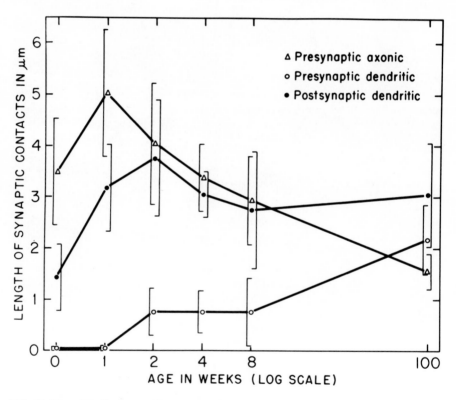

FIG. 11. Mean length of synaptic contacts of interneuron processes present in 200 μm² of LGN neuropil as a function of postnatal age. Vertical segments represent standard deviations. Note that after an initial increase, the axonal presynaptic sites (triangles) decrease progressively with age, whereas the changes in dendritic presynaptic sites (open circles) are opposite in direction attaining a higher value at maturity. Means are significantly different except at 100 weeks of age. Postsynaptic dendritic sites (solid circles) reach a peak at 2 weeks and stabilize at a lower value from the 8-week stage on.

(surface) of interneuron dendrites and axons exhibiting presynaptic specializations, as well as the mean percentage of dendritic surface showing
postsynaptic sites. It is apparent that presynaptic membranes occupy about
2.6% of the total surface of interneuron processes and that this proportion
is fairly similar in the newborn and the fully mature monkey. The relative
contribution of presynaptic axonal and dendritic sites, however, changes
drastically during development. Figure 11 is a semilogarithmic plot of the
mean length and standard deviation of synaptic membranes belonging to
interneuron profiles present in 200 μm^2 of neuropil as a function of postnatal
age. It is clear that after an initial increase to a peak of 5 μm at 1 week, the
length of axonal sites diminishes steadily, and in the fully mature monkey
is only 1.6 μm, representing only a 45% of the value at birth. In contrast,
the presynaptic dendritic sites are practically absent in the newborn and
in the 1-week-old animal. They attain a meaningful length at 2 weeks, and
remain fairly stable at least until 8 weeks of age. Thereafter the length of
presynaptic dendritic specializations increases to reach mean values higher
than those of axonal sites in the mature specimen. The difference, however,
is not significant.

The postsynaptic dendritic sites are well developed at birth. They attain a
peak mean length of close to 4 μm at 2 weeks, and decline thereafter,
stabilizing at about 3 μm after 8 weeks of age (Fig. 11). The percentage of
interneuron dendrites surface occupied by postsynaptic sites does not vary
significantly during development (Table 1).

DISCUSSION

The present findings indicate that dendrites of interneurons in the LGN
of monkeys are not fully mature at birth. Although the dendritic arborization
is present, and the appendages or varicosities contain synaptic vesicles,
the profiles are exclusively postsynaptic until the end of the second postnatal
week. Only at this time do the dendrites also become presynaptic, adopting
the characteristic triadic arrangement that is typical of the mature animal
(Hámori et al., 1974). These developmental features may be an expression
of inherent properties of these neurons, or they may be dependent on postnatal experiences. Visual deprivation studies are needed to answer this
question.

The observation that the differentiation and increase of dendritic/pre-
synaptic sites occur simultaneously with the reduction in the amount of
axonal presynaptic specializations may signify that some of the functions of
the latter processes are taken over by the dendrites. This suggestion is
supported by the relative constancy of the percentage of interneuron processes surface occupied by presynaptic thickenings from birth to maturity.
It should be noted, however, that the primary role of presynaptic dendrites
is most probably different from that of the axon: (1) Their sphere of influence

is considerably larger (Hámori et al., 1974); and (2) they participate in the triadic units, whereas the axon makes individual contacts on principal cell somata, dendrites, and even axon hillocks (Famiglietti and Peters, 1972). Speculation as to the possible functional significance of this topographic separation between interneuron dendrites and axons was advanced by Hámori et al. (1974). The proposed model suggested three possible interneuron actions, i.e., local inhibition limited to the triadic arrangement, inhibition at a short distance through an axonal mechanism, and inhibition at a long distance by way of the presynaptic dendrites. The triadic unit has been interpreted as a device for the inhibitory phasing of the principal cell discharge (Andersen and Eccles, 1962) resulting from the release of the interneuron inhibitory transmitter by excitation of this cell through the same retinal afferent responsible for the initial tonic activity of the principal cell. The present results would predict that such phasing occurs only after the second postnatal week. This hypothesis awaits electrophysiologic testing. It is noteworthy that infant monkeys trained from the first day of life to discriminate white from black, horizontal from vertical stripes, and a triangle from a circle attained a criterion level of performance at 10, 21, and 25 days, respectively (Zimmermann, 1961). It is tempting to conclude that presynaptic dendritic activity and phasing of neuronal discharges may not be indispensable for brightness, or perhaps total luminous flux discrimination, but could be required for more complex types of visually guided behavior.

SUMMARY

The most characteristic synaptic arrangement in the LGN is the triadic unit, in which a retinal terminal is presynaptic to a principal cell (P cell) and to a Golgi interneuron (I cell) dendrite, which contains synaptic vesicles and is in turn presynaptic to the same P-cell element. The ontogenetic differentiation of these "presynaptic dendrites" was studied in monkey LGN by standard and quantitative electron microscopy. The dendrites and axonal arborization of I cells are well developed in the newborn monkey. Scattered synaptic vesicles are present in the dendrites, but these profiles exhibit only postsynaptic sites. The dendrodendritic synapse of the triadic arrangement is missing, although contacts between P-cell and I-cell dendrites can be observed. Conversely, the I-cell axons in the newborn establish numerous synapses with dendrites and perikarya of P cells. At about 2 weeks of age, presynaptic sites appear in the I-cell dendrites, resulting in the formation of synaptic triads. Parallel to the development of "axonal" properties in the dendrites, the number of true I-cell axonal profiles decreases sharply. These transformations become progressively more frequent with age, and beyond 8 weeks the LGN ultraarchitectonics approaches that of the mature animal. The percentage of the surface of interneuron processes occupied by presynaptic sites is similar at all developmental stages at about the 2.6% level. The relative contribution of presynaptic dendrites and of axons changes, however, so that the actual length of contacts in the mature monkey is only one-half that of the newborn for the axonal sites, and over 50 times longer for the dendritic sites. The correlation of these findings with electrophysiologic and behavioral references suggests that some but not all axonal functions may be taken over by the dendrites, that the possible inhibitory phasing of P-cell discharge would appear only after the second postnatal week, and that the triadic arrangement may not be indispensable for brightness or total luminous flux discrimination but could be required for more complex forms of visually guided behavior.

ACKNOWLEDGMENT

This work was supported by USPHS Grant MH-02261 from the National Institute of Mental Health.

REFERENCES

Andersen, P., and Eccles, J. C. (1962): Inhibitory phasing of neuronal discharge. *Nature,* 196:645–647.

Famiglietti, E. V., Jr., and Peters, A. (1972): The synaptic glomerulus and the intrinsic neuron in the dorsal lateral geniculate nucleus of the cat. *J. Comp. Neurol.,* 144:285–334.

Famiglietti, E. V., Jr. (1970): Dendro-dendritic synapses in the lateral geniculate nucleus of the cat. *Brain Res.,* 20:181–191.

Guillery, R. W. (1966): A study of Golgi preparations from the dorsal lateral geniculate nucleus of the adult cat. *J. Comp. Neurol.,* 128:21–50.

Hámori, J., Pasik, T., Pasik, P., and Szentágothai, J. (1974): "Triadic" synaptic arrangements and their possible significance in the lateral geniculate nucleus of the monkey. *Brain Res.,* 80:379–393.

Le Vay, S. (1971): On the neurons and synapses of the lateral geniculate nucleus of the monkey, and the effects of eye enucleation. *Z. Zellforsch.,* 113:396–419.

Lieberman, A. R., and Webster, K. E. (1972): Presynaptic dendrites and a distinctive class of synaptic vesicle in the rat dorsal lateral geniculate nucleus. *Brain Res.,* 42:196–200.

Lieberman, A. R. (1973): Neurons with presynaptic perikarya and presynaptic dendrites in the rat lateral geniculate nucleus. *Brain Res.,* 59:35–59.

Morest, D. K. (1971): Dendrodendritic synapses of cells that have axons: The fine structure of the Golgi type II cell in the medial geniculate body of the cat. *Z. Anat. Entwicklungsgesch.,* 133:216–246.

Pasik, P., Pasik, T., Hámori, J., and Szentágothai, J. (1973): Golgi type II interneurons in the neuronal circuit of the monkey lateral geniculate nucleus. *Exp. Brain Res.,* 17:18–34.

Ralston, H. J., and Herman, M. D. (1969): The fine structure of neurons and synapses in the ventrobasal thalamus of the cat. *Brain Res.,* 14:77–97.

Scheibel, M. E., Davies, T. L., and Scheibel, A. B. (1972): An unusual axonless cell in the thalamus of the adult cat. *Exp. Neurol.,* 36:512–518.

Szentágothai, J. (1963): The structure of the synapse in the lateral geniculate body. *Acta Anat.,* 55:166–185.

Szentágothai, J., Hámori, J., and Tömböl, T. (1966): Degeneration and electron microscope analysis of the synaptic glomeruli in the lateral geniculate body. *Exp. Brain Res.,* 2:283–301.

Wong, M. T. T. (1970): Somato-dendritic and dendrodendritic synapses in the squirrel monkey lateral geniculate nucleus. *Brain Res.,* 20:135–139.

Zimmermann, R. R. (1961): Analysis of discrimination learning capacities in the infant rhesus monkey. *J. Comp. Physiol. Psychol.,* 54:1–10.

Advances in Neurology, Vol. 12, edited by
G. W. Kreutzberg, Raven Press, New York
© 1975.

Neuronal Growth Cone Relationships and Their Role in Synaptogenesis in the Mammalian Central Nervous System

G. D. Pappas, G. Q. Fox, E. B. Masurovsky, E. R. Peterson, and S. M. Crain

Department of Neuroscience and the Rose F. Kennedy Center for Research in Mental Retardation and Human Development, Albert Einstein College of Medicine, Bronx, New York 10461

Several recent studies have suggested that synaptic remodeling may occur in the adult mammalian central nervous system (CNS) under various experimental conditions (e.g., Raisman and Field, 1973; Nakamura, Mizuno, Konishi, and Soto, 1974; see also Bernstein, *this volume*). It is not clear from those studies whether the formation of new synapses occurs first on the growth cones of the new neuritic outgrowths.

In the development and differentiation of the fetal rat spinal cord (Vaughn and Grieshaber, 1973; Vaughn, Henrikson, and Grieshaber, 1974) as well as of the chick embryo (Skoff and Hamburger, 1974) synaptic formation is preceded by identifiable growth cones. Electron-microscopic examination of early postnatal kitten (2 to 17 days) medullary raphe nuclei (n. pallidus, n. obscurus, and n. magnus) has revealed the presence of both dendritic and axonal growth cones (Fox, Pappas, and Purpura, 1975*a,b*). Because these neurons have well-established dendritic trees at birth, the formation of dendritic growth cones as primary dendrites from the medium-sized neurons of these nuclei is interpreted as an unusual secondary growth process (Fox et al., 1975*a,b*). A substantial population of axosomatic and axodendritic synapses with the usual fine structural features can be found in the newborn kitten. Synapses are present on large dendrites as well as on spines, and axosomatic synapses occur on the cell bodies and sometimes on somatic spines. The fine structural characteristics are of "mature" tissue. In contrast, the dendritic growth cones possess a pleomorphic vesicle population. These vesicles are partially derived from tubular endoplasmic reticulum (ER) present at first in the cell body and then in the growth cone and dendritic shaft (Fig. 1). Axonal growth cones have also been observed. In the surrounding well-developed neuropil we have not found presynaptic processes that can be identified as dendritic. In addition, these newly formed processes which we designate as "axonal" are not found to originate directly from cell bodies. Many of these axons are found to be presynaptic to den-

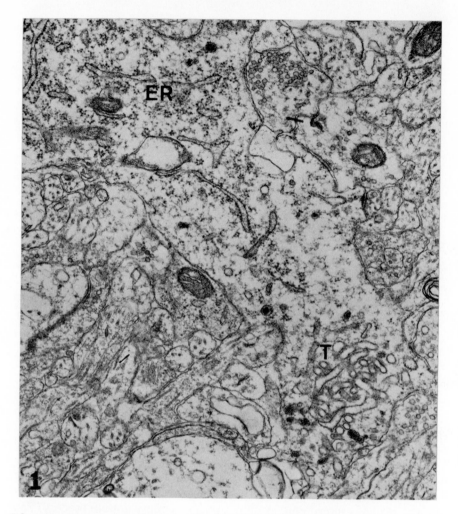

FIG. 1. Electron micrograph of a section from the medullary raphe nucleus (n. pallidus) of a 4-day-old kitten. A dendritic process, rich in elements of the ribosome-studded endoplasmic reticulum, ER, contains at its growth-tip smooth-surfaced tubular elements, T. Many pleomorphic vesicles, some with dense contents, can be seen in the process as well as at the tip. (×26,000.)

drites ("mature or newly formed") as well as to neuronal cell bodies (Fig. 2). Their vesicle populations are also pleomorphic, many having a dense core, and some of the large vesicles having an excentric dense core. Whereas the dendritic growth cones are clearly seen to be direct outgrowths from the neuron cell body, the origin of the axonal growth cones has not been traced. None of the direct outgrowths from the cell body has been observed to be a presynaptic process. It is suggested, therefore, that axonal growth cones are derived from sprouting or branching of existing axons.

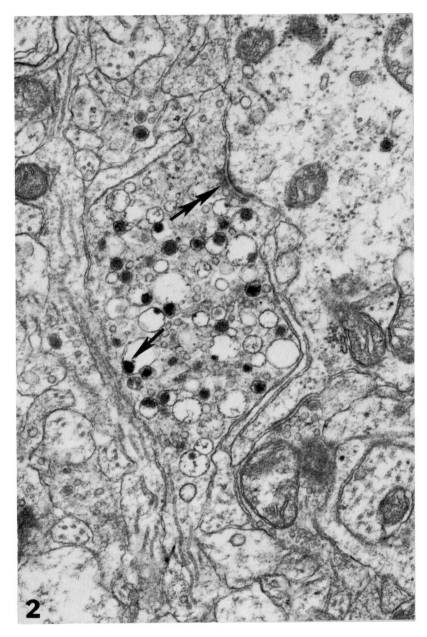

FIG. 2. Electron micrograph of a section from the medullary raphe nucleus (n. pallidus) of a 4-day-old kitten. An axonal growth cone is in synaptic contact with a neuronal soma (*double arrow*). Axonal growth cones are characterized as having various-sized vesicles, many of which have a dense core. The dense core is excentric in the larger ones (e.g., *arrow*). (×35,000.)

Nerve tissue culture preparations have played an important role in our ongoing studies of synaptogenesis in relation to function. In our earlier work with newborn mouse cerebral neocortex, synaptic junctions were rarely found at explanation (Pappas, 1966; see also Model, Bornstein, Crain, and Pappas, 1971). After several days in culture, complex bioelectric activities were recorded suggesting development of functional synaptic networks (Crain and Bornstein, 1964). Electron-microscopic examination of these older explants showed an abundance of axodendritic and some axosomatic synapses. These electron-micrographic studies of cerebral cultures (Pappas, 1966; see also Crain, Raine, and Bornstein, 1975b) and similar analyses of fetal rat spinal cord explants (Bunge, Bunge, and Peterson, 1967) have established that the onset of complex bioelectric activities (Crain and Bornstein, 1964; Crain and Peterson, 1967) is correlated with the formation of clear-cut synaptic junctions in vitro (see Crain, 1974a, 1975). The morphologic characteristics of neuritic outgrowth has been studied in a number of embryonic or neonatal nerve tissues (cf. Tennyson, 1970; Yamada et al., 1971; Bunge, 1973; Vaughn and Grieshaber, 1973). In embryonic chick spinal cord in situ, Skoff and Hamburger (1974) have suggested that neuritic outgrowths identified by growth cones are responsible for the formation and the onset of synaptogenesis. Early neuritic outgrowth and synapse formation in cultures of 13- to 14-day fetal mouse spinal cord with attached dorsal root ganglia are now under study in our laboratory (e.g., Peterson, Masurovsky, and Crain, 1974). Emphasis is being placed on the patterns of synapse distribution and other ultrastructural features in dorsal (and contiguous central) regions of the spinal cord.

In these studies cross sections (0.5 to 1 mm thick) of fetal mouse spinal cord with meningeal covering and attached dorsal root ganglia were explanted onto collagen-coated coverslips with a drop of nutrient fluid (Peterson, Crain, and Murray, 1965; Peterson and Crain, 1972; Masurovsky and Peterson, 1973). The culture preparations were incorporated into a Maximow slide assembly and incubated at 34.5°C. Within 24 hr, neuropil begins to form over the surface of the explant, and a fine neuritic outgrowth is observed from boundaries of the spinal cord and dorsal root ganglia. It is not possible, however, to distinguish or resolve by light microscopy growth cone processes within the relatively thick, multilayered regions of the spinal cord in these cultures. Therefore, representative specimens were selected and fixed for electron microscopy at 1, 2, and 3 days in vitro (as well as at later intervals) using as primary fixatives either buffered glutaraldehyde alone (Model et al., 1971; Pappas, Peterson, Masurovsky, and Crain, 1971) or a combination of glutaraldehyde with paraformaldehyde, acrolein, and dimethyl sulfoxide (DMSO) similar to that of Skoff and Hamburger (1974). Subsequent to the usual postfixation in buffered OsO_4 and embedding in Epon 812, thin sections were stained with 50% ethanolic uranyl acetate and lead citrate for examination in a Philips 300 electron microscope.

Some of the cultures were tested with microelectrodes shortly before fixation to evaluate the degree to which functional synaptic network activity could be elicited with electric stimuli and pharmacologic agents (for details of electrophysiologic techniques, see Crain, 1973).

The distal regions of the newly formed processes display ultrastructural features typical of growth cones. In cultures only 24 hr old, morphologic specializations resembling synaptic contacts can be seen, although they are rare. By two days *in vitro* some pre- and postsynaptic entities can be identified. Neuritic processes containing bulbous growth cones can be found to be both pre- and postsynaptic elements. It is not possible, however, to make a clear-cut distinction in these early cultures between axonal and dendritic growth cones. In the profiles observed in thin sections most of the neuritic processes from which growth cones emerge do not contain the fine structural characteristics associated with mature dendrites, i.e., ribosomes (scattered or in clusters), ribosome-studded ER and Golgi elements. Ideally, the differentiation of axonal and dendritic growth cones should be based primarily on precise location within the neuraxis or identifiable interconnections or both (cf. Tennyson, 1970; Vaughn and Grieshaber, 1973), as well as serial section analysis of growth cone origin (Skoff and Hamburger, 1974). In the culture material, however, exact location, identifiable interconnections, or the accurate tracing of all cells of the origin of their process has not yet been feasible. Neuritic processes identified as having growth cones and being presynaptic are common. In Fig. 3, a characteristic bulbous ending, with a fine flocculent material and few, if any, organelles, can be seen to have clusters of vesicles forming presynaptic contacts with processes which contain microtubules, elements of the smooth tubular ER, and a more dense-appearing cytoplasm. The neuritic shafts, a short distance before the bulbous growth cone terminals, also form presynaptic relationships with other processes (Fig. 4). In the latter cases, however, the cytoplasmic characteristics of both the pre- and postsynaptic processes are essentially identical (i.e., the presynaptic region also contains microtubules, mitochondria, and tubular ER). Some growth cones occur as presynaptic elements in junctions with cell bodies (Fig. 5), although these are not as common as those formed with neurites. Growth cones may also be presynaptic to filopodia-like structures (Figs. 6 and 7), as on motor neuron dendrites *in situ* (Vaughn et al., 1974).

In addition to growth cones themselves forming synaptic contact with cell bodies, possible transitional "bouton-like" endings containing organelles (Fig. 8) and having a more dense cytoplasm form synaptic contact with both a neuritic process and a cell body. Also, neuritic shafts form synapses on neuronal cell bodies, as well as on adjacent neuritic processes (Fig. 9). Some profiles of presynaptic processes cannot readily be classified as originating from growth cones (see A, B, Fig. 10). Large irregular bulbous processes with few organelles can sometimes be found to be presynaptic (Fig. 11) or postsynaptic (e.g., to processes A and B, Fig. 10).

The appearance of growth cones as a postsynaptic element can be slightly

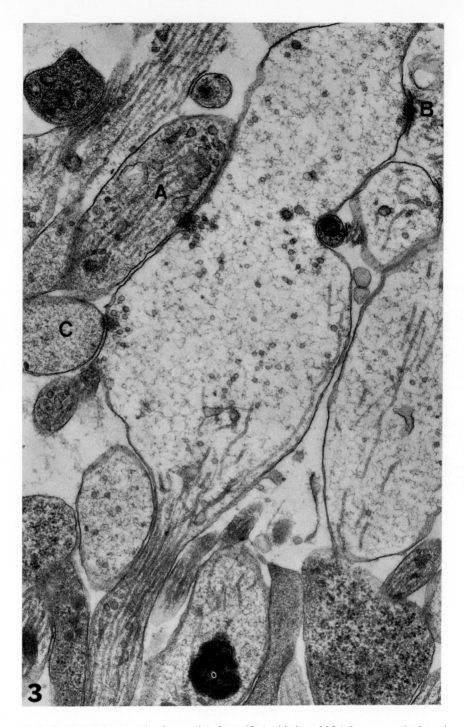

FIG. 3. Electron micrograph of a section from 13- to 14-day-old fetal mouse spinal cord 2 days *in vitro*. A characteristic pleomorphic bulbous growth cone ending with fine flocculent material containing few organelles forms presynaptic contacts with two types of processes. One type contains microtubules, as well as other organelles (A and B), whereas the other (C) has a fine fibrillar appearance. Note that the shaft of the growth cone is filled with microtubules and some elements of the smooth tubular ER. (×32,000.)

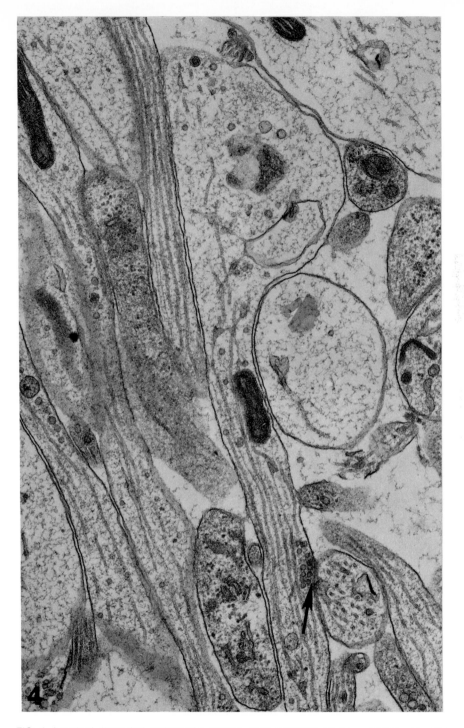

FIG. 4. A typical distended ending of a growth cone containing a few vesicles, vacuoles, and inclusions. The shaft contains microtubules, tubular ER and a mitochondrion. The shaft is presynaptic to another neurite (*arrow*). Taken from a 2-day-old culture. (×32,000.)

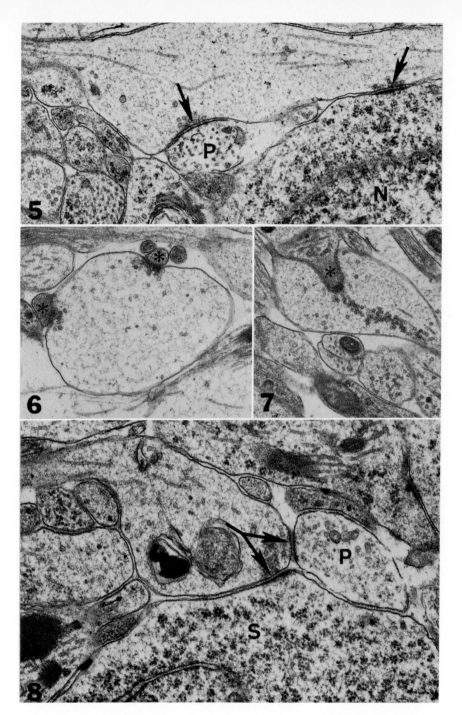

FIG. 5. A portion of a growth cone is found to be presynaptic (*arrows*) to a cell body and to a neuritic process, P. A small portion of the nucleus, N, of the cell can be seen (2 days *in vitro*). (×25,000.)

FIG. 6. A cross section of a growth cone is shown to be presynaptic to two filopodia-like processes (*asterisks*) (2 days *in vitro*). (×20,500.)

FIG. 7. An oblique section through a filopodia-like process (*asterisk*). A portion of a growth cone as a presynaptic element partially envelops this process (2 days *in vitro*). (×20,500.)

FIG. 8. A bouton-like ending is forming synaptic contact (*arrows*) with a soma, S, as well as a neuritic process, P (2 days *in vitro*). (×25,500.)

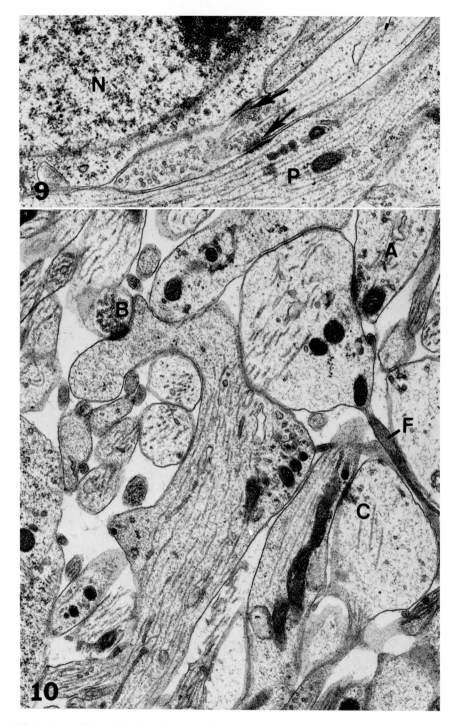

FIG. 9. A neuritic shaft is forming synaptic contact (*arrows*) with a cell body and another process, P. N, nucleus (2 days *in vitro*). (×25,500.)

FIG. 10. Two different processes (A and B) are presynaptic to growth cones. One growth cone can be seen to have a filopodial extension (F). A growth cone (C) similar to that which has the filopodial extension appears to be presynaptic (2 days *in vitro*). (×20,500.)

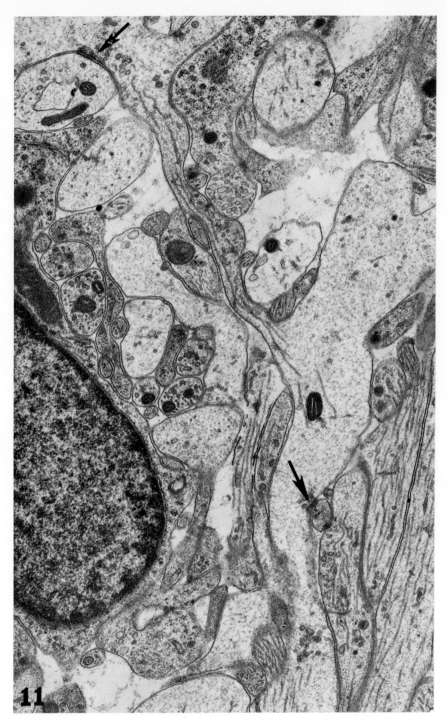

FIG. 11. Section of portion of a large very irregular process which forms presynaptic contacts (*arrows*) with two smaller processes. In the more attenuated portions of this varicose process microtubules and vesicles can be found (2 days *in vitro*). (×20,500.)

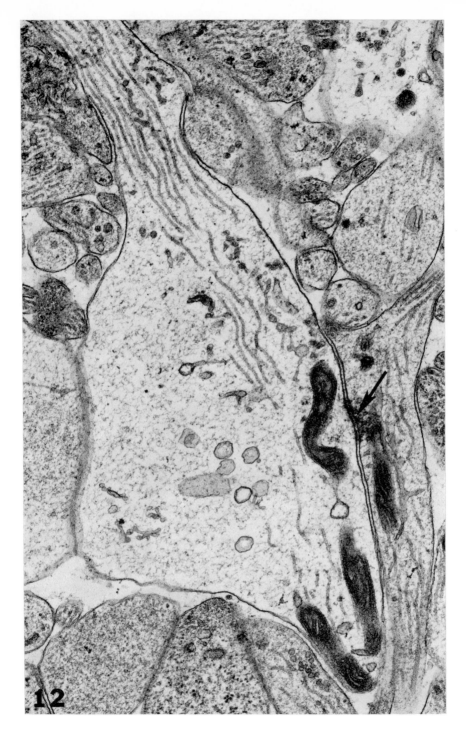

FIG. 12. A large bulbous process containing some microtubules, mitochondria, vesicles, and a few elements of the tubular ER. This growth cone forms a postsynaptic relationship with another process (*arrow*). Most of the previous growth cone processes (e.g., Figs. 3 to 9 and C in Fig. 10) are shown to be presynaptic (2 days *in vitro*). (×32,000.)

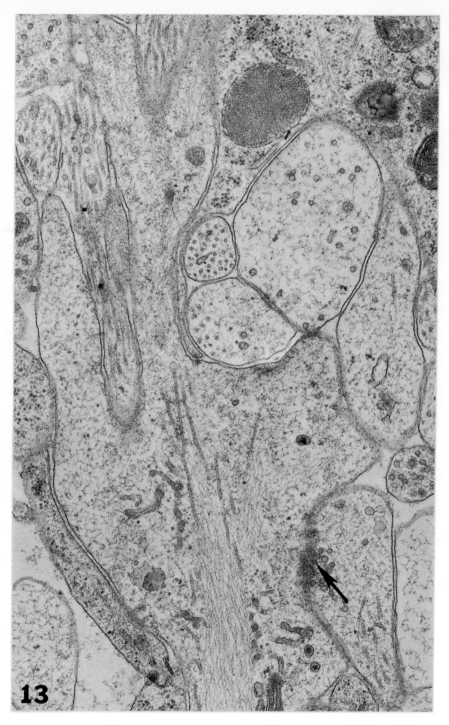

FIG. 13. A portion of a pleomorphic process containing fine fibrils, some microtubules, elements of the tubular ER and a few dense core vesicles is found to be the postsynaptic element to a process containing similar organelles (*arrow*) (2 days *in vitro*). (×32,000.)

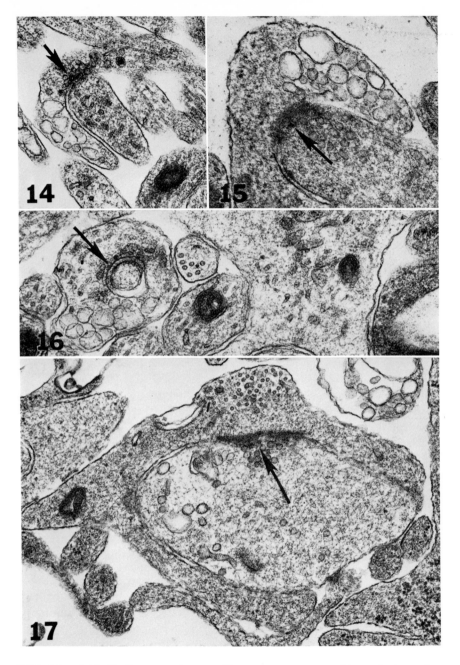

FIGS. 14 and 15. Similar appearing neuritic processes, presumably newly formed, are found to be presynaptic in Fig. 14 (*arrow*) and postsynaptic in Fig. 15 (*arrow*). Figure 14, 3 days *in vitro*. (×40,500.) Figure 15, 2 days *in vitro*. (×51,500.)

FIGS. 16 and 17. "Wrap-around" neuritic processes can be found to be presynaptic (Fig. 16, *arrow*) and postsynaptic (Fig. 17, *arrow*). Figure 16, 3 days *in vitro*. (×51,500.) Figure 17, 2 days *in vitro*. (×38,500.)

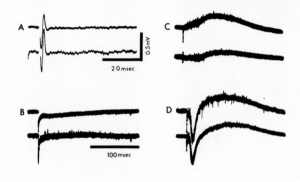

18

FIG. 18. Onset of complex synaptic network functions in fetal mouse spinal cord explants (13 to 14 days *in utero;* 1 to 3 days *in vitro*). (A) Simple early-latency spike potentials evoked in two sites of cord explant (at 1 day *in vitro*) by single stimulus applied to third site. No signs of complex discharges were detected following these spikes, both in balanced salt solution (BSS) and after addition of pharmacologic agents (see below). (B) Long-lasting repetitive spike barrages and small-amplitude slow-wave responses elicited in two sites of cord explant at 2 days *in vitro,* but only after introduction of bicuculline (10^{-5} M) and caffeine (10^{-3} M); see text. Note change in time calibration; afterdischarges lasted more than 1 to 2 sec. (C) Similar long-lasting repetitive spike barrages, but accompanied by much larger amplitude negative slow-wave responses, evoked in two sites of another cord explant at 2 days *in vitro* (tissue obtained from slightly more mature fetus than in B). These complex discharges were observed only after introduction of strychnine (10^{-5} M) and caffeine (10^{-5} M). (D) Still more elaborate diphasic slow-wave potentials and spike barrages evoked in two sites in cord explant at 3 days *in vitro* after addition of strychnine (10^{-5} M). Smaller-amplitude slow-wave potentials and shorter spike barrages (as in C) could also be elicited in this explant in BSS (prior to strychnine). These response patterns already include many of the basic features characteristic of complex synaptic network discharges of cord explants observed during the following weeks *in vitro.* (*Note:* Time and amplitude calibrations apply to all succeeding records, *until otherwise noted;* upward deflection indicates negativity at active recording electrode, and onset of stimuli is indicated by first sharp pulse or break in base line of each sweep.) Recordings were made with saline-filled pipettes with 3- to 5-μm tips and stimuli were applied with similar pipettes with 10-μm tips. (From Crain et al., 1975a.)

different from presynaptic ones in that there may be more organelles present (i.e., mitochondria, tubular ER, vacuoles, fibrillae, and some microtubules), but there are no readily identifiable ribosomes (Figs. 12 and 13). Similar to the neuritic outgrowths described by Skoff and Hamburger (1974) in embryonic chick spinal cord *in situ,* the neuritic outgrowths in our mouse cord explants show extremely irregular varicosities, with large bulbous inflated areas, and they are followed by very attenuated regions. Attenuated or narrowed areas are often characterized by prominent arrays of microtubules.

The neuritic outgrowths which form presynaptic contacts with other processes can be found at times to wrap around smaller processes (Figs. 14 and 16). Conversely, processes that are found to be wrapped around other neurites can be postsynaptic (Figs. 15 and 17).

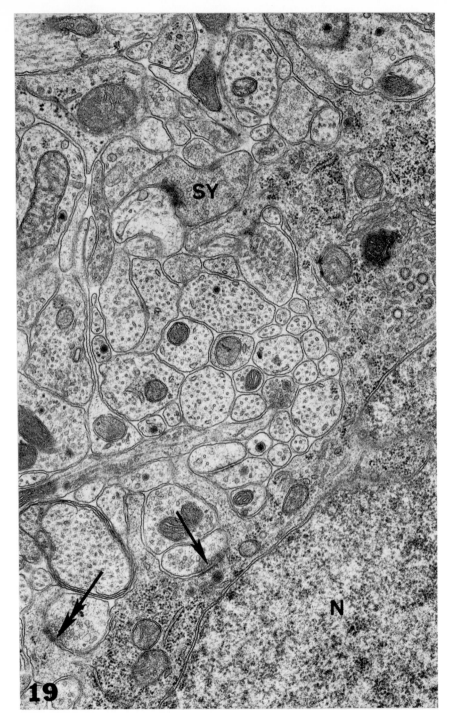

FIG. 19. Section of a 43-day-old culture of 13- to 14-day mouse fetal spinal cord. The neuron and surrounding compact neuropil appear "mature." Synapses (SY) can be found in the neuropil, as well as on the soma (*arrow*) and at a somatic spine (*double arrow*). N, nucleus. (×27,000.)

Skoff and Hamburger (1974) attempt to distinguish axonal and dendritic growth cones by their shape and their cytoplasmic components. In their summation analysis, however, they remark that *dendritic* growth cones are "specified" as *post*-synaptic elements. Would it follow, then, that *axonal* growth cones should be thought of or "specified" as *pre*-synaptic elements? In our embryonic spinal cord cultures it has not been possible to rigorously apply suggested morphologic criteria for unambiguously distinguishing axonal processes from dendritic ones (*vide supra*). Hence, we have morphologically similar neuritic shafts and growth cones varying only in that some are presynaptic and others are postsynaptic.

This chapter is concerned primarily with explants of 13- to 14-day fetal mouse spinal cord during the developmental period corresponding with the inception of synaptogenesis. The electron microscopy showing clear-cut synaptic profiles at 2 days *in vitro*, described previously, correlates with the observed onset of characteristic evoked slow-wave potentials and repetitive spike-barrages indicative of synaptic network activity in the same 2-day cord explants (Fig. 18 B, C versus A; Crain et al., 1975a). The earlier onset of complex network discharges in these 13- to 14-day fetal *mouse* spinal cord explants as compared to our previous studies of fetal *rat* cord explants (Crain and Peterson, 1967) may be related, in part, to species differences, but it may also be caused by application of more effective pharmacologic agents in the mouse cord experiments (e.g., caffeine and bicuculline; see Crain and Bornstein, 1974; Crain, 1974b, 1975). Formation of functional synaptic networks by 2 days after explantation of 14-day fetal mouse cord correlates well with evidence of spinal reflex activity as early as 16 days in the rat *in utero*. In dorsal horn regions of the spinal cord, *clusters* of synapses are encountered rather frequently, whereas in other regions of the cord synapses appear to be distributed more diffusely. Dorsal root ganglia and spinal cord neurons continue to differentiate in culture and develop organotypic synaptic network structures and functions (e.g., Fig. 18D; Crain et al., 1975a). The morphologic characteristics of "mature" spinal cord, i.e., perikarya with well-differentiated and regionalized organelles, and compact neuropil with typical synaptic profiles can be readily observed in older cultures (Fig. 19).

ACKNOWLEDGMENTS

This work was supported in part by grants from the National Institute of Neurological Diseases and Stroke, NS-07512, NS-11431, NS-06545 and from the Alfred P. Sloan Foundation.

REFERENCES

Bunge, M. B. (1973): Fine structure of nerve fibers and growth cones of isolated sympathetic neurons in culture. *J. Cell Biol.*, 56:713–735.

Bunge, M. B., Bunge, R. P., and Peterson, E. R. (1967): The onset of synapse formation in spinal cord cultures as studied by electron microscopy. *Brain Res.*, 6:728–749.

Crain, S. M. (1973): Microelectrode recording in brain tissue cultures. In: *Methods in Physiological Psychology, Vol. 1: Bioelectric Recording Techniques: Cellular Processes and Brain Potentials*, edited by R. F. Thompson and M. M. Patterson, pp. 39–75. Academic Press, New York.

Crain, S. M. (1974a): Tissue culture models of developing brain functions. In: *Studies on the Development of Behavior and the Nervous System, Vol. 2: Aspects of Neurogenesis*, edited by G. Gottlieb, pp. 69–114. Academic Press, New York.

Crain, S. M. (1974b): Selective depression of organotypic bioelectric activities of CNS tissue cultures by pharmacologic and metabolic agents. In: *Drugs and the Developing Brain*, edited by A. Vernadakis and N. Weiner, pp. 29–57. Plenum, New York.

Crain, S. M. (1975): Early onset of inhibitory functions during synaptogenesis in fetal mouse brain cultures. In: *Golgi Centennial Symposium*, edited by M. Santini. Raven Press, New York.

Crain, S. M., and Bornstein, M. B. (1964): Bioelectric activity of neonatal mouse cerebral cortex during growth and differentiation in tissue culture. *Exp. Neurol.*, 10:425–450.

Crain, S. M., and Bornstein, M. B. (1974): Early onset in inhibitory functions during synaptogenesis in fetal mouse brain cultures. *Brain Res.*, 68:351–357.

Crain, S. M., and Peterson, E. R. (1967): Onset and development of functional interneuronal connections in explants of rat spinal cord-ganglia during maturation in culture. *Brain Res.*, 6:750–762.

Crain, S. M., Peterson, E. R., Masurovsky, E. B., and Pappas, G. D. (1975a): Early formation and development of functional synaptic networks in organotypic cultures of fetal mouse spinal cord with attached dorsal root ganglia. (*In preparation.*)

Crain, S. M., Raine, C. S., and Bornstein, M. B. (1975b): Early formation of synaptic networks in cultures of fetal mouse cerebral neocortex and hippocampus. *J. Neurobiol. (In press.)*

Fox, G. Q., Pappas, G. D., and Purpura, D. P. (1975a): Fine structure of growth cones in medullary raphe nuclei in the postnatal cat. *Brain Res. (In press.)*

Fox, G. Q., Pappas, G. D., and Purpura, D. P. (1975b): Morphology and fine structure of the feline neonatal medullary raphe nuclei. *Brain Res. (In press.)*

Masurovsky, E. B., and Peterson, E. R. (1973): Photo-reconstituted collagen gel for tissue culture substrates. *Exp. Cell Res.*, 76:447–448.

Model, P. B., Bornstein, M. B., Crain, S. M., and Pappas, G. D. (1971): An electron microscopic study of the development of synapses in cultured fetal mouse cerebrum continuously exposed to xylocaine. *J. Cell Biol.*, 49:362–371.

Nakamura, Y., Mizuno, N., Konishi, A., and Soto, M. (1974): Synaptic reorganization of the red nucleus after chronic deafferentation from cerebellorubral fibers: An electron microscope study of the cat. *Brain Res.*, 82:298–301.

Pappas, G. D. (1966): Electron microscopy of neuronal junctions involved in transmission in the central nervous system. In: *Nerve as a Tissue*, edited by K. Rodahl and B. Issekutz, Jr., pp. 49–87. Harper, New York.

Pappas, G. D., Peterson, E. R., Masurovsky, E. B., and Crain, S. M. (1971): The fine structure of developing neuromuscular synapses in vitro. *Ann. NY Acad. Sci.*, 183:33–45.

Peterson, E. R., and Crain, S. M. (1972): Regeneration and innervation in cultures of adult mammalian skeletal muscle coupled with fetal rodent spinal cord. *Exp. Neurol.*, 36:136–159.

Peterson, E. R., Crain, S. M., and Murray, M. R. (1965): Differentiation and prolonged maintenance of biologically active spinal cord cultures (rat, chick and human). *Z. Zellforsch. Mikrosk. Anat.*, 66:130–154.

Peterson, E. R., Masurovsky, E. B., and Crain, S. M. (1974): Enhanced survival and selective 'hypertrophy' of dorsal root ganglia after exposure of fetal rodent spinal cord-ganglion explants to nerve growth factor. *J. Cell Biol.*, 63:265a.

Raisman, G., and Field, P. (1973): A quantitative investigation of the development of collateral reinnervation after partial deafferentation of the septal nuclei. *Brain Res.*, 50:241–264.

Skoff, R. P., and Hamburger, V. (1974): Fine structure of dendritic and axonal growth cones in embryonic chick spinal cord. *J. Comp. Neurol.*, 153:107–148.

Tennyson, V. M. (1970): The fine structure of the axon and growth cone of the dorsal root neuroblast of the rabbit embryo. *J. Cell Biol.*, 44:62–79.

Vaughn, J. E., and Grieshaber, J. A. (1973): A morphological investigation of an early reflex pathway in developing rat spinal cord. *J. Comp. Neurol.*, 148:177–210.

Vaughn, J. E., Henrikson, C. K., and Grieshaber, J. A. (1974): A quantitative study of synapses on motor neuron dendritic growth cones in developing mouse spinal cord. *J. Cell Biol.,* 60:664–672.

Yamada, K. M., Spooner, B. S., and Wessells, N. K. (1971): Ultrastructure and function of growth cones and axons of cultured nerve cells. *J. Cell Biol.,* 49:614–635.

Advances in Neurology, Vol. 12, edited by
G. W. Kreutzberg, Raven Press, New York
© 1975.

Differentiation of Dendrites in the Transplanted Neuroblasts in the Mammalian Brain

Gopal D. Das

Department of Biological Sciences, Purdue University, West Lafayette, Indiana 47907

Embryologic development of the central nervous system is characterized by various well-defined events, some of which are the times of origin of different neurons, their paths of migration, the growth of axons, and specific cytoarchitectural patterns in different regions of the brain. These and other events, for a given neural structure, appear to be rigidly regulated within the temporal and spatial dimensions. These observations have provided a basis for the acceptance of the idea, which has acquired axiomatic significance, that the developmental events underlying neuroembryogenesis are predetermined. Other concepts, such as neuronal specification and genetic programming, in fact, convey this very notion.

Perhaps most significant of the various developmental events that take place during neuroembryogenesis is the morphologic differentiation of neurons and their dendrites. Each nerve cell, at the end of its differentiation, acquires its own unique somatic appearance and dendritic organization. As a matter of fact, it was the uniqueness of the dendritic arborization that provided Ramón-Moliner (1968) with a basis for classification of nerve cells, and this according to him represents a dendroarchitectonic approach to the neuronal classification. In the context of these observations the question may be posed: Is the basic dendritic pattern of a neuron predetermined? In an attempt to obtain a more direct and positive answer to this question, we have employed the technique of transplantation of embryonic neuroblasts in heterologous neural structures in the brains of the neonate animals. The somatic and dendritic differentiation of the transplanted neuroblasts is studied from a developmental viewpoint. This chapter analyzes the pattern of differentiation of dendrites of the neuroblasts destined to differentiate into the pyramidal cells of neocortex following their transplantation in the cerebellum of neonate animals.

MATERIALS AND METHODS

Laboratory-bred Wistar albino rats were used in this study. Adult female rats were placed with male animals overnight for mating. Those animals that showed sperm-positive smears were taken to provide the embryos as donors for transplantation. The day on which smears were sperm-positive was considered day 1 of gestation. On day 8 of gestation the pregnant animals were anesthetized with Nembutal. Laparotomy was performed on these animals, and both uterine horns were exposed. For transplantation purposes only one embryo at a time was removed; each was quickly dissected to remove the neuronal tissue from the dorsal aspect of the developing neocortex. This tissue was transplanted into the cerebellum of 10-day-old host animals.

The host animals also were obtained from the laboratory-bred Wistar albino strain. Ten-day-old animals were used as the recipients of the neural transplants. After the animals were anesthetized with ether an incision was made to expose the region of the cisterna magna. An incision, about 1 mm long, was made in the meningeal membranes overlying the cisterna magna, and the cerebrospinal fluid was allowed to flow out freely. After a few seconds the neural tissue obtained from the embryos was transplanted into the cerebellum of the host animals. The technique of transplantation is presented in detail elsewhere (Das, 1975). After transplantation the incision was sutured and covered with 6% celloidin, and the animals were returned to their cages.

Animals were sacrificed at 6 hr and at 1, 2, 3, 6, 15, 20, 30, and 60 days postsurgery for nissl as well as Golgi preparations. For the study of nissl-stained material, animals were perfused with 10% neutral Formalin after they were deeply anesthetized; the brains obtained from these animals were processed for histology in the standard manner. The blocks containing cerebellum were cut serially in the sagittal plane at 8 μm thickness, and every fourth section was saved. The sections were stained with cresyl violet. For Golgi study the animals were anesthetized and sacrificed. The unfixed brains obtained from these animals were processed for silver impregnation according to the Golgi–Cox method. This material was used for the analysis of growth and differentiation of the neuronal dendrites in the transplants. Some animals that survived for 30 days after transplantation were used for electron microscopy, for which the animals were deeply anesthetized and perfused with 6% buffered glutaraldehyde. Following perfusion the cerebellar regions containing the transplants were removed and placed in 6% buffered glutaraldehyde for 2 hr at 4°C. From this material blocks of 1 mm thickness were prepared, which were washed in phosphate buffer at 4°C, postfixed in 1% buffered osmium tetroxide for 1½ hr, dehydrated, and embedded in epon-araldite. This material was cut serially into ultrathin sections on Porter-Blum MT-2 ultramicrotome. The sections were stained with uranyl acetate and lead citrate, and were studied under a Philips-300 electron microscope.

FIG. 1. (a) Transplant, tr, in the anterior region of the host cerebellum, cb. The portion of transplant indicated by arrows is shown at a higher magnification in (b). Six-hr survival, CV stain. (×28.) (b) The transplant is largely composed of the neuroepithelium, ne. On its outer aspects lies a thin layer of neuroblasts, nb, possibly formed on days 16–17 of gesta-

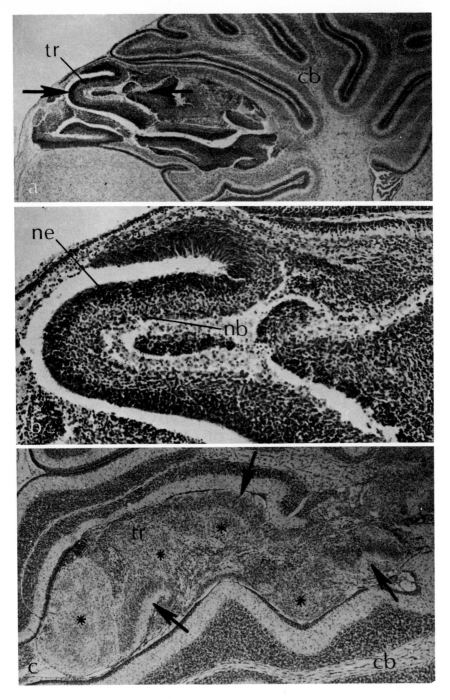

tion. Six-hr survival, CV stain. (×115.) (c) The transplant, tr, has acquired a differential histogenetic character. Some regions show laminated cytoarchitecture (*arrows*) and other nuclear organization (*). The postnatal neurogenesis and emergence of cytoarchitecture in the host cerebellum, cb, appear to progress independent of the transplant. Six-day survival, CV stain. (×45.)

OBSERVATIONS

Nissl-Stained Material

In the cerebellum of animals that were sacrificed 6 hr after the transplantation, the transplanted neural tissue could be readily identified (Fig. 1a). Although in no transplant was the entire neocortex of the embryo found intact, at the same time the transplants were not observed to be fragmented into numerous small pieces. They appeared as large chunks of the embryonic neural tissue (Fig. 1a). These large chunks of transplants were largely composed of the embryonic neuroepithelium, and lying on its outer aspect a thin layer of neuroblasts could be distinguished (Fig. 1b). It is possible that these neuroblasts were formed on days 16–17 of gestation. During subsequent stages of development the transplants were seen to undergo a variety of degenerative and regenerative changes, the details of which will be presented in a subsequent paper. The portion of the host cerebellum that was displaced by the transplants also underwent some degenerative and subsequent regenerative and reorganizational changes. These findings also will be reported elsewhere. However, 6 days after transplantation the transplants were observed to have occupied a large volume in the host cerebellum (Fig. 1c). At this stage neuroepithelium was not seen, and the transplants were composed of nerve cells (Fig. 1c). Various types of nerve cells with different morphologic characteristics could be distinguished. The most striking feature of these transplants was the presence of subregions showing different forms of cytoarchitectural organization. Some subregions showed laminated cytoarchitecture and other nuclear organization (Fig. 1c). It was interesting to observe that the host cerebellum surrounding the transplants appeared to follow its own course of postnatal neurogenesis and development of cerebellar cytoarchitecture. Presence of a heterologous neural tissue in the host cerebellum did not appear to affect these histogenetic activities. In no instance was any form of mixture or blend of transplanted neural tissue and the host cerebellum noticed.

An analysis of the transplants during following periods of development showed that the neuronal elements of the transplants achieved morphologic differentiation, spaced apart from one another, and that they were embedded in neuropil. The host cerebellum surrounding the transplants showed normal growth and development (Fig. 2a). Within the transplants differential patterns of cytoarchitectural organization, observed earlier, were found to persist. Long discontinuous patches of laminated structures were observed to contain neurons of different shapes in different layers (see arrows in Fig. 2a). These laminated structures were composed of two or three layers of distinctly identifiable nerve cells and a layer of neuropil, identical to the molecular layer of neocortex, on the superficial aspect. The nerve cells in the deep layers of such structures of the transplant appeared pyramidal in shape bearing an identical morphology to those seen in the neocortex.

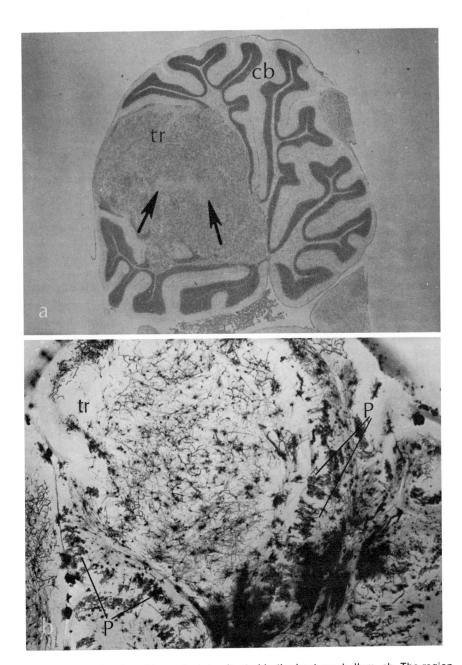

FIG. 2. (a) Fully developed transplant, tr, situated in the host cerebellum, cb. The region indicated by arrows shows laminated cytoarchitecture containing pyramidal cells identical to those seen in the neocortex. Thirty-day survival, CV stain. (×10.) (b) Transplant, tr, in Golgi–Cox preparation, surrounded by Purkinje cells, P, of the host cerebellum. The transplant shows rudimentary form of laminated cytoarchitecture containing no evidence of Purkinje cells. Thirty-day survival, Golgi–Cox. (×28.)

Those brains that were processed for the Golgi–Cox method of silver impregnation further supported the observations made on nissl-stained material. Layered arrangement of the nerve cells and morphologic identity of the pyramidal neurons could be established clearly (Fig. 2b). Cytoarchitectural segregation between the host cerebellum and the transplanted neural tissue was markedly visible in such preparations. Furthermore, this material revealed that despite such cytoarchitectural segregation many axons and their processes traversed between the host cerebellum and the transplanted neocortex. To this extent, it must be emphasized that the cytoarchitectural segregation between the transplants and the host neural tissue did not amount to absolute anatomic separation; that is, the transplanted neural tissue, despite its cytoarchitectural autonomy, had its connections with other regions of the host nervous system, albeit they were not the connections generally found in the case of normally located cerebral cortex.

Golgi–Cox Preparations

In the brains of host animals that survived for 30 days after the transplantation, a variety of neurons with different patterns of dendritic arborization, including pyramidal cells, could be seen in the transplants (Fig. 2b). Because the pyramidal cells of cerebral cortex are the focus of attention, the following analysis of differentiation of dendrites will be based exclusively upon this type of neuron. At the earliest stage of differentiation, that is, 3 days after the transplantation, the pyramidal cells along with their apical dendrites appeared like long club-shaped entities. Their somata merged smoothly into the tapering apical dendrites. This morphologic characteristic suggested that the apical dendrites, also the primary dendrites, were the first to emerge, and that they were not clearly demarcated from the perikaryon. These features of early growth of the apical dendrites could also be noticed in the transplants that survived for 6 days following transplantation (Fig. 3a). Moreover, at this stage of development it was observed that the apical dendrites, at their basal level very close to the perikaryon, had fine-caliber processes, and at their apical level had bifurcated into two smaller dendritic processes (see arrows and d in Fig. 3a). Furthermore, the apical dendrites of the pyramidal cells were found to course in well-defined bundles. This attribute of bundle-forming was

FIG. 3. (a) Pyramidal cells of the transplant in early stages of differentiation. The somata and the apical dendrites together show club-shaped morphology of these neurons. The apical dendrites tend to form a bundle, particularly at the distal ends, db. One apical dendrite shows characteristic bifurcation, d, before its terminal end. Two pyramidal cells show a very thin process, bp, emerging from the basal portions of the somata. Small arrows point to the fine-caliber processes emerging from the basal portion of the apical dendrites. Six-day survival, Golgi–Cox. (×280.) (b) A well-differentiated pyramidal cell. This nerve cell shows characteristic pyramidal shape identical to that found in the neo-

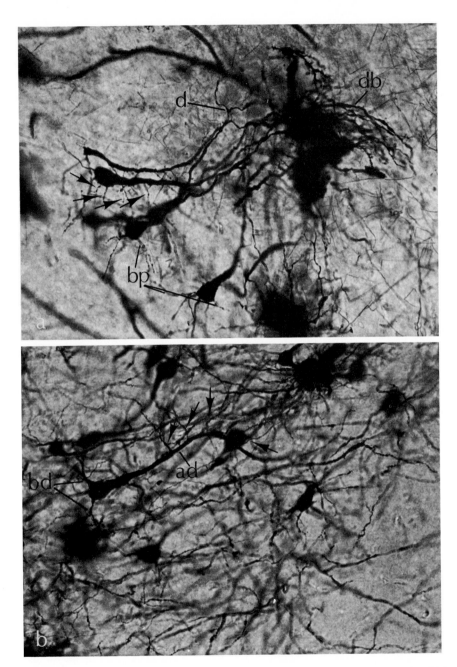

cortex. Its curved apical dendrite, ad, has acquired secondary branches (*arrows*), which are farther removed from the perikaryon. There is no evidence of fine-caliber processes on the apical dendrite close to the cell body found in earlier stages of differentiation. Along its basal aspect two stout basal dendrites, bd, in the place of many fine-caliber processes are seen. Fifteen-day survival, Golgi–Cox. (×280.)

more conspicuously noticed in the case of collaterals of the apical dendrites immediately after their bifurcation (see db in Fig. 3a). A few cases showed very thin basal processes emerging from the basal portions of the nerve cells (see bp, Fig. 3a).

The pyramidal cells in the brains of the host animals that survived for 15 days after transplantation were found to have acquired their characteristic pyramidal shape (Fig. 3b). The perikarya were not yet distinctly demarcated from the apical dendrites. The apical dendrites had grown thicker and longer, and had acquired well-defined secondary branches along their main shafts (see arrows, Fig. 3b). Neither at this stage nor at the later stages of development were the fine-caliber processes at the basal level of the apical dendrites, observed earlier, noticed. The secondary branches emerging from the apical dendrites were further distally removed from the region in which the fine-caliber processes were seen earlier, which suggests that the second-ary branches were *de novo* entities and not the thickened fine-caliber proc-esses. It is possible that the fine-caliber processes during the differentiation of the apical dendrites were resorbed. Along the basal aspects of the pyramidal cells thick basal dendrites, in the place of fine processes observed earlier, were found to emerge (see bd, Fig. 3b). These basal dendrites too had acquired secondary and tertiary branches. From this material it could not be determined whether the fine processes along the basal aspects of the pyramidal cells, seen at the earlier stages of development, had been resorbed or differentiated into the thick basal dendrites.

During further stages of differentiation of the pyramidal cells and their dendrites in the transplants, the somata of the pyramidal cells were seen to have acquired a distinct shape, which helped delineate a perikaryon from its apical dendrite (Fig. 4a,b). The apical dendrites had grown longer and seemed to follow a curved rather than straight course. The secondary branches emerging from the apical dendrites had acquired tertiary branches (see arrows and 3, Fig. 4a). The basal dendrites also were observed to give rise to secondary and tertiary branches (see bd, Fig. 4a,b). In some cases fine-caliber processes were seen to emerge from the perikaryon between the points of origin of the apical and basal dendrites (see p, Fig. 4a). In the transplants with longer survival intervals instead of these fine proc-esses various well-defined short dendrites were observed to arise from the perikarya of the pyramidal cells (see p, Fig. 4b). Whether these fine proc-esses were resorbed before the emergence of the new dendrites or whether

FIG. 4. (a) A differentiated pyramidal cell. Its apical dendrite, ad, follows a curved course. The secondary branches (*arrows*) are seen to have acquired tertiary branches (3). From the basal portion of this neuron three basal dendrites, bd, appear to emerge. An inde-pendent process, p, is seen to emerge from the soma and follow a course similar to that of the apical dendrite. Twenty-day survival, Golgi–Cox. (×280.) (b) A differentiated py-ramidal cell sending its apical dendrite, ad, into the molecular layer of the host cerebellum, where it bifurcates (*arrow*) and the two branches follow a course parallel to the molecular

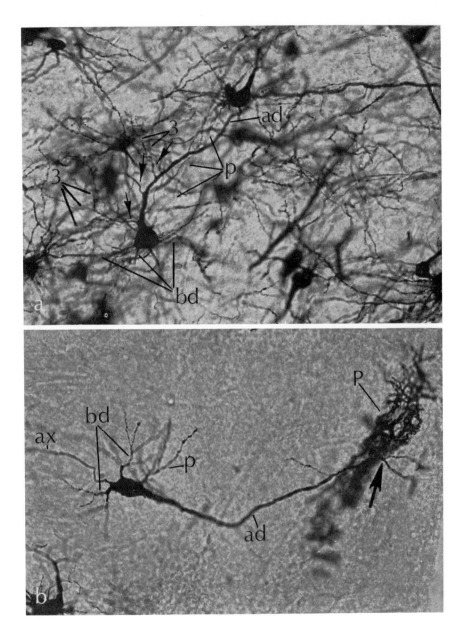

layer. Close to the point of bifurcation of the apical dendrite is the Purkinje cell, with clearly identifiable dendritic processes, P. The basal dendrites, bd, are seen to give rise to secondary and tertiary branches. A dendritic process, p, with its secondary and tertiary branches, is observed to arise from the lateral aspect of the perikaryon of the pyramidal cell. Axon, ax, is seen to emerge from the base of the pyramidal cell and appears oriented in the direction opposite to that of the apical dendrite. Twenty-day survival, Golgi–Cox. (×280.)

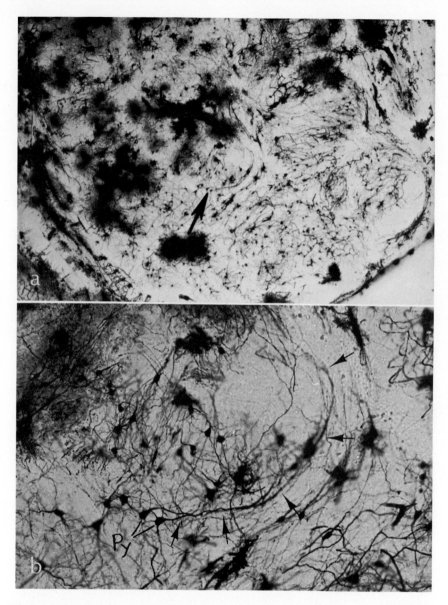

FIG. 5. (a) A low-power view of the transplant. Two pyramidal cells (arrows) are shown at a higher magnification in (b). Differential histogenetic patterns in the transplant may be noted. Thirty-day survival, Golgi–Cox. (×28.) (b) Two pyramidal cells, Py, are sending their long apical dendrites (arrows) along a curved path following the contour of a histogenetically differentiated portion of the transplant. Thirty-day survival, Golgi–Cox. (×115.)

they themselves differentiated into the dendrites could not be established clearly.

Generally, the dendritic processes of all the neurons, including those of the pyramidal cells, were confined within the limits of the transplants. But in a few cases it was observed that the apical dendrites had extended their distal collaterals into the molecular layer of the host cerebellum (see ad, Fig. 4b). Such findings further confirmed the facts that the transplants and the host neural tissue were not absolutely separated, and that they had a continuity of neuropil.

The above-described data showed that the basic dendritic pattern and the sequence of differentiation of dendrites of the transplanted pyramidal cells remained unaltered following the transplantation. However, two other attributes of dendritic growth and differentiation appeared to be influenced by the changes wrought upon the cytoarchitectural organization within the transplants. First, the apical dendrites appeared to follow a curved path (Figs. 3a,b; 4a,b; 5a,b; and 6). This was observed to be related to the different subregions with differential cytoarchitectural organization present in the transplants. As a rule, the apical dendrites in their course of following the contour of a subregion in the transplant acquired a curved appearance (Fig. 5a,b). When the pyramidal cells formed an integral part of a subregion of the transplant their apical dendrites remained relatively straight (see c, Fig. 6). Second, the length of the apical dendrites seemed to vary considerably among pyramidal cells of the same size. In many instances the apical dendrites of the pyramidal cells were of normal size and were confined within the bounds of the subregion of the transplant, but in some cases the apical dendrites appeared to be excessively long and followed the contours of the subregions (Fig. 5a,b). Such morphologic changes associated with both the direction and the length of the dendrites were not observed in either the basal dendrites or in those arising from the lateral aspects of the perikarya.

Finally, the formation of bundles by the apical dendrites appeared to be related to the clustering of the pyramidal cells. Regardless of where the pyramidal cells were located in the transplant, their apical dendrites formed compact bundles and coursed in such bundles for their entire length provided the pyramidal cells themselves were clustered together (see a, Fig. 6). In those cases in which single or isolated pyramidal cells were observed, their apical dendrites did not show any tendency to form bundles with neighboring apical dendrites. In a few cases some aberrations of bundles of dendrites were seen. A commonly encountered aberration was arrangement of the apical dendrites in an hourglass formation (see b, Fig. 6). Such hourglass formations by the apical dendrites, when reconstructed in a developmental sequence, were found to be the result of some abrupt topographic changes in the path of the apical dendrites much before their termination. Such anatomic changes in their milieu caused the apical

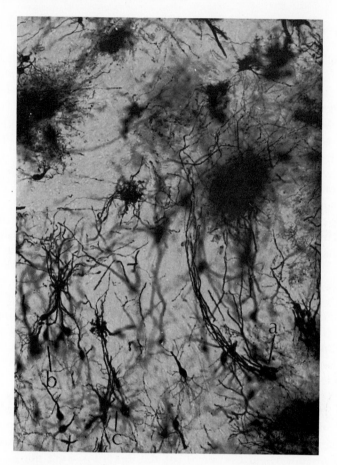

FIG. 6. Clusters of pyramidal cells forming distinct bundles of dendrites. Pyramidal cells in cluster (a) have long apical dendrites, all of which are coursing together in a curved path. Those in cluster (b) first come together to form a bundle and then diverge, thus acquiring an hourglass appearance. In cluster (c) the apical dendrites are seen to form a bundle, but histologic sectioning prevents their entire course from being followed. Thirty-day survival, Golgi–Cox. (×115.)

dendrites to diverge and fan out, rather than continue to course straight in bundles. These observations indicated that formation of bundles by the apical dendrites of the pyramidal cells may not be predetermined, and that this characteristic may be dependent upon clustering of the pyramidal cells and other developmental events in the neural tissue.

Electron Microscopic Observations

The pyramidal cells could readily be identified in electron microscopic preparations by their large size and by their typical pyramidal morphology (Fig. 7). Large masses of rough endoplasmic reticulum in their cytoplasm

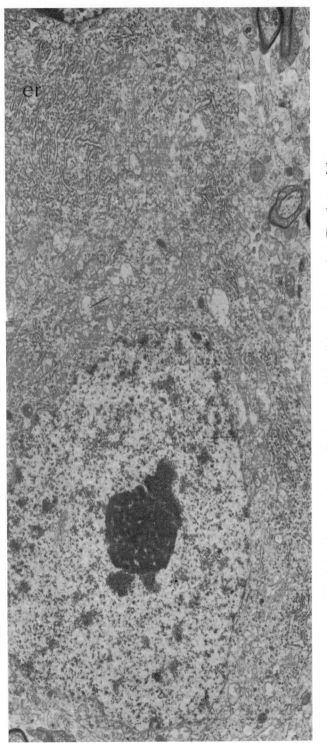

er

FIG. 7. An electron micrograph of a pyramidal cell from the transplant. The shape of the nucleus as well as of the soma strongly indicate the pyramidal morphology of the neuron. Large areas of cytoplasm are seen occupied by closely packed rough endoplasmic reticulum, er. Thirty-day survival. (×7,000.)

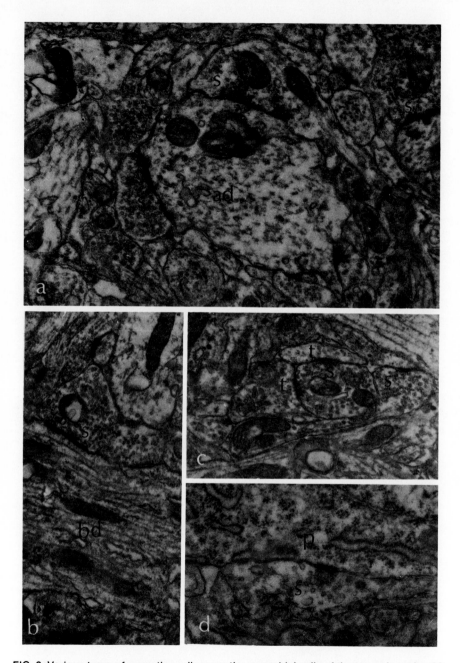

FIG. 8. Various types of synaptic endings on the pyramidal cells of the transplant after 30-day survival. (a) Axodendritic synapses, s, closer to the distal region of the apical dendrite, ad. (×17,750.) (b) Axodendritic synapse, s, on a basal dendrite, bd. (×15,000.) (c) Synaptic endings, s, on the spines or thorns, t, of the dendrites. (×15,000.) (d) Axosomatic synapse, s, on the perikaryon, p, of a pyramidal cell. (×22,500.)

were observed to be the conspicuous organelles, which indicated the possible presence of large nissl bodies as seen in basophilic preparations for light microscopy. In relation to these pyramidal cells, axodendritic synapses on their apical (Fig. 8a) as well as basal (Fig. 8b) dendrites were noticed. The apical dendrites were observed to be richly invested with spines or thorns, and they also received synaptic endings (Fig. 8c). Although axosomatic synapses were observed in all the cases studied (Fig. 8d), they were relatively fewer in number than the axodendritic synapses. The exact source of these synaptic endings, whether axodendritic or axosomatic, could not be determined.

DISCUSSION

Earlier studies on the transplantation of postnatally developing neural tissue obtained from the cerebellum indicated that such transplantations in the brains of the neonate animals could be achieved successfully (Das and Altman, 1971, 1972; Das, 1973). Recently, it was shown that the neuroblasts of embryonic origin could also be successfully transplanted into the developing cerebellum of the neonate animals (Das, 1975). Although in that study the transplanted neuronal elements could be conclusively identified with the aid of ³H-thymidine autoradiography, it was observed that they had achieved somatic differentiation and cytoarchitectural organization in a manner identical to that achieved in their normal locations—that is, during differentiation the transplanted neuroblasts did not transform into neurons resembling those of the host cerebellum, but they did differentiate and achieve cytoarchitectural organization according to their predetermined course. These findings suggested that the unique morphologic differentiation of different types of neurons and the distinct cytoarchitectural patterns that they would achieve could be employed as a means of unequivocal identification of the transplanted elements. The findings reported in the present study support this conclusion. In the fully differentiated transplants various laminated structures and nuclear masses could be identified, representing the cortical tissue and the subcortical nuclei, respectively. Out of this complex structure in the transplants, only the pyramidal cells of the neocortex were evaluated for the purpose of this study. Our objective was to identify the large pyramidal cells of the cerebral cortex, to analyze the pattern of their dendritic differentiation, and, in electron microscopic preparations, to demonstrate their synaptic endings.

The large pyramidal cells could be readily identified, as early as 3 to 6 days after the transplantation, in the nissl-stained material as well as in the Golgi–Cox preparations. In the nissl-stained material they were seen to lie in the deeper layers of the laminated structures, showing a rudimentary pyramidal morphology and appearing larger than other globular nerve cells in the vicinity. In Golgi–Cox preparations they appeared as club-shaped cells.

This morphologic peculiarity was observed to be due to the fact that the apical dendrites and the associated somata had not yet differentiated to the point at which the boundary between the two could be properly defined. One smoothly merged into and continued with the other without any indentations. However, after 15 days of transplantation the somata and the apical dendrites of the pyramidal cells could be adequately distinguished. These changes may have been largely due to the growth in the volume of the pyramidal cells. These morphologic changes and the fact that other neurons in the transplants did not show the presence of single long apical dendrites helped to identify the pyramidal cells of neocortex in the transplants without any error.

Dendritic differentiation of the pyramidal cells in the cerebral cortex was described by Purpura, Shofer, Housepian, and Noback (1964), and Åström (1967). Data presented in this study closely agree with their findings. In essence, the apical dendrites are first to arise, and they are followed by the basal dendrites. After the emergence of the primary dendritic branches, the secondary and tertiary branches are seen to sprout and grow. This basic sequence of dendritic differentiation seems to have remained unaltered in the case of the transplanted neural tissue. In addition, the basic pattern of dendritic arborization of the pyramidal cells also remained unaffected, for the pyramidal cells and their dendroarchitecture in the transplants appeared identical to those seen in the normal neocortex. These observations suggest that these two attributes of the differentiating pyramidal cells of the neocortex, namely, sequence of dendritic differentiation and the pattern of dendritic arborization, are predetermined. The exact nature of the factors or forces that contribute to the predetermination of these aspects of dendritic differentiation of the pyramidal cells is not known. Phrases such as genetic programming and stability of differentiation do not provide a satisfactory explanation, although they do seem to carry the illusionary connotation.

In this chapter it has been shown that before the emergence of the secondary and tertiary dendrites from the apical dendrites, a number of fine-caliber processes are present at their basal level that are absent at later stages of dendritic differentiation. It is possible that these fine-caliber processes are resorbed during differentiation, although there is no direct evidence in support of this. Ramón y Cajol (1909, 1911) and Morest (1969) also have commented on the possibility of resorption of such fine-caliber processes associated with the differentiating dendrites. Out of these observations two major questions arise: Are the emergence and pattern of fine-caliber processes also predetermined? Do the fine-caliber processes grow thick and differentiate into dendrites, or do they simply undergo resorption to allow for the emergence of *de novo* dendrites? At this stage of our knowledge there are no definite answers to these questions. It is possible that information from related fields such as cell biology and developmental biology will provide some insight into these problems.

Differentiation of dendrites also involves direction of their course and the length they attain. The observations made in the present study show that these two attributes of the apical dendrites of the pyramidal cells in the transplants were greatly altered. Under normal conditions in the growing neocortex a multitude of other developmental changes occur simultaneous to the differentiation of the dendrites of the pyramidal nerve cells. Some of these developmental changes involve growth and differentiation of dendrites of other neurons in different layers of neocortex, growth and penetration of axons from outside and inside the neocortex, and evolution of a laminated cytoarchitecture. It is possible that these developmental changes provide a continually evolving anatomic milieu for the differentiating apical dendrites of the pyramidal cells, thus regulating their direction and extent of growth. In the transplants these developmental events themselves were altered, and they in turn contributed to the alterations in the direction and in the length of the apical dendrites of the pyramidal cells.

In addition to the above described attributes of the differentiation of dendrites of the pyramidal cells, it has been observed that the apical dendrites and their collaterals at distal ends showed a strong tendency to form bundles. This property observed in the transplants of the neocortex is also noticed under normal conditions. In their studies on the cerebral cortex, Fleischhauer, Petsche, and Wittkowski (1972) and Peters and Walsh (1972) showed that the apical dendrites of the pyramidal cells tend to be organized in bundles. Our observations have shown that it is not only the apical dendrites but also their collaterals at distal ends that are organized in bundles. On the basis of these observations it may appear that this aggregate behavior of the apical dendrites is also predetermined. However, closer investigation of the findings made in the present study reveals that dendritic bundles may have been formed because some pyramidal cells clustered together during their differentiation; this and other developmental changes may have contributed to the formation of bundles. In fact, neither the normative studies nor the present study on transplantation of neocortex provides a conclusive support to one or the other hypothesis. More experimental studies are required to determine whether formation of bundles by the apical dendrites is predetermined or largely influenced by other developmental events taking place in their vicinity.

Finally, the data in the present study have shown that the transplanted pyramidal cells and their dendrites receive synaptic endings, the source of which is unknown. This suggests that these transplanted neural elements may also be physiologically active. These ultrastructural findings indicate the possibility that the synaptic endings on the pyramidal cells and on their dendrites may have had some trophic influences on their differentiation, but such trophic influences must have been nonspecific. In all likelihood, a transplant of cortical tissue growing in cerebellum will receive afferents from those sources that are associated with the cerebellum and not the cerebral cortex. Furthermore, in the brains of the host animals which contain their own intact and growing cerebral cortex, it is unlikely that the neuronal structures—particularly the thalamic nuclei, which provide afferents to the cerebral cortex—would also provide afferents to the transplants in the cerebellum following a totally new path in the brain. Therefore, although a neuron and its dendrites may require some trophic influences for their morphologic differentiation, they need not necessarily be specific.

Viewing these cytologic changes in the transplants comprehensively, one may feel tempted to conclude that transplanted neural tissue in the brains of neonate rats and rabbits is not at all different from tissue culture of neural slabs. However, no matter how forcefully made, this comparison remains invalid because transplantation of neural tissue involves not only the growth and differentiation of the transplants, but also their anatomic integration with the brains of the host animals. Moreover, the transplants grow and differentiate in an environment composed of neural tissue, cerebrospinal fluid, and vascular elements of a living organism. Therefore, studies employing the technique of transplantation of neural tissue have a far more valuable significance for neuroembryology in that they can contribute to our understanding of the growth and differentiation of neuroblasts, differentiation of dendrites, growth of axons, intercellular relationships, and the emergence of cytoarchitectural organization. With this technique it is possible to analyze the extent to which these neuroembryogenetic events are predetermined in a living system.

SUMMARY AND CONCLUSIONS

Neocortical tissue obtained from the 8-day old rat embryos was transplanted into the cerebellum of 10-day-old rats. Within these transplants various subregions were seen, some with laminated cytoarchitecture and others with nuclear organization. The laminated structures were found to contain the pyramidal nerve cells of the neocortex. The differentiation of dendrites of these pyramidal cells was studied in Golgi–Cox preparations. The sequence of dendritic growth and differentiation and the pattern of dendritic arborization were found to be very similar to those seen in the pyramidal cells of the neocortex. These two attributes of dendritic differentiation of the pyramidal cells were therefore considered to be predetermined. However, the course and the length of the apical dendrites were found to be greatly altered; therefore, these two characteristics were evaluated and found to be influenced by the milieu immediately surrounding the transplanted neuronal elements. Furthermore, the apical dendrites were found to form bundles. It was not possible to establish whether or not this characteristic of dendritic organization was predetermined. Electron microscopic evaluation revealed the presence of axodendritic and axosomatic synapses on the pyramidal cells. These observations suggested that the transplanted neuronal elements may be physiologically active, and that if trophic influences mediated by the synaptic endings had contributed to the differentiation of the pyramidal cells and their dendrites, they could not have been specific in nature.

REFERENCES

Åström, K.-E. (1967): On the early development of the isocortex in fetal sheep. In: *Developmental Neurology, Progress in Brain Research, Vol. 26,* edited by C. G. Bernhard and J. P. Schadé, pp. 1–59. Elsevier, Amsterdam.

Das, G. D. (1973): Transplantation of cerebellar tissue in the cerebellum of neonate rabbits. *Brain Res., 50:*170–173.

Das, G. D. (1975): Transplantation of embryonic neural tissue in the mammalian brain. I. Growth and differentiation of neuroblasts from various regions of the embryonic brain in the cerebellum of neonate rats. *T.-I.-T. J. Life Sci.,*

Das, G. D., and Altman, J. (1971): The fate of transplanted precursors of nerve cells in the cerebellum of young rats. *Science,* 173:637–638.

Das, G. D., and Altman, J. (1972): Studies on the transplantation of developing neural tissue in the mammalian brain. I. Transplantation of cerebellar slabs into the cerebellum of neonate rats. *Brain Res.,* 38:233–249.

Fleischhauer, K., Petsche, H., and Wittkowski, W. (1972): Vertical bundles of dendrites in the neocortex. *Z. Anat. Entwicklungsgesch.,* 136:213–223.

Morest, D. K. (1969): The growth of dendrites in the mammalian brain. *Z. Anat. Entwicklungsgesch.,* 128:290–317.

Peters, A., and Walsh, T. M. (1972): A study of the organization of apical dendrites in somatic sensory cortex of the rat. *J. Comp. Neurol.,* 144:253–268.

Purpura, D. P., Shofer, R. J., Housepian, E. M., and Noback, C. R. (1964): Comparative ontogenesis of structure–function relations in cerebral and cerebellar cortex. In: *Progress in Brain Research, Vol. 4: Growth and Maturation of the Brain,* edited by D. P. Purpura and J. P. Schadé, pp. 187–221. Elsevier, Amsterdam.

Ramón y Cajal, S. (1909, 1911): *Histologie du système nerveux de l'homme et des vertébrés, Vols. I* and *II,* translated by L. Azoulay. [Reprinted by Instituto Ramón y Cajal del C.S.I.C., Madrid, 1952–1955.]

Ramón-Moliner, E. (1968): The morphology of dendrites. In: *The Structure and Function of Nervous Tissue, Vol. I: Structure. I,* edited by G. H. Bourne, pp. 205–267. Academic Press, New York.

Advances in Neurology, Vol. 12, edited by
G. W. Kreutzberg, Raven Press, New York
© 1975.

Dendritic Growth *In Vitro*

A. Privat

Laboratoire de Culture de Tissu Nerveux INSERM, U-106, Hôpital Port-Royal, Paris 75014, France

The use of *in vitro* models for the study of the nervous system has been diversely appraised since the early work by Harrison (1910) on neurite elongation and growth cones. Since then, most of the attention has been focused on axonal growth, both in *in vitro* and *in vivo* studies of maturation of the neuron and elongation of its processes (Lewis, 1950; Nakai, 1959; Pomerat, Hendelman, Raiborn, and Massey, 1967; Del Cerro and Snider, 1968; Bray, 1970, 1973*a,b;* Bunge and Bray, 1970; Tennyson, 1970; Yamada, Spooner, and Wessels, 1970*a,b;* Kawana, Sandri, and Akert, 1971; Bunge, 1973).

Dendritic growth has been illustrated in a few *in vivo* studies, namely by Morest (1969) with Golgi techniques, by Sotelo and Palay (1968) at the ultrastructural level, and more recently by Hinds and Hinds (1972) and by Vaughn, Henrikson, and Grieshaber (1974).

An increasing body of evidence is accumulating in favor of the role of dendrites (as postsynaptic elements) in the setup of neural connectivity (Sotelo, 1973) and, as a tridimensional receptor, in the modulation of the afferent input to the cell (Rall, 1970; Llinás and Nicholson, 1971). These two properties served as guidelines in our *in vitro* study.

We attempted first to illustrate both the ultrastructure of dendritic growth cones in the outgrowth of organized cultures of rat cerebellum and the early synapse formation in this region; second, in the particular case of the Purkinje cell dendrite (PCD), to determine to what extent dendritic — and spine — growth was dependent on the presence of afferent boutons.

MATERIALS AND METHODS

Preparation of Cultures

Newborn germfree rats (IFFA, CREDO) are sacrificed by exsanguination; the cerebellum is quickly dissected and separated into 10 sagittal slices. Each slice is explanted onto a collagen-coated coverslip and sealed into the Maximow assembly with a drop of nutrient composed of 30% freshly collected human serum, 30% minimal Eagle medium, 40% balanced salt solution (BSS), and supplemented with glucose to a final concentration of 6%. The cultures are then washed and refed twice a week.

In addition, almost 100 cultures were fed from explantation inward with the same medium in which 20 μg/ml methylazoxymethanol acetate (MAM) was added. This drug is a derivative of cycasin, a drug that has been shown to inhibit the proliferation of granule neurons (Hirano, Dembitzer, and Jones, 1972).

Examination Technique

More than 1,000 cultures were used for these studies, each of which was examined daily under phase and interference microscopes. For transmission electron microscopy, three sets of cultures were considered.

Set 1. About 50 cultures with a well-developed outgrowth zone were selected with the phase microscope, and were fixed at various intervals from days 1 to 10 *in vitro*. The cultures were fixed in glutaraldehyde and postfixed in osmium tetroxide (for details see Privat, Drian, and Mandon, 1973).

Set 2. Cultures 20 to 30 days *in vitro* (DIV) were selected according to the usual criteria of good health (Murray, 1965), and regions corresponding to the presumptive cerebellar cortex selected on 1 μm toluidine blue-stained plastic sections were used for ultrathin sectioning.

Set 3. Cultures treated with MAM, which were selected and processed in the same way as the second set.

RESULTS

Outgrowth Zone

Within 24 to 48 hr after explantation, numerous cells migrate from the explant (Privat et al., 1973), and growth cones are readily found. These appear in increasing number until days 5 to 6 when they begin to decrease in number. At that time, the outgrowth zone appears almost as a monolayer, with flat fibroblasts supporting various kinds of neuroblasts and macrophages (Fig. 1).

Dendritic growth cones were tentatively identified at the ultrastructural level by the presence of synapses upon them (Fig. 2). [The axon, pre-synaptic to these growth cones, often shows growth cone appearance, too (Figs. 3 and 4).] They appear as varicose tips, studded with numerous short, spine-like microvilli, the so-called filopodia; the varicosity contains a large number of mitochondria, some glycogen in the form of B-particles, some multivesicular bodies, a few microtubules, and several cisternae of smooth reticulum.

The filopodia show a finely filamentous matrix, and the only organelle is the frequent cistern of smooth endoplasmic reticulum (ER) (Figs. 3 and 4). They differ from axonal growth cones, the varicosities of which appear

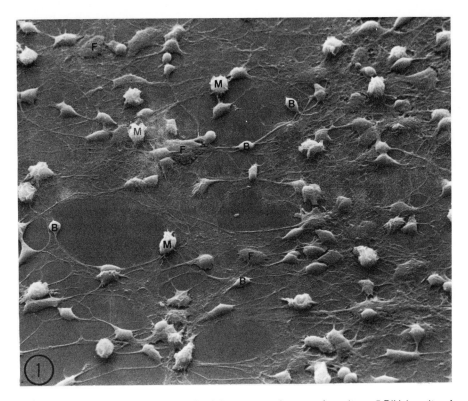

FIG. 1. Scanning electron micrograph of the outgrowth zone of a culture, 5 DIV. In spite of the low magnification, it is possible to identify on their tridimensional appearance macrophages, M, fibroblasts, F, bipolar cells, B. (×750.)

to be more discrete, with filopodia that are longer and slender, and less numerous.

The tridimensional appearance of these growth cones is shown with some detail on scanning electron micrographs (Figs. 5 and 6). Their shape and size differ from one cell to another, and even for the same cell. Nevertheless, the varicose appearance, irradiated with short filopodia, is a constant feature.

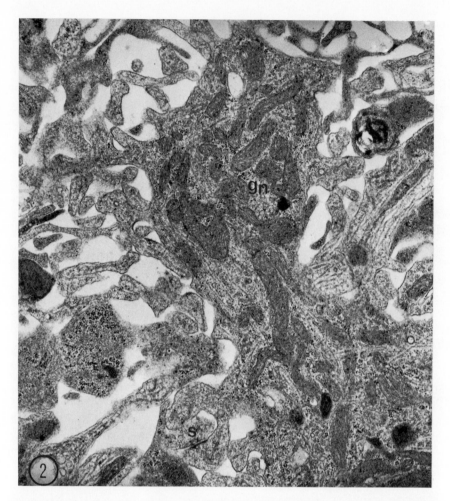

FIG. 2. Transmission electron micrograph, 10 DIV. Large growing tip probably belongs to a Purkinje dendrite. Spines are numerous and one of them bears a synapse, s. The center of the varicosity is occupied by mitochondria and glycogen granules, gn. (×20,000.)

EXPLANT ZONE

Purkinje Dendrites of Standard Cultures

In 20 to 30 DIV cultures, Purkinje cells appeared fully differentiated as no obvious difference, either qualitative or quantitative, was noted in older cultures. The dendritic arborization was found to consist of a few large trunks, studded with numerous spines. Such a dendrite is illustrated in Fig. 7, in which the extracellular space has been filled with horseradish peroxidase. On that rather thick section, the outline of these spiny ex-

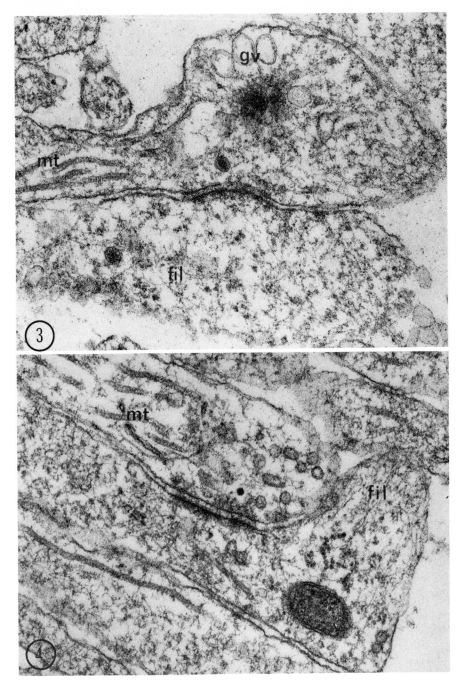

FIG. 3. Transmission electron micrograph, 4 DIV. Contact between the growing tip of an axon, containing microtubules, mt, and growth vesicles, gv, and a dendritic spine containing filaments, fil, as usual in growing spines. The contact is asymmetric, with postsynaptic density and dense cleft. Synaptic vesicles are absent. (×85,000.)

FIG. 4. Transmission electron micrograph, 4 DIV. This contact between an axon and a dendritic spine, containing microtubules, mt, and filaments, fil, features a postsynaptic density, discrete dense presynaptic dense projections, a densification of the cleft, and a few synaptic vesicles, as seen in Gray's type I synapses. (×8,500.)

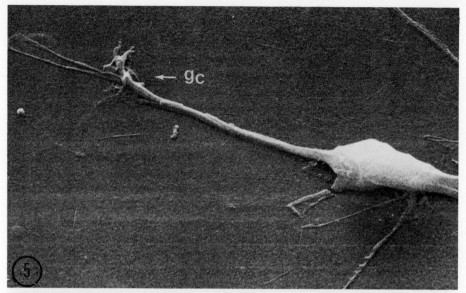

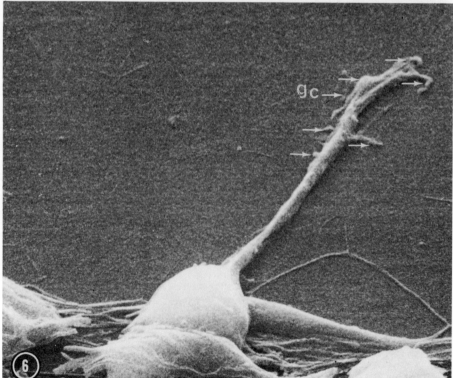

FIG. 5. Scanning electron micrograph, 4 DIV. The large process of a bipolar cell, presumed to be a dendrite, ends up with a slight varicosity of the growth cone, gc, provided with numerous spine-like filopodia. (×4,500.)

FIG. 6. Five DIV. The large process of a bulbous cell ends up with a growth cone, gc, the varicosity of which is studded with several short filopodia (↗). Several other filopodia are seen more proximal, thus illustrating the notion of "terminal segment" of Morest (1969). Scanning electron micrograph. (×5,000.)

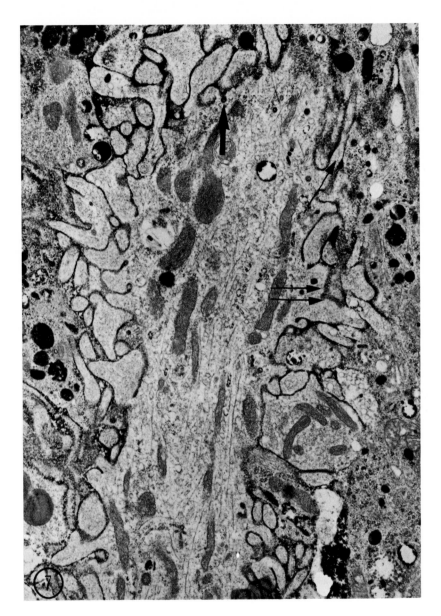

FIG. 7. 20 DIV. This culture has been incubated with peroxidase, which has penetrated and completely filled the extracellular space. On this rather thick section (120 nm) the numerous spines are well outlined, and their variety of shapes and sizes is obvious. Notice the presence of peroxidase-positive vacuoles of various sizes. Arrows indicate that some of them are formed by local pinocytosis. (×18,000.)

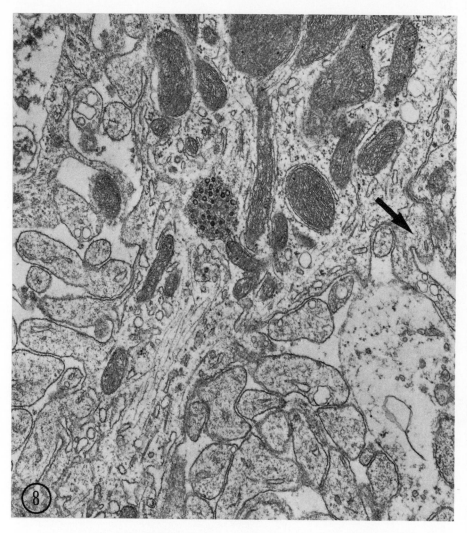

FIG. 8. 24 DIV. The large dendritic trunk of a Purkinje cell is studded with numerous spines, all of which are naked. Notice the various shapes and sizes of these spines, one of which is bifurcated (↗). (×28,000.)

pansions is sharply delineated. They vary greatly in shape and size from the long, slender expansion (single arrow) to the large branched one (double arrow). That several of these spines are devoid of any synaptic contact appears clearly in Fig. 8, in which another dendritic trunk is seen at higher magnification. Here again, some typical features of these dendrites are quite apparent: the abundance of mitochondria, the presence of multivesicular bodies, and of cisternae of smooth ER, which frequently also invade the spines; the latter always have a more-or-less fuzzy appearance, owing to the presence of a fibrous material.

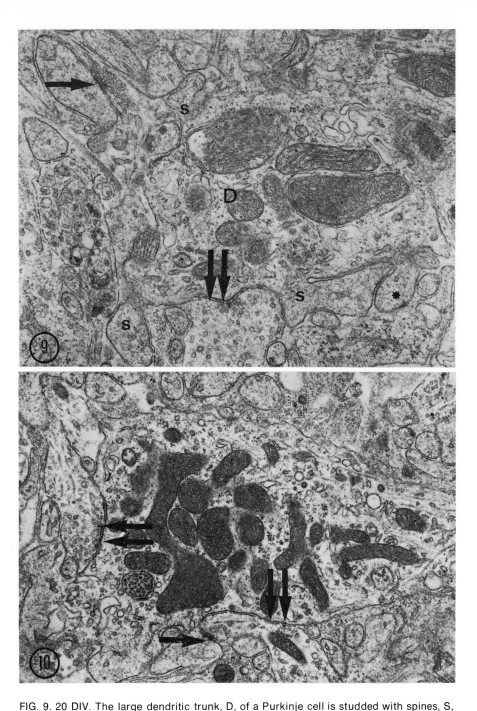

FIG. 9. 20 DIV. The large dendritic trunk, D, of a Purkinje cell is studded with spines, S, some of which are naked. Two types of synapses are found: the axospinous synapse (single arrow) of Gray's type I, and the true axodendritic (double arrow) of Gray's type II; one spine (*) has an isolated postsynaptic density. (×20,000.)

FIG. 10. 20 DIV. Large, possibly terminal varicosity of a Purkinje dendrite. The two types of synapses featured in Fig. 9 are represented. Notice that the bouton at the lower center makes a type I synapse with a spine, and type II with the shaft. (×20,000.)

Two types of synapses are found on these dendrites, according to their location. Axospinous synapses are of the "asymmetric" type (Gray's type I) with a short "active" zone and a coarse postsynaptic thickening. The vesicles are spherical, and the general appearance of the bouton is that of a parallel fiber. Other synapses occur on the smooth surfaces of dendrites; their "active" zone is longer, and the postsynaptic thickening is thin. They all have the character of "symmetric" synapses (Gray's type II), their vesicles vary from spherical to flattened, and they are usually pleomorphic. These boutons may be attributed to the axons of stellate cells (Figs. 9 and 10).

Occasionally a spine may be seen (Fig. 9) to bear a postsynaptic density devoid of any bouton, but they are very rare, compared to what appear to be completely naked spines.

In conclusion, it appears that despite the absence of mossy and climbing fibers, the PCD is able to grow outward, and to differentiate dendritic spines.

Purkinje Dendrites in Cultures Treated with MAM

These cultures, as seen in the living state with the phase microscope, are characterized by two features not found in standard cultures. First, the extent of the outgrowth zone and the number of cells are drastically reduced; this corresponds to the absence of granule cells, as it has been found that these cells constituted the bulk of the migrating elements, in our culture conditions. Second, the number of myelinated fibers is definitely higher when compared to the control.

Purkinje cells are readily found in these cultures, and their dendritic tree is not very different from that of control cultures. More precisely, large dendritic trunks are studded with numerous spines, as is the perikaryon. The characteristic feature of these dendrites resides in the nature of the synapses found on their surfaces. In the absence of parallel fibers, most of the synapses found on the dendrites are constituted of large boutons, filled with flattened vesicles, showing several "active" zones, either on the spines or on the shaft of the dendrites; these flattened vesicles are intermingled with thin profiles of smooth reticulum. Mitochondria and microtubules are two other common features of these boutons (Fig. 11).

Similar boutons are also found to synapse upon somatic spines of the Purkinje cell (Fig. 12), where the other type of synapse commonly found originates from the few basket cells unaffected by MAM.

These large boutons, according to the common opinion (Larramendi, 1969; Palay and Chan-Palay, 1974), share the ultrastructural features of recurrent collaterals of the Purkinje cell axon.

Thus, in this model, it appears that in the absence of the two principal afferent systems, namely the climbing and parallel fibers, the Purkinje

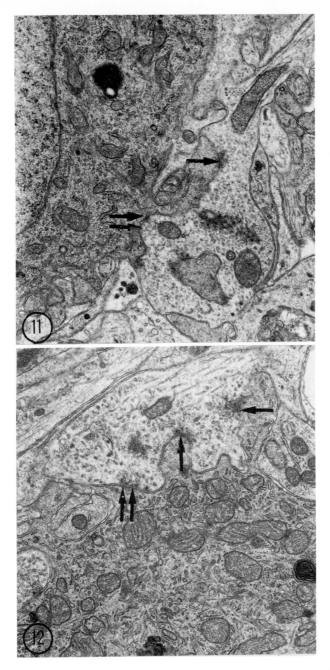

FIG. 11. 19 DIV. Culture treated with MAM. Dendrite of a Purkinje cell with spines (single arrow) and shaft (double arrow) contacted by a large bouton similar to that of Fig. 12. (×20,000.)

FIG. 12. 19 DIV. Culture treated with MAM. Perikaryon of a Purkinje cell with spines (single arrow) and soma (double arrow) contacted by a large bouton that shows characteristic features of the Purkinje recurrent axon collateral. (×20,000.)

dendrite is able to undergo differentiation, and especially to show the specific postsynaptic structures, i.e., spines. In the absence of the normal afferents, these sites are occupied by the only important type of axon present in the cultures — the Purkinje axon collateral.

DISCUSSION

More than 80 years ago (1890), Ramón y Cajal and von Lenhossek independently described for the first time "growth cones" at the tip of growing nerve expansions in embryonic material. At that time these growing tips were described by Ramón y Cajal (1890) as "club- or cone-shaped thickenings from whose base arose at times spines and fine appendices." Later, with the help of neurofibrillar methods, Ramón y Cajal (1906) was able to show that the neurofibrillar framework did not occupy the whole cone, and took the form of a lance, or the tip of a brush. Bud- and olive-shaped forms were attributed to "slow" cones, or "arrested fibers." In any case, Ramón y Cajal (1928) made a clear-cut distinction between active growing tips, club- or cone-shaped, and large bulbous tips, thought to be degenerative in nature.

Harrison (1910) elegantly illustrated for the first time the *in vitro* behavior of growing nerve fibers, and again he stressed the presence of "filopodia" upon actively moving growing tips.

Since then, Lewis (1950), Nakai (1959), and especially Pomerat et al. (1967) have illustrated the *in vitro* aspects of growth cones. The main conclusions that arose from these studies concerned the variety of shape and sizes of growth cones, according to the tissue under examination, and even in the same tissue. Emphasis was placed on the activity of filopodia; most often, the only mention as to the nature of the process involved refers to "neurites," and sometimes to axons.

More recently, Morest (1969) illustrated the morphology of dendritic growth cone in Golgi-stained material, pointing to the variability of their shapes, and the constant presence of filopodia, along the whole "distal segment" (cf. Figs. 5 and 6).

Ultrastructural study of growth cones by Bodian (1966) in the spinal cord and del Cerro and Snider (1968) and Kawana et al. (1971) in the cerebellum made no clear mention of filopodia, and described growth cones as varicosities filled with numerous electron-lucent vacuoles. Conversely, Tennyson (1970) *in vivo,* Yamada et al. (1970a or b, 1971), Bunge and Bray (1973b), Bunge (1973), and Privat et al. (1973), *in vitro,* pointed to the presence of filopodia containing a filamentous material while the varicosity contained the following organelles: cisternae of smooth ER, vacuoles, mitochondria, and eventually a few microtubules.

Dendritic growth cones have been studied with the electron microscope by Sotelo and Palay (1968) in the lateral vestibular nucleus of the adult rat, by Hinds and Hinds (1972) in the neonatal mouse olfactory bulb, by Hayes and Roberts (1973) in the amphibian embryo spinal cord, by Vaughn et al. (1974) in the mouse spinal cord, and by Privat et al. (1973 and Figs. 2, 5, and 6) in the rat cerebellum *in vitro*—like "neuritic" growth cones, they affect a large variety of shapes and sizes, and some of their organelles lack mitochondria from some varicosities, glycogen is seldom found, and the extent of smooth ER may vary. A general consensus (for details see Bray, 1973*b;* Bunge, 1973) is nonetheless reached as to the role of filaments in the active process of movement of filopodia and as to that of smooth ER in the building of new membrane. The model theory elaborated by Bray (1973*b*) to account for the complex interaction between filopodia, vacuoles, filaments, and tubules, may then be applied to both axonal and dendritic growth cones.

The possible association of dendritic growth cones with early synapse formation was hypothesized by Morest (1969) and was visualized among others by Hinds and Hinds (1972), Hayes and Roberts (1973), Tennyson, Mytilineou, and Barrett (1973), Privat, Drian, and Mandon (1974), and Vaughn et al. (1974). The systematic observation of such a conjunction led Vaughn et al. (1974) to determine the possible role of synaptogenesis in the induction of dendritic growth. Such a mechanism was accounted, in the detailed analysis of Kornguth and Scott (1972), for the growth of the Purkinje cell dendrite. In this case, the climbing fibers, first synapsing upon the soma, then upon the dendrites, were thought to be responsible for the outgrowth of the latter. A somewhat similar explanation was formulated by Hamori (1973) for the differentiation of dendritic spines in an agranular cerebellum: the activation provided by synaptic contacts of climbing fibers could elect spine formation over the whole dendritic tree. Our present results with tissue culture (Privat et al., 1973, 1974; Calvet, Drian, and Privat, 1974; Privat and Drian, 1974) allow some clarification of this problem. Although early synapse formation may occur upon growing PCD (Figs. 2, 9, and 10), this does not seem necessary to elect dendritic growth. Indeed, when climbing (Figs. 7 and 8) and parallel fiber activity (Figs. 11 and 12) are absent before the outgrowth of PCD (Crepel, 1972), their growth is not precluded, and spines can develop as well. It is only later, in the second model (Privat and Drian, *in preparation*) that synaptic sites on these spines are occupied by Purkinje axon collaterals. Therefore, it appears that neither climbing fibers nor parallel fibers are necessary for the PCD to grow and that parallel fibers were not necessary, for the outgrowth of tertiary spines was already well documented by several works upon agranular cerebella (Herndon, Hirano, Sotelo, *this volume*). That these afferents have a definitive responsibility in the tridimensional development of PCD is evidenced by the fact that in agranular cerebella, as well as in our cultures, the dendritic tree is markedly different from the normal; spiny branchlets are absent, the primary dendritic trunks are studded with spines (Fig. 7), and their direction appears to be random.

Therefore, the high degree of sophistication attained by the dendritic arborization of at least one class of neuron, the Purkinje cell, appears to be the result of several influences. First, a genetic factor is involved, which promotes the growth as well as the differentiation of receptive surfaces. Second, the microenvironment, and essentially the putative afferent axons, appear to act as growth modulators, possibly through the action of gradients (Herndon, *this volume*). That the Purkinje cell is in some way a unique example has been suggested by Hirano and Dembitzer (1974); conversely, in the visual pathway, dendritic spines on pyramidal cells are apparently reduced in number when the animals (mice) are reared in the dark (Valverde, 1967, 1968). In any case, it is not known at present whether the decreased number of spines is caused by agenesis or by destruction.

CONCLUSION

The *in vitro* study of dendritic growth has provided some information about the mechanism of dendritic elongation with correlative light, transmission, and scanning electron microscopy. In addition, it has been possible, with the use of two different models of cultivated cerebellum, to delineate more precisely than with *in vivo* models, the relative importance of genetic and epigenetic factors responsible for the adult dendritic configuration.

ACKNOWLEDGMENTS

This study has been made possible through a grant from I.N.S.E.R.M. (ATP 6). The constant help and advice of Dr. J. E. Gruner is gratefully acknowledged as well as the excellent collaboration of Miss M. J. Drian.

REFERENCES

Bodian, D. (1966): Development of fine structure of spinal cord in monkey fetuses. I. The motoneuron neuropil at the time of onset of reflex activity. *Johns Hopkins Med. J.*, 119:129–133.

Bray, D. (1970): Surface movements during the growth of single explanted neurons. *Proc. Natl. Acad. Sci. USA*, 65:905–910.

Bray, D., (1973*a*): Branching patterns of sympathetic neurons in culture. *J. Cell Biol.*, 56:702–712.

Bray, D. (1973*b*): Model for membrane movements in the neural growth cone. *Nature*, 244:93–96.

Bunge, M. B. (1973): Fine structure of nerve fibers and growth cones of isolated sympathetic neurons in culture. *J. Cell Biol.*, 56:713–735.

Bunge, M. B., and Bray, D. (1970): Fine structure of growth cones from cultured sympathetic neurons. *J. Cell Biol.*, 47:241a.

Calvet, M. C., Drian, M. J., and Privat, A. (1974): Spontaneous electrical patterns in cultured Purkinje cells grown with an antimitotic agent. *Brain Res.*, 79:285–290.

Crepel, F. (1972): Maturation of cerebellar Purkinje cells. I. Postnatal evolution of the Purkinje cell spontaneous firing in the rat. *Exp. Brain Res.*, 14:463–471.

del Cerro, M., and Snider, R. S. (1968): Studies on the developing cerebellum. I. Ultrastructure of the growth cones. *J. Comp. Neurol.,* 133:341–362.

Harrison, R. G. (1910): The outgrowth of the nerve fibers as a model of protoplasmic movement. *J. Exp. Zool.,* 9:787.

Hayes, B. P., and Roberts, A. (1973): Synaptic junction development in the spinal cord of an amphibian embryo. An electron microscope study. *Z. Zellforsch. Microsk. Anat.,* 137:251–165.

Hinds, J. W., and Hinds, P. L. (1972). Reconstruction of dendritic growth cones in neonatal mouse olfactory bulb. *J. Neurocytol.,* 1:169–187.

Hirano, A., and Dembitzer, H. M. (1974): Observations on the development of the weaver mouse cerebellum. *J. Neuropathol. Exp. Neurol.,* 33:354–364.

Hirano, A., Dembitzer, H. M., and Jones, M. (1972): An electron microscopic study of cycasin induced cerebellar alteration. *J. Neuropathol. Exp. Neurol.,* 31:113–125.

Kawana, E., Sandri, C., and Akert, R. (1971): Ultrastructure of growth cones in the cerebellar cortex of the neonatal rat and cat. *Z. Zellforsch. Mikrosk. Anat.,* 115:284–298.

Larramendi, L. M. H., and Lemkey-Johnston (1970): The distribution of recurrent Purkinje collateral synapses in the mouse cerebellar cortex: An electron microscope study. *J. Comp. Neurol.,* 138:451–482.

Lenhossek, Von (1890): Zur Kenntnis der ersten Entstehung der Nervensellen und Nervenfasern bei Vogelembryo. *Verh. X. Med. Kongr. Berlin.*

Lewis, W. H. (1950): Motion pictures of neurons and neuroglia in tissue culture. In: *Genetic Neurology,* edited by P. Weiss, Vol. 5. Chicago Univ. Press, Chicago, Illinois.

Llinás, R., and Nicholson, C. (1971): Electrophysiological properties of dendrites and somata in alligator Purkinje cells. *J. Neurophysiol.,* 34:532–551.

Morest, D. K. (1969): The growth of dendrites in the mammalian brain. *Z. Anat. Entwicklungsgesch.,* 128:290–317.

Murray, M. R. (1965): Nervous tissue *in vitro.* In: *Cells and Tissues in Culture,* edited by E. N. Willmer. Academic Press, New York.

Nakai, J., and Kawasaki, Y. (1954): Studies on the mechanism determining the course of nerve fibers in tissue culture. I. The reaction of the growth cone to various obstructions. *Z. Zellforsch. Mikrosk. Anat.,* 51:108–122.

Palay, S. L., and Chan-Palay, V. (1974): Cerebellar cortex—Cytology and organization. Springer-Verlag, New York, pp. 50–61.

Pomerat, C. R., Hendelman, W. J., Raiborn, C. W., and Massey, J. F. (1967): *Dynamic Activities of Nervous Tissue in Vitro.* In: *The Neuron,* edited by H. Hyden. Elsevier, Amsterdam.

Privat, A., and Drian, M. J. (1974): Première analyse ultrastructurale de la plasticité des circuits cerebelleux in vitro. *C.R. Acad. Sci. D.* 278:659–662.

Privat, A., Drian, M. J., and Mandon, P. (1973): The outgrowth of rat cerebellum in organized culture. *Z. Zellforsch. Mikrosk. Anat.,* 146:45–67.

Privat, A., Drian, M. J., and Mandon, P. (1974): Synaptogenesis in the outgrowth of rat cerebellum in organized culture. *J. Comp. Neurol.,* 153:291–308.

Rall, W. (1970): Cable properties of dendrites and effects of synaptic location. In: *Excitatory Synaptic Mechanism,* edited by P. Andersen and J. P. Jansen. Trönsö Univ. Press, Oslo and Bergen.

Ramón y Cajal, S. (1890): A quelle époque apparaissent les expansions des cellules nerveuses. *Anat. Anz.,* 5.

Ramón y Cajal, S. (1906): Genesis de las fibras nerviosas en el embrion. *Trab. Inst. Cajal Invest. Biol.,* 4.

Ramon y Cajal, S. (1928): *Degeneration and Regeneration of the Nervous System,* Vol. 1. Hafner, New York.

Sotelo, C. (1973): Permanence and fate of paramembranous synaptic specialization in "mutants" and experimental animals. *Brain Res.,* 62:345–351.

Sotelo, C., and Palay, S. L. (1968): The fine structure of the lateral vestibular nucleus in the rat. I. Neurons and neuroglial cells. *J. Cell Biol.,* 36:151–174.

Tennyson, V. M. (1970): The fine structure of the axon and growth cone of the dorsal root neuroblast of the rabbit embryo. *J. Cell Biol.,* 44:62–79.

Tennyson, V. M., Mytilineou, C., and Barrett, R. E. (1973): Fluorescence and electron microscopic studies of the early development of the substantia nigra and area ventralis tegmenti in the fetal rabbit. *J. Comp. Neurol.,* 149:233–258.

Valverde, F. (1967): Apical dendritic spines of the visual cortex and light deprivation in the mouse. *Exp. Brain Res.,* 3:337–352.

Valverde, F. (1968): Structural changes in area striata of the mouse after enucleation. *Exp. Brain Res.,* 5:274–292.

Vaughn, J. E., Henrikson, C. R., and Grieshaber, J. A. (1974): A quantitative study of synapses in motor neuron dendrite growth cones in developing spinal cord. *J. Cell Biol.,* 60:664–672.

Yamada, K. M., Spooner, B. S., and Wessels, N. K. (1970a): Axon growth: Role of microfilaments and microtubules. *Proc. Natl. Acad. Sci. USA,* 66:1206.

Yamada, K. M., Spooner B. S., and Wessels, N. K. (1970b): Ultrastructure and function of growth cones and axons of cultured nerve cells. *J. Cell Biol.,* 49:614–635.

Advances in Neurology, Vol. 12, edited by
G. W. Kreutzberg, Raven Press, New York
© 1975.

Application of Network Analysis to the Study of the Branching Patterns of Dendritic Fields

M. Berry, T. Hollingworth, E. M. Anderson, and R. M. Flinn

*Departments of Anatomy and Pathology, Medical School, University of Birmingham,
Birmingham B15 2TJ, England*

The dendritic arrays of neurons share the fundamental property of channeling the flow of material or information or both through a network of branches much as a river system. The geographic sciences have evolved a methodology closely linked with graph theory for describing and quantitating rivers and roadways (Haggett and Chorley, 1969) that is directly applicable to the study of the branching patterns of dendritic trees. The three-dimensional dendritic array of neurons is extremely complex, but some simplification can be achieved by ignoring such geometric components as the orientation, course, and length of individual segments, thereby reducing the pattern of branching of the array to a series of lines successively added to preexisting lines to form a simple tree-like structure rooted to the perikaryon. The theory of such systems, which only takes account of the pattern of branching, is called graph theory and is part of a branch of mathematics known as topology (Berge, 1958; Busacker and Saaty, 1965).

Mathematically the simplified tree-like arrangement of the dendritic array may be viewed as a plane graph composed of points – designated "vertices" – interconnected by lines – designated "arcs." Vertices at the outermost tips of the dendritic tree each connect one arc and are called "pendant vertices"; the respective "pendant arcs" are the terminal segments. Vertices connecting three arcs are the sites of branching, and both arcs and pendant arcs form the "segments" of the dendritic array. Moreover, the dendritic network has a functional orientation in that it is an afferent system that channels information toward a spike-generating area at the "root point" and hence is composed of "true" or directed arcs. The "sink" of an arc is defined as the next consecutive arc nearest the root point. Each sink drains two arcs. The latter are called the "sources" of each sink. The connectivity of a dendritic tree is defined as the mode of interconnection of arcs and pendant arcs in the network and is not used in the context of synaptic geometry. Branching patterns may be established by a variety of growth processes. This chapter describes the topologies of networks generated by monochotomous, dichotomous, and trichotomous branching. The large number of topologically distinct networks, which are possible with only small numbers of pendant arcs, precludes the application of many of the above considerations to all but the smallest dendritic arrays.

A less precise topologic approach to the quantification of large networks is to apply a method of ordering to the system by the assignment of a relative order of magnitude to all arcs. Several such methods have been adopted by geographers and have been applied to river systems. Horton (1945) introduced a method of ordering that led him to some important conclusions concerning the average configuration of streams in the network of a given basin. Of these only the first, which has become known as the Law of Stream Numbers is relevant to this discussion. This law states that "the number of streams of different order in a given drainage basin tends closely to approximate to an inverse geometric series in which the first term is unity and the ratio is the bifurcation ratio." Horton (1945) attempted to explain his law in hydrophysical terms, and Woldenberg (1966) considered it to be the outcome of allometric growth, i.e., relative growth of a part of the system being a constant fraction of the relative growth of the whole system. Others have suggested a graph-theoretical explanation. Consequently Scheidegger (1967) argued that a given river system represents nothing more than one particular example of a large number of possible arborescences with the same number of pendant vertices; he assumed that in nature every possible arborescence is equally possible. Such ideas fit better the fact that observed correlations between bifurcation ratios and environmental variables are poor. Computer simulation techniques have been employed (Shreve, 1966; Scheidegger, 1967; Liao and Scheidegger, 1968) to study large numbers of possible arborescences and such models have been compared with observed network patterns, both of which support the contention that natural networks arise as a result of random processes. These graph-theoretical explanations allow the application of methods of ordering to other naturally occurring networks, such as dendritic arrays, with the advantage over current methods of dendritic analysis of defining the entire system in quantitative topologic terms. Moreover, geometric parameters such as dendritic lengths are readily incorporated. With such information at hand it is possible that the elucidation of the integrative functions of the dendritic tree may be more attainable than by the use of traditional techniques of dendritic field analysis (Berry, Anderson, Hollingworth, and Flinn, 1972*a;* Berry, Hollingworth, Flinn, and Anderson, 1972*b,* 1973) and that the mode of growth of networks can be elucidated (Hollingworth and Berry, 1975).

MATERIALS AND METHODS

Topology

Branching patterns were constructed for different modes of growth from a single pendant arc. The position of the root point remained identical throughout. All topologic branching patterns, which were transformations of each other by rotation or reflexion about one or more vertices in two dimensions, were regarded as being topologically similar in three dimensions (see Figs. 1, 4, and 5).

Monochotomous Branching

Monochotomous branching occurs on segments only, and, with the addition of each new branch, the number of pendant arcs is increased by one. Figure 1 (row 1) illustrates this mode of branching and gives examples of some of the topologic types produced and their frequency of occurrence, if branching occurs on random segments.

Dichotomous Branching

Dichotomous branching can occur on segments and pendant vertices. This form of branching on segments increases the number of pendant arcs by two, but if branching is confined to pendant vertices only one pendant arc is effectively added. The resulting topologic branching patterns are illustrated in Fig. 1 (row 2).

Trichotomous Branching

The number of pendant arcs increases by two when trichotomous branching is confined to pendant vertices and by three by trichotomous branching on segments. The topologic types that may be generated by this form of branching are illustrated in Fig. 1 (row 3).

Hypotheses of Growth

The frequency of topologic types that are produced at each stage of branching is a function of the mode of growth of the network. For monochotomous, dichotomous, and trichotomous branching as defined above, we have worked out the frequencies of topologic types that occur over the first stages of branching when arcs are added randomly to existing arcs (segmental hypotheses) or added randomly to pendant vertices (terminal hypotheses). There is no evidence that dendrites grow by such stochastic branching, but these two alternative hypotheses are the easiest to test and will provide a guide to the deviation, if any, in the growth of dendritic networks from a purely random process. Figure 1 illustrates how the frequencies of topologic branching patterns may be worked out when these hypotheses are applied to each form of growth.

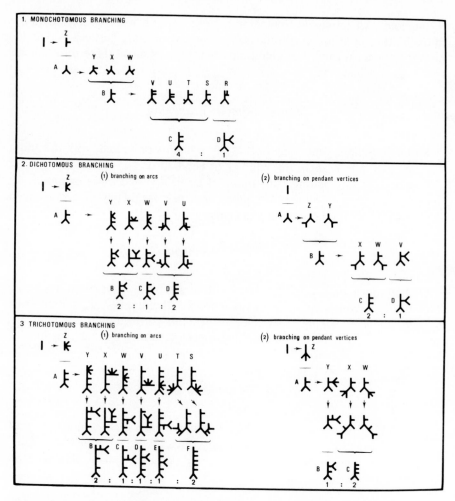

FIG. 1. Topologic branching patterns formed by monochotomous, dichotomous, and trichotomous branching. The root point of each pattern is the uppermost pendant vertex. (1) Monochotomous branching can occur only on arcs. Beginning with a single arc, the addition of another arc produces the topologic type Z. Type Z is represented in the standard format described in this chapter as A. The addition of one arc singly to any of the three arcs of A produces types Y, X, and W, which are resolvable into a standard type B. The addition of an arc singly to any of the five arcs of type B produces types U, V, T, S, and R, which are resolvable into two standard types C and D. If growth occurs by the addition of an arc to any of the five segments of type B, then the distribution of types C and D in the population will be 4:1, respectively. (2) Dichotomous branching can occur on arcs or pendant vertices. When this type of branching is constrained to arcs, the addition of one dichotomous branch to a single arc produces type Z. If subsequent growth occurs at the node this pattern may be transformed into type A. The addition of dichotomous branches singly to any of the five arcs of type Z produces types Y, X, W, V, and U. If growth occurs at the nodes of these types, topologic types B, C, and D are formed. If growth occurs by the addition of a dichotomous branch to any of the five segments of type A, randomly, then the distribution of types B, C, and D in the population will be 2:1:2, respectively. When dichotomous branching takes place on the pendant vertex of a single arc, type A is produced. The addition of dichotomous branches singly to the two pendant

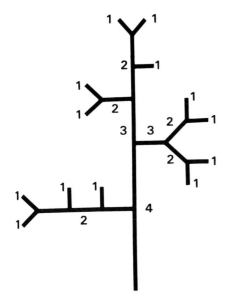

FIG. 2. Diagrammatic representation of the method of Strahler ordering. Terminal segments are assigned order 1. The confluence of order 1 branches forms order 2 branches; the confluence of order 2 forms order 3 branches, etc.; collateral branches converging on branches of higher order do not change the order of the branch into which they drain but divide it into segments.

Ordering of Topologic Branching Patterns

Horton's (1945) original concept of stream order contains a geometric element (angles); the simpler version by Strahler (1953) was chosen. According to this method all pendant arcs are first order and the junction of two first-order arcs produces a second-order arc. Second-order arcs receive only first-order arcs at their vertices. The junction of two arcs of second order produces an arc of third order. Third-order arcs may receive first- and second-order arcs at their vertices. Thus, the junction of an arc of order n with an arc of similar order produces a resultant arc of order $n + 1$. The method is shown diagrammatically in Fig. 2. A series of consecutive arcs

vertices of type A produces the patterns Z and Y, which are resolvable into a standard type B. The addition of a dichotomous branch singly to the three pendant vertices of type B produces type X, W, and V, which are resolvable into types C and D. If the addition of such branches is a random process, types C and D will be distributed in a population in the ratio of 2:1, respectively. (3) Trichotomous branching may occur on arcs or pendant vertices. The addition of a trichotomous branch to a single arc produces type Z, and if growth occurs at the node the standard type A is produced. The addition of a trichotomous branch singly to the seven arcs contained in type A produces the standard topologic types B, C, D, E, and F. If the addition of branches to arcs occurs randomly types B, C, D, E, and F will be distributed in a population in the ratio of 2:1:1:1:2, respectively. Trichotomous branching on the pendant vertex of a single arc produces type Z, and subsequent growth at the node produces the standard type A; the addition of trichotomous branches produces types Y, X, and W, and growth at the nodes produces the standard topologic types B and C. If branches are added randomly to vertices, then the types B and C will be distributed in the population in the ratio of 1:2, respectively. Note that it is assumed that only the node giving rise to the new branch is active and that the shaft from which the node springs is passive. If, however, both shaft and branch are active, branching patterns and frequencies will be different from those given here for trichotomous branching.

(or segments) of identical Strahler order is termed a "branch." A "daughter branch" or "collateral" is defined as any branch of $n - 1$ Strahler order or less that drains into a "parent branch" of Strahler order n.

Computer Simulation of Branching Patterns

Monochotomous Branching on Random Segments

Starting from a simple three-arc tree, with two pendant arcs and a third arc, representing the first part of the dendritic tree between the perikaryon and the first bifurcation, a network with the required number of pendant vertices was generated. If the tree had $2n - 1$ segments (i.e., arcs including pendant arcs), then a number k was chosen between 1 and $2n - 1$ using a random number generator. A list of segment numbers was kept and the tree branched monochotomously on the kth segment in this list, thereby generating a new pendant arc. The list of pendant arcs was updated, n was increased by 1, and the process was repeated until the required number of pendant vertices was obtained.

Dichotomous Branching on Random Pendant Vertices

Networks were generated in a manner similar to that described for monochotomous branching except that if there was a total of n pendant arcs, then k was randomly chosen between 1 and n and the network branched on the vertex of the kth pendant arc. The number of pendant arcs in the network increased by 1 with the addition of each branch.

Dichotomous Branching on Random Segments

The method of branching here was the same as that described above, but instead of a single pendant arc being added at random segments, a simple three-arc tree was added. The number n of pendant arcs increases by two with the addition of each branch.

Trichotomous Branching on Random Pendant Vertices

Branching patterns were generated as in dichotomous patterns by the addition of a simple five-arc tree at random pendant vertices. The number of pendant arcs in the network increased by two with the addition of each branch.

Trichotomous Branching on Random Segments

Networks were grown as described above, but instead of the addition of a single pendant arc to random segments, a simple five-arc tree was added, thereby increasing the number of pendant arcs in the tree by three.

Absolute Bifurcation Ratios

The mean bifurcation ratios of successive Strahler orders may be calculated for each complete group of topologic types common to a given number of pendant arcs (i.e., each complete pendant arc series) if the frequency of occurrence of each type is known. These ratios have been called absolute bifurcation ratios. Because a characteristic distribution of types is generated by each model, absolute bifurcation ratios may be used to test hypotheses of growth.

RESULTS

Monochotomous Branching

The table of possible topologic types of tree with from one to nine pendant arcs obtained by monochotomous branching on segments is given in Fig. 3.

It has been deduced (Berge, 1958) that for n pendant vertices the number m of topologically distinct structures theoretically possible is given by the expression

$$m = \frac{1}{(2n-1)} \binom{2n-1}{n-1} = \frac{1}{(2n-1)} \binom{2n-1}{n} \qquad (1)$$

When $n = 6$, 42 such structures are possible; these are shown in Fig. 4.

However, with respect to the topology of dendritic trees, it has already been stated that all types that are transformations of each other by rotation or reflexion about one or more vertices in two dimensions may be regarded as being topologically similar in three dimensions; this is because such differences are imposed by the position of the observer and may therefore be arbitrary (see Fig. 5).

The 42 branching patterns seen in Fig. 4 may be resolved into six topologically distinct types (Fig. 5) by application of this latter principle.

The number of topologic branching patterns that are possible in a given complete nth pendant arc series (for definition see previous section of Materials and Methods) can be calculated using the recursive function defined by the following formulas (Etherington, 1937) and

$$f(1) = 1$$

$$m = f(n) = \frac{1}{2} \sum_{r=-1}^{n-1} f(r) \cdot f(n-r) + \frac{1}{2} f\left(\frac{n}{2}\right) \times \left((n+1) \bmod 2\right) \qquad (2)$$

are listed in Table 1.

The distribution of types in each complete pendant arc series can be calculated for a given hypothesis of growth. The distribution of topologic types when branching occurs on random segments is given in Fig. 3. When

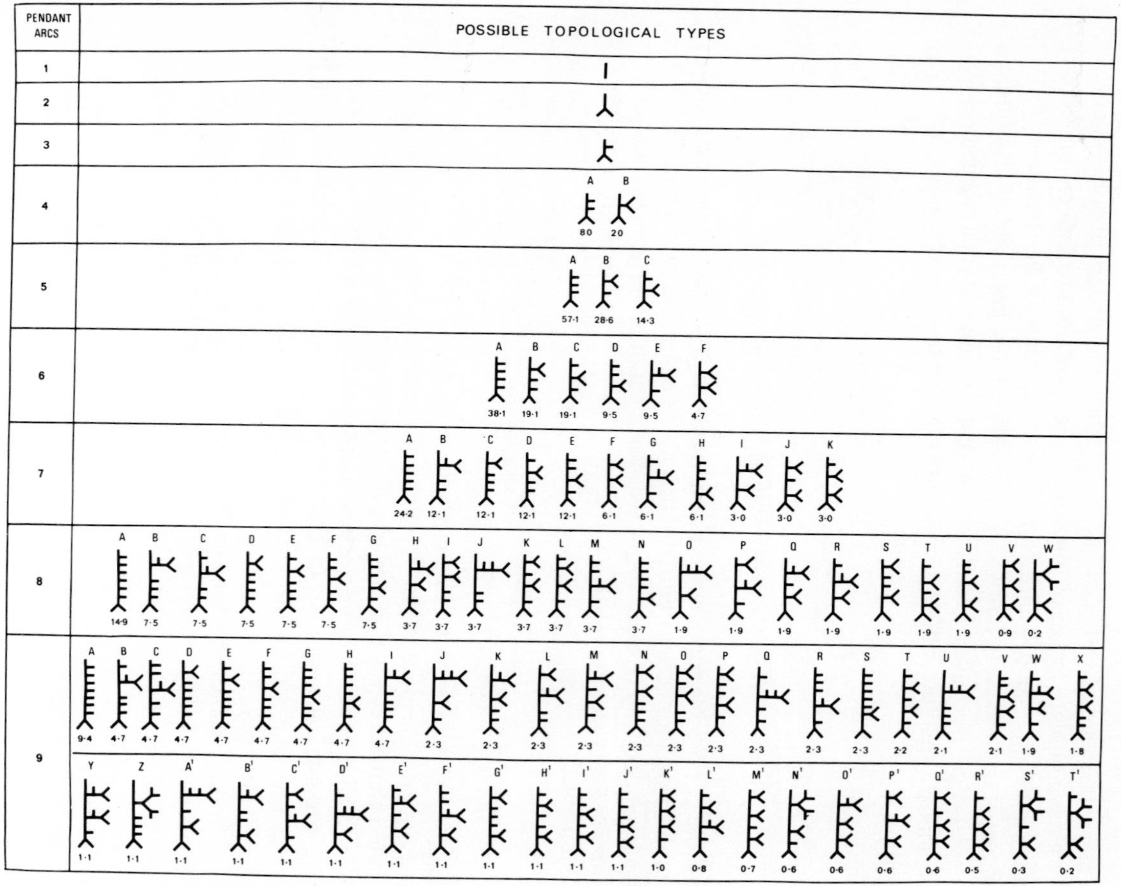

FIG. 3. Possible topologic types generated by monochotomous branching on segments in networks with from one to nine pendant arcs are listed together with the frequency of occurrence (%) of types when branching occurs on random segments. The letter associated with each topologic type may be used for identification.

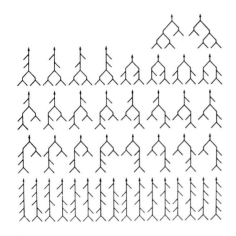

FIG. 4. Possible topologic types in networks with six pendant arcs in which mirror images and right and left distinctions are included—the arrow indicates the root point of the network (Shreve, 1966.)

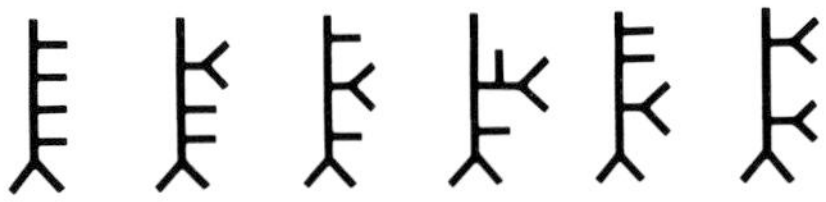

FIG. 5. Topologic types from networks with six pendant arcs after equating mirror images and right and left distinctions shown in Fig. 4.

monochotomous branching occurs on random pendant arcs the networks generated are indistinguishable from those grown by dichotomous branching on random pendant vertices (see below). The preceding arguments apply to trees that grow by the addition of one arc only with the formation of each branch.

Dichotomous Branching

Dichotomous branching on pendant vertices gives rise to the same number of complete pendant arc series as monochotomous branching on segments (Fig. 6), as only one pendant arc is added with each branch. The distribution of topologic types in each series is different. The distribution of topologic branching patterns when dichotomous branching occurs on random pendant vertices is given in Fig. 6.

When dichotomous branching occurs on segments, two different groups of topologic branching patterns occur. In one group four arcs stem from each vertex; this pattern is thus clearly distinguishable from all other forms of branching (Fig. 1). In the other group growth at the vertex transforms each branch into a form topologically identical to the patterns achieved by monochotomous segmental branching and dichotomous branching on pendant vertices (see Fig. 1). However, because two pendant arcs are added with each branch, even-numbered pendant arc series are not possible with this form of growth (Fig. 7). The topologic branching patterns that occur in odd pendant arc series are the same as those that occur in the odd series of monochotomous segmental and dichotomous branching on pendant

TABLE 1. *Number of unique topologic branching patterns in networks with from 1 to 17 pendant arcs*

Number of pendant arcs	1	2	3	4	5	6	7	8	9	10	11	12	13	14	15	16	17	n
Number of topologic types in the network	1	1	1	2	3	6	11	23	46	98	207	451	983	2,179	4,850	10,905	24,631	see Eq. (2)

Note the exponential rise in the number of topologic types so a small network with as few as 17 pendant arcs has the potential of producing 24,631 different branching patterns. For the method of calculation of the number of possible topologic types see Eq. (2).

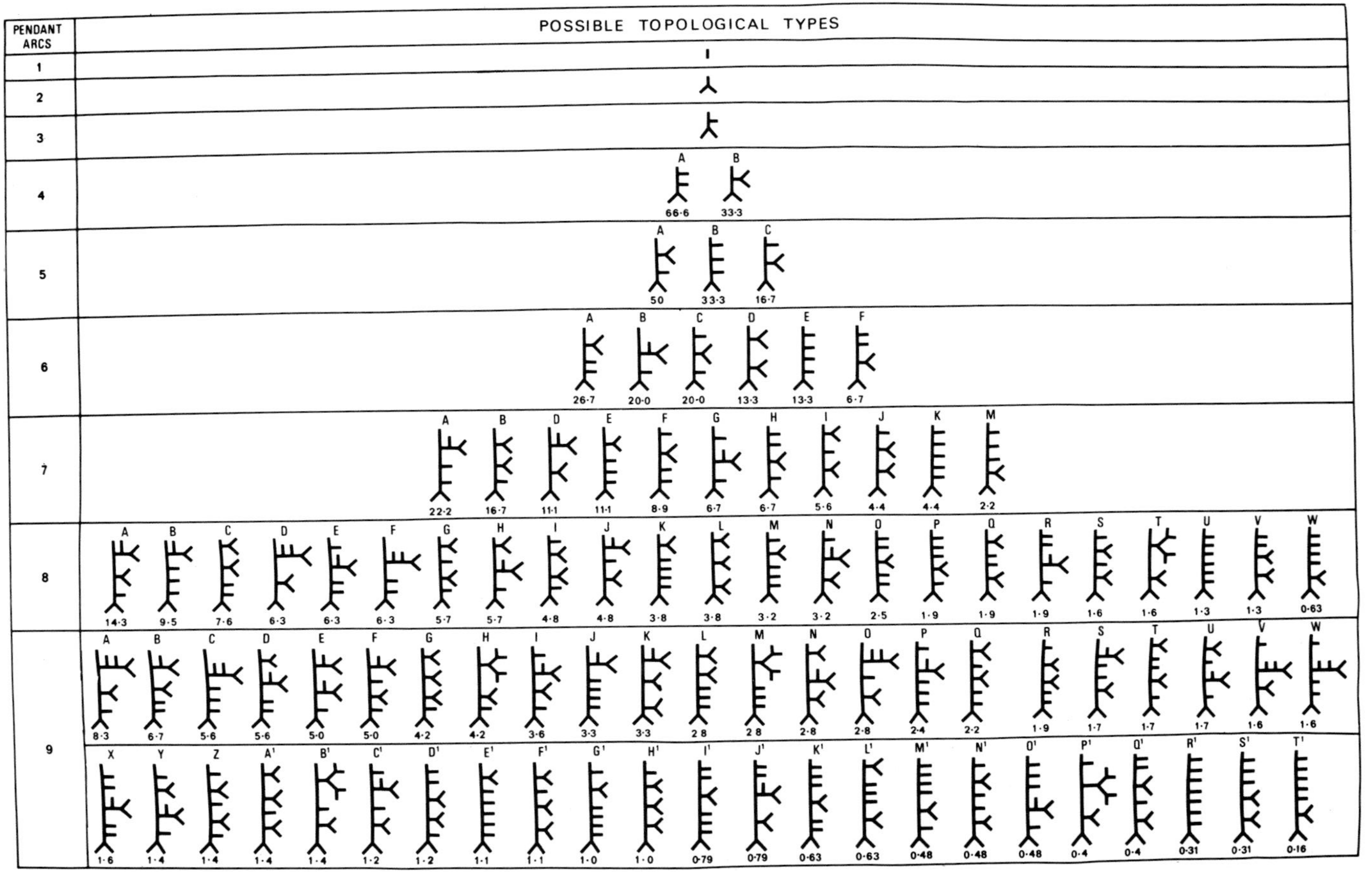

FIG. 6. Possible topologic types generated by dichotomous branching on pendant vertices in networks with from one to nine pendant arcs. When branching occurs on random pendant vertices the frequencies of occurrence of types are those listed. The letters associated with each topologic type may be used for identification.

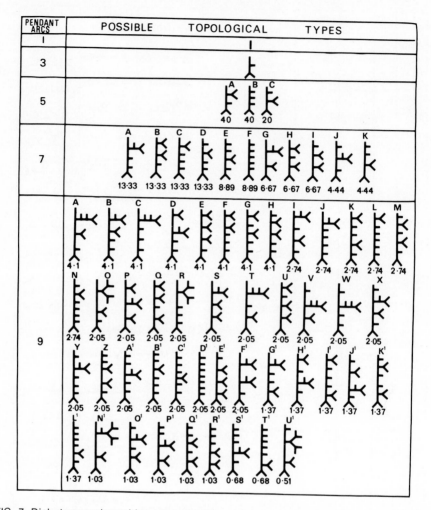

FIG. 7. Dichotomous branching on segments generates the topologic types shown. Because two arcs are added with each branch, even-numbered pendant arc series are missing. The frequency of topologic types when branching occurs on random segments is shown. The letters associated with each topologic type may be used for identification.

vertices, but their distribution is different. The distribution of topologic branching types when dichotomous branching occurs on random segments is given in Fig. 7.

Trichotomous Branching

Trichotomous branching on pendant vertices produces two distinct groups of topologic branching patterns. One group is characterized by having four arcs converging on each vertex (Fig. 1). In the other group,

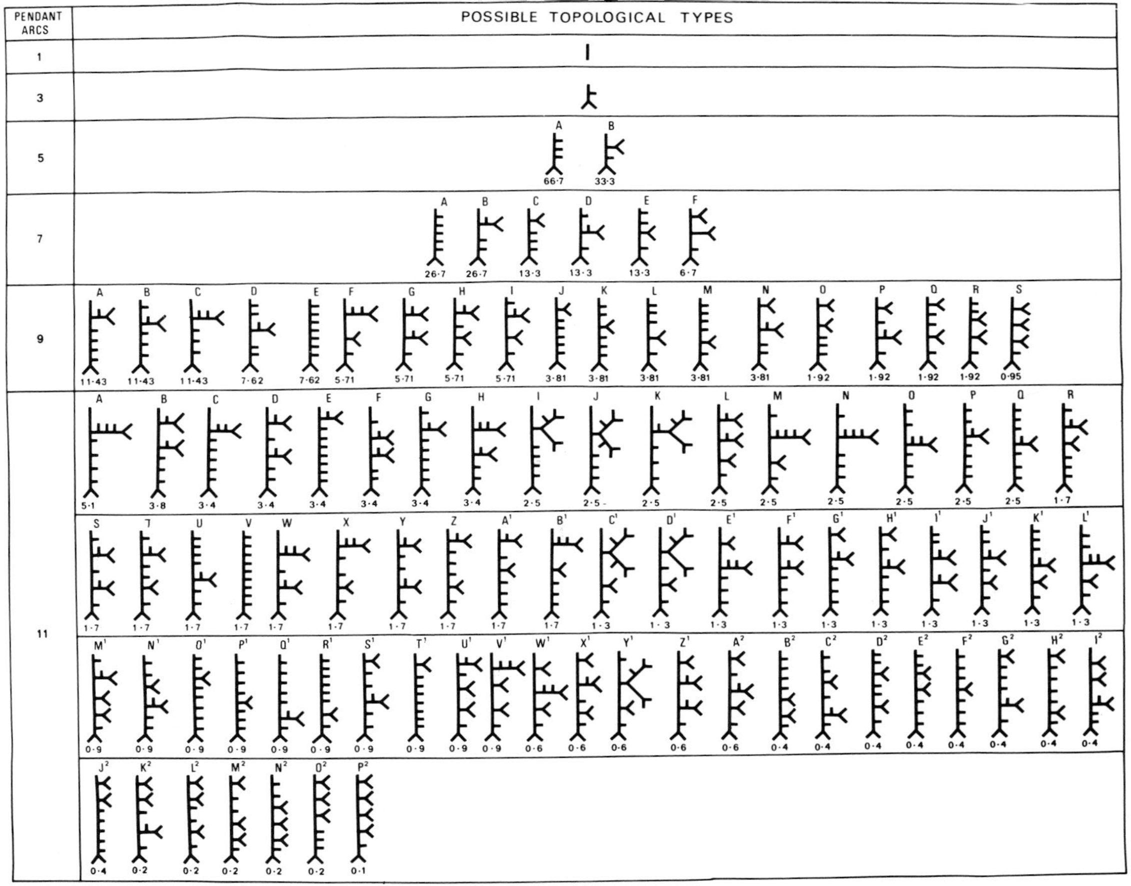

FIG. 8. Trichotomous branching on pendant vertices produces the topologic types listed. Because two arcs are added with each branch even-numbered pendant arcs series are absent. The frequencies of occurrence of types are given when branching occurs on random pendant vertices.

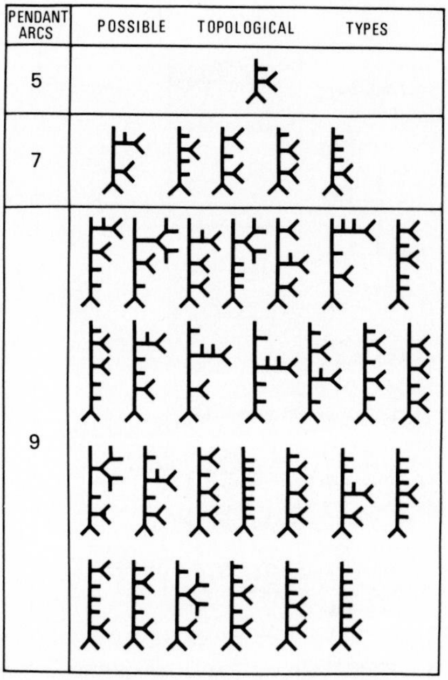

FIG. 9. The maximum number of topologically distinct branching patterns in the pendant arc series of systems growing by the addition of one arc only at each branch is given in Table 1, and the topologic types in the 1st to 9th pendant arc series are listed in Figs. 3 and 6. Trichotomous branching on pendant vertices is unable to generate the full complement of the above topologic types, and those that are missing from the 5th, 7th and 9th pendant arc series are shown.

growth at the vertices again transforms the branching pattern into a form that is indistinguishable from other arrays sharing the feature of having three arcs converging at each node. In common with dichotomous segmental branching trichotomous branching on pendant vertices generates two pendant arcs with the addition of each branch, and thus only odd pendant arc series are possible. This form of growth may, however, be distinguished from dichotomous segmental growth because the number of topologic branching patterns is reduced in each odd pendant arc series and their distribution is different (Fig. 8). The distribution of topologic types for trichotomous branching occurring on random pendant vertices is shown in Fig. 8. The topologic branching patterns that are missing from the 5th, 7th, and 9th pendant arc series are shown in Fig. 9.

Trichotomous branching on segments produces two groups of topologic branching patterns. The vertices of one group all have five arcs converging into them, but growth at the vertices of the other group produces a branching pattern that is indistinguishable from other forms in which three arcs stem from each vertex. In this latter group three pendant arcs are added with the addition of each branch, and therefore only the 1st, 4th, 7th, 10th, etc., pendant arc series are formed by this mode of growth. The numbers of topologic branching types in these pendant arc series is not the same as occurs in all forms of monochotomous and dichotomous branching or in trichotomous branching on pendant vertices. The distribution of topologic branching patterns in each pendant arc series is also characteristic. The

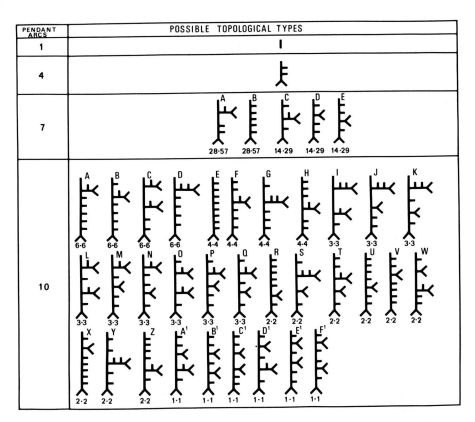

FIG. 10. Trichotomous branching on segments generates the topologic types shown. Because three arcs are added with each branch, the 2nd and 3rd, 5th and 6th, 8th and 9th, etc., pendant arc series are missing. The frequencies of topologic types that occur when branching occurs on random segments are listed. The letter associated with each topologic type may be used for identification.

FIG. 11. The maximum number of topologically distinct branching patterns in the pendant arc series of systems growing by the addition of one arc only at each branch is given in Table 1, and the topological types in the first to ninth pendant arc series are listed in Figs. 3 and 6. Trichotomous branching on segments is unable to generate the full complement of the above topologic types, and those that are missing from the 4th and 7th pendant arc series are shown.

distribution of topologic branching patterns when trichotomous branching occurs at random segments is given in Fig. 10.

The topologic branching patterns missing from each pendant arc series in relationship to monochotomous, all forms of dichotomous, and trichotomous branching on pendant vertices are listed in Fig. 11.

Absolute Bifurcation Ratios

Each topologic branching pattern in a complete pendant arc series may be ordered by the Strahler method. By summing the products of the frequency and the total number of each Strahler order from each topologic type in a series, the absolute bifurcation ratio between adjacent orders in that series may be calculated. Pendant arc series with a common number of Strahler orders are contained in the same order rank (see Tables 2–6). The attainment, by the kth order rank, of $k+1$, $k+2$, . . . $k+n$ order rank occurs in a stepwise progression. The progression is characterized by the

TABLE 2. *Absolute bifurcation ratios of networks exhibiting monochotomous branching on random segments*

No. pendant arcs	1 (%)	Ratio 1:2	2 (%)	Ratio 2:3	3 (%)	Ratio 3:4	4 (%)	Overall bifurcation ratio (slope of linear regression)	Order rank
1	100 (100)								1
2	200 (66.6)	2	100 (33.3)					2 ⎫	
3	300 (75.0)	3	100 (25.0)					3 ⎭	2
4	400 (74.1)	3.3	120 (22.2)	6	20 (3.7)			4.5 ⎫	
5	500 (72.9)	3.5	142.9 (20.8)	3.3	42.9 (6.3)			3.4 ⎪	
6	600 (72.4)	3.6	166.6 (20.1)	2.69	61.9 (7.5)			3.1 ⎬	3
7	699.3 (72.4)	3.7	190.7 (19.8)	2.52	75.7 (7.8)			3.0 ⎭	
8	801.6 (72.7)	3.7	215.8 (19.6)	2.5	85.5 (7.8)	427.5	0.2 (0.02)	13.2 ⎫	
9	892.8 (73.0)	3.8	237.3 (19.4)	2.6	90.9 (7.4)	82.6	1.1 (0.09)	8.2 ⎭	4

See Results and Fig. 5 for full explanation.

TABLE 3. *Absolute bifurcation ratios of networks exhibiting dichotomous branching on random pendant vertices*

No. pendant arcs	1 (%)	Ratio 1:2	2 (%)	Ratio 2:3	3 (%)	Ratio 3:4	4 (%)	Overall bifurcation ratio (slope of linear regression)	Order rank
				Strahler orders					
1	100 (100)								1
2	200 (66.6)	2	100 (33.3)					2 ⎫	
								⎬	2
3	300 (75.0)	3	100 (25.0)					3 ⎭	
4	400 (70.6)	3	133.4 (23.5)	4	33.3 (5.9)			3.5 ⎫	
5	500 (66.8)	3	166.7 (23.3)	2.5	66.7 (9.9)			2.7	
6	600 (67.7)	3	200 (22.6)	2.3	86.7 (9.8)			2.6 ⎬ 3	
7	700 (68.0)	3	233.4 (22.7)	2.4	95.6 (9.3)			2.7	
8	800 (68.5)	3	266.6 (22.8)	2.7	100.2 (8.5)	62.6	1.6 (0.1)	7.1	
9	904.2 (68.4)	3	300.5 (22.7)	2.8	109 (8.2)	12.4	8.8 (0.6)	4.4 ⎭	

See Results and Fig. 6 for full explanation.

accumulation of orders of the highest Strahler category in successive pendant arc series in the kth-order rank to a critical magnitude after which the next consecutive pendant arc series is the first in the $k+1$ order rank. Order ranks contain few pendant arc series when the number of pendant arcs is small, but the number of series within order ranks becomes large with increasing numbers of pendant arcs. Pendant arc series at the beginning and end of a given order rank are called "immature" and "mature" pendant arc series, respectively. The bifurcation ratio between first and second Strahler orders increases steadily over pendant arc series. In most cases the ratio stabilizes to an established bifurcation ratio that is characteristic for a given pattern of growth. The established bifurcation ratio (1) for dichotomous branching on random terminal vertices is three and forms in the 3rd pendant arc series; for dichotomous branching on random segments it is 3.1 and is formed in the fifth pendant arc series; (2) for trichotomous

TABLE 4. *Absolute bifurcation ratios of networks exhibiting dichotomous branching on random segments*

	Strahler orders								
No. pendant arcs	1 (%)	Ratio 1:2	2 (%)	Ratio 2:3	3 (%)	Ratio 3:4	4 (%)	Overall bifurcation ratio (slope of linear regression)	Order rank
1	100 (100)								1
3	300 (66.7)	3	100 (33.3)					3	2
5	500 (69.4)	3.1	160 (22.2)	2.7	60 (8.3)			2.9 ⎫	
7	700 (69.0)	3.1	224 (22.1)	2.5	91 (9.0)			2.8 ⎭	3
9	906.54 (69.6)	3.1	290.64 (22.3)	2.8	102.24 (7.8)	28.5	3.59 (0.28)	5.8	4

See Results and Fig. 7 for full explanation.

TABLE 5. *Absolute bifurcation ratios of networks exhibiting trichotomous branching on random pendant vertices*

	Strahler orders								
No. pendant arcs	1 (%)	Ratio 1:2	2 (%)	Ratio 2:3	3 (%)	Ratio 3:4	4 (%)	Overall bifurcation ratio (slope of linear regression)	Order rank
1	100 (100)								1
3	300 (66.7)	3	100 (33.3)					3	2
5	500 (75.0)	3.8	133.3 (20.0)	4.0	33.3 (5.0)			3.9 ⎫	
7	700 (73.4)	3.9 ·	180 (18.9)	2.5	73.3 (7.7)			3.1 ⎬	3
9	899.7 (73.9)	4.0	224.7 (18.5)	2.4	92.4 (7.6)			3.1 ⎭	
11	1102.2 (74.6)	4.0	273.2 (18.5)	2.7	100.8 (6.8)	168	0.6 (0.04)	13.3	4

See Results and Fig. 8 for full explanation.

TABLE 6. *Absolute bifurcation ratios of networks exhibiting trichotomous branching on random segments*

No. pendant arcs	1 (%)	Ratio 1:2	2 (%)	Ratio 2:3	3 (%)	Ratio 3:4	4 (%)	Overall bifurcation ratio (slope of linear regression)	Order rank
				Strahler orders					
1	100 (100)								1
4	400 (80)	4	100 (20)					4	2
7	700.1 (74.2)	4.1	171.45 (18.2)	2.4	71.44 (7.6)			3.1 ⎫	3
10	1001.0 (74.6)	4.1	245.3 (18.3)	2.6	95.7 (7.1)			3.2 ⎬	

See Results and Fig. 10 for full explanation.

branching on random pendant vertices it is 4.0, and is formed in the 9th pendant arc series, and for trichotomous branching on random segments it is 4.1, and formed on the 7th pendant arc series (see Tables 3, 4, 5, and 6). An established ratio is not formed between the first and second Strahler orders by monochotomous branching on random segments by the 9th pendant arc series.

The absolute bifurcation ratio between the second and third Strahler orders does not become established over the third-order rank. Characteristically, the ratio in the immature pendant arc series is large, but progressively diminishes to a small value in the mature series. In the fourth-order rank the ratio appears to increase progressively in size and may, in some cases, becomes established within this order rank (see Table 3, for example). The ratio between the third and fourth Strahler orders is always large in the immature series of the fourth-order rank because the number of fourth Strahler orders is, initially, always small relative to the number of third Strahler orders.

The effect of these changes on the absolute bifurcation ratios in complete pendant arcs series in a given order rank is reflected in the overall bifurcation ratios (Tables 3, 4, 5, and 6), which show large deviations from the established bifurcation ratio. Except for the second-order rank, overall bifurcation ratios show a uniform deviation from the established ratio in that they are larger in mature series and progressively smaller in immature series.

The percentage frequency of occurrence of categories of adjacent Strahler orders exhibiting an established bifurcation ratio approximates to a constant

TABLE 7. Bifurcation ratios between Strahler orders of large networks grown by computer simulation

Mode of growth	Size of network (order)	No. of examples	Strahler orders													Overall bifurcation ratio (slope of regression line)
			1	Ratio 1:2	2	Ratio 2:3	3	Ratio 3:4	4	Ratio 4:5	5	Ratio 5:6	6	Ratio 6:7	7	
Monochotomous branching on random arcs	5th	40	356 ± 72	4.0	89 ± 18	3.9	23 ± 5	4.1	5.6 ± 1.6	5.6	1					4.3
	6th	59	423 ± 89	4.0	106 ± 22	3.9	27 ± 6	3.8	7.1 ± 1.9	3.1	2.3 ± 0.5	2.3	1			3.4
	7th	1	513	3.9	132	3.9	34	3.1	11	2.8	4	2	2	2.0	1	2.8
Dichotomous branching on random pendant vertices	6th	49	350 ± 72	3.0	117 ± 25	3.1	38 ± 9	3.2	12 ± 3	3.4	3.5 ± 0.9	3.5	1			3.2
	7th	51	434 ± 70	3.0	145 ± 23	3.0	48 ± 8	3.0	16 ± 3	2.8	5.7 ± 1	2.6	2.2 ± 0.4	2.2	1	2.8
Dichotomous branching on random arcs	5th	4	393 ± 31	3.0	131 ± 13	3.7	35 ± 3	3.7	9.5 ± 1.7	9.5	1					4.3
	6th	86	451 ± 62	3.0	151 ± 20	3.8	40 ± 6	3.6	11 ± 2	3.7	3 ± 1	3	1			3.4
	7th	10	463 ± 36	3.0	156 ± 16	3.6	43 ± 5	3.3	13.4 ± 1.8	2.6	5 ± 1	2.5	2	2		2.8
Trichotomous branching on random pendant vertices	5th	1	369	4.1	90	3.3	27	3.4	8	8	1					4.2
	6th	73	442 ± 62	3.9	113 ± 16	3.1	36 ± 6	3.3	11 ± 2	2.8	3.6 ± 0.9	3.6	1			3.3
	7th	26	474 ± 65	4.0	120 ± 11	3.2	38 ± 4	2.9	13 ± 2	2.6	4.6 ± 0.7	2.3	2	2	1	2.8
Trichotomous branching on random arcs	5th	3	361 ± 10	4.0	90 ± 5	3.6	25 ± 2	3.6	7 ± 1	7.0	1					4.2
	6th	90	447 ± 57	4.0	112 ± 15	3.5	32 ± 5	3.6	9.0 ± 2.0	3.3	2.7 ± 0.7	2.7	1			3.4
	7th	7	476 ± 47	4.0	122 ± 13	3.2	23 ± 5	2.9	13 ± 2	2.6	5 ± 1	2.5	2	2	1	2.8

Note the agreement between the bifurcation ratio of the smaller Strahler orders with the established bifurcation ratio shown in Tables 2–6 for each form of growth. Note also the disparity between the established ratios and the overall bifurcation ratios for each mode of growth and the constancy of the overall bifurcation ratios of networks of a given size, regardless of their mode of growth. See text for explanation.

value. For example, in those exhibiting an established bifurcation ratio of 3, approximately 66.6% of their Strahler orders are order 1, 22.2% are order 2, 7.4% order 3, etc.; in those exhibiting a ratio of 4, approximately 75.0% are order 1, 18.75% order 2, 4.69% order 3, etc.

Computer Simulation of Large Networks

Because the number of topologic branching patterns in pendant arc series grows according to functions as expressed in Eq. (2), it becomes difficult to work out bifurcation ratios from ordering topologic types in pendant arc series beyond about the 10th pendant arc series. Computer simulation is therefore useful both for estimating the established bifurcation ratio when stabilization has not occurred in the early pendant arc series, as is the case in monochotomous branching on random segments (Table 2), and for assessing the degree of deviation that overall bifurcation ratios exhibit from the established ratio in large networks.

It can be seen that networks formed by the addition of single branches to random segments have an established bifurcation ratio approximating to 4, but those with a single branch added at terminal segments only (dichotomous branching on pendant vertices) the established bifurcation ratio approximates to 3.

Networks adding two pendant arcs by dichotomous branching at random segments have an established bifurcation ratio approximating to 3, but a ratio approximating to 4 if branching is trichotomous at pendant vertices. Trichotomous branching on random segments generates a network with an established bifurcation ratio approximating to 4.

In every case the ratio between adjacent small Strahler orders bears the closest similarity to the established ratio for a given form of growth, and the greatest disparity is seen in the higher Strahler orders (Table 7). The overall bifurcation ratio may thus show considerable deviation from the established bifurcation ratio. For a given size of network the overall bifurcation ratio is similar for each mode of growth (Berry and Bradley, *submitted*).

DISCUSSION

Horton's Law

Horton's original observations have been interpreted in both stochastic and deterministic terms. Whereas workers such as Horton (1945), Gregory (1966), Eyles (1968), and Woldenberg (1966) have interpreted the data deterministically viewing the relationship between the numbers of streams of successive orders as the outcome of various constraints imposed upon the system, e.g., geologic factors, growth, and stream rejuvenation, a stochastic approach has been made by Shreve in particular (1963, 1966),

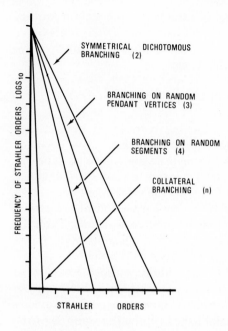

FIG. 12. Graphic illustration of some of the possible bifurcation ratios (numbers in parentheses) of bifurcating arborescences growing by the addition of one arc with each branch. n, Number of pendant arcs. See text for full explanation.

Scheidegger (1968a,b) and Smart, Surkan, and Considine (1967), who have considered the relationships between stream orders to be the outcome of a random process. However, it is clear from an analysis of the topology of branching patterns that the approximate inverse geometric series formed by the frequencies of Strahler orders is a fundamental property of branching networks, and that the overall bifurcation ratio of large networks is a parameter that is determined by the natural history of the network; it includes such factors as the mode of growth or the pattern of loss of branches or both and the size of the network. As a general rule the overall bifurcation ratio becomes more closely approximated to the established bifurcation ratio the larger the network becomes.

Because different modes of growth can generate networks with the same bifurcation ratio, it might appear that this parameter cannot be used to analyze growth. However, when the established bifurcation ratio is studied in conjunction with an analysis of topologic branching patterns, this ratio becomes specified to one form of growth. For example, systems growing by the addition of one pendant arc with each branch, have established bifurcation ratios ranging between 2 and n—the total number of pendant arcs in the network (Fig. 12). A ratio of 2 is found in an arborescence grown by symmetric, synchronous dichotomous branching at pendant vertices; a ratio of 3 by dichotomous branching on random pendant vertices or by monochotomous branching on random pendant arcs; a ratio of 4 by monochotomous branching on random segments; and a ratio approximating to n (the total number of pendant arcs) is found in a completely collateral system

(Fig. 12) as there is one branch of Strahler order 2 and there are *n* Strahler 1 segments.

It has been shown that other modes of growth produce bifurcation ratios of approximately 3 and 4, but these can be distinguished from the above by the occurrence of unique frequencies of the topologic types, and the characteristic absence of certain patterns in pendant arc series formed by other modes of growth.

The Strahler Method of Ordering

Several criticisms can be leveled against the Strahler system of ordering. For example, the technique may impose numerical constraints on branching networks that are too rigid so that artifactual results may be produced. This objection can be investigated by testing the same hypothesis using different ordering systems or by employing a technique that is independent of a system of ordering. In the former instance, Smit, Uylings, and Veldmaat-Wansink (1972) came to a conclusion similar to that of Hollingworth and Berry (1975) about the growth of basal dendrites, using a centrifugal system of ordering. The topologic analysis conforms with the latter criterion, and the results of Hollingworth and Berry (1975) obtained by this method also support the contention that the constraints of the Strahler system are minimal.

The technique does, however, ascribe a hierarchy of orders to the networks that appears inappropriate for the analysis of growth; this is because an array must be reordered each time a pendant arc is added, as a result of which there is no consistency of order for established branches during the growth of the network. Accordingly, it would appear more logical to order a dendritic network from the soma outward to avoid reordering the entire tree after the growth of new branches, and to allow comparison of growth rates of parts of the whole of the dendritic array. Coleman and Riesen (1968) devised a centrifugal system of ordering whereby first-order dendrites arise from the cell body, second-order dendrites arise from the first branching point, third-order dendrites from second branching point, etc. (see Fig. 13); the method has subsequently been used by Smit et al. (1972) and Greenough and Volkmar (1973) to study branching patterns in cortical dendrites. It has been claimed that this method has the advantage over a centrifugal system of ordering such as the Strahler method by assigning the same order to daughter branches and of not relying upon the identification of terminal segments before ordering can commence. However, there appears to be no special advantage to assigning daughter branches to the same order—on the contrary, such practice implies certain properties about growth for which there may be no evidence (Fig. 13). Smit et al. (1972) have argued that it is impossible to order a network by the Strahler method if branches are missing or incomplete. However, any

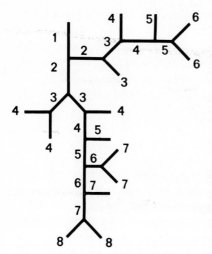

FIG. 13. Centrifugal method of ordering networks by Coleman and Riesen (1968). Although terminal segments are not identified by this method Smit et al. (1972) have subordered the system so that terminal and intermediate segments are designated. Daughter branches of a given order may arise together if dichotomous branching occurs on pendant arcs only. If branching occurs on segments, for example, then segments of a given order need not be formed at the same time. Note also that segments of a given order, *n*, are equivalent by this method in as much as they are preceded by $n - 1$ consecutive branches from first-order segments outwards. It may be incorrect, however, to infer that orders were established sequentially until the mode of growth of the networks has been worked out.

ordering system is subject to the same criticism because an ordering method offers a means of numerically recording the topology of an observed network and can make no assumption about parts of the network that are missing. Therefore, in practice, when an ordering system is applied to the study of dendritic branching, it is subject to the limitations that plague this field of research, e.g., the resolving power of the light microscope (Schadé, Van Backer, and Colon, 1964), the vagaries of the Golgi–Cox technique (Mitra, 1955; Nobach and Pupura, 1961; Schadé et al., 1964; Stell, 1965; Van der Loos, 1965, Beresford, 1966; Schadé and Caveness, 1968; Smit and Colon, 1969; Blackstad, 1970; Ramon-Moliner, 1970), and artifacts imposed both by histologic sectioning and by projection with the microscope (Berry et al., 1972).

Because the dendritic tree is made up of true or directed arcs that conduct information toward the soma, the Strahler ordering method is suited to the study of the structural basis of integration of electrophysiologic events within the dendritic network. Growth and conduction are operating in diametrically opposite directions; consequently, it may be more meaningful to study both using a reversed Strahler ordering method. This technique orders networks inward by the conventional Strahler method to establish the integrative pattern of branches after which the magnitude of the orders of each branch is transformed so that the branch of highest order, which drains into the soma, is ascribed order 1, the next lowest Strahler order branches order 2, etc. By this means established branches obtain a consistency of order so that analysis of growth is more easily undertaken and information about connectivity is retained.

Yet another disadvantage of the Strahler system of ordering is the fact that the method defines only the branches and not the segments of the tree thereby giving only general information about connectivity. One method of overcoming this objection is to note the number and order of daughter branches, or collaterals, that drain into parent branches of each order. If this is done it is possible to see more clearly how dendrites are joined together within the array (Hollingworth and Berry, 1975).

Absolute Bifurcation Ratios

The analysis of the absolute bifurcation ratios of networks with small numbers of pendant arcs offers a means of comparing branching patterns in small systems. Overall bifurcation ratios cannot be used because they appear to reflect only the size of the network and not the mode of growth. In small networks monochotomous branching on random segments differs from all the other forms of growth studied by exhibiting a greater variability of the overall bifurcation ratios of successive pendant arc series and by failing to achieve an established bifurcation ratio in any of the initial order ranks.

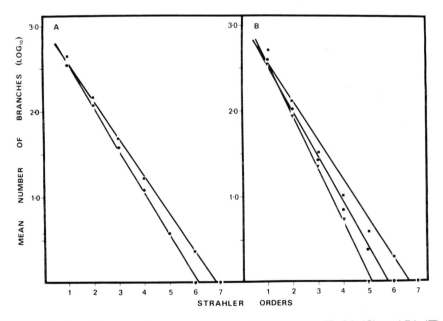

FIG. 14. Graph of the mean frequency of Strahler orders in 5th-(▼), 6th-(●), and 7th-(■) order networks. (A) Dichotomous branching on random pendant vertices; (B) monochotomous branching on random segments. (A) 6th-order networks: intercept, 3.08, slope −0.51, r, −1.0; 7th-order networks: intercept, 3.02, slope −0.45, r, −0.99. (B) 5th-order networks: intercept, 3.20, slope −0.63, r, −0.99; 6th-order networks: intercept, 3.07, slope −0.53, r, −0.99; 7th-order networks: intercept, 2.99, slope −0.45, r, −0.99.

This study of absolute bifurcation ratios illustrates that it is the established bifurcation ratio only that is the reliable index of growth. Therefore, comparison in large networks is meaningful using only the bifurcation ratios of small Strahler orders because it is these ratios that will most closely approximate to the established ratio. Moreover, comparison between overall bifurcation ratios is unlikely to be reliable as the degree of variability of the overall bifurcation ratio of a given network is accounted for by the frequency of occurrence of the network in the appropriate pendant arc series and the degree of "maturity" of the series in the respective order rank.

Analysis of Large Networks

It is possible to apply a topologic analysis to large networks by noting the topology of patterns at the periphery of the tree, e.g., the topology of network with from four to nine pendant vertices. Such an analysis will define the mode of growth of the network if the same mode of branching has occurred throughout growth and if no additional factors such as losses of segments or remodeling have disturbed the branching pattern (Berry and Bradley, *submitted*).

Another means of studying the growth of large branching arrays is to compare the inverse geometric series formed by the frequency of occurrence of Strahler orders with that of a network grown by computer in which the mode of branching is defined. It is stressed, however, that the growth of networks can only be compared by this method if the bifurcation ratios between the smallest Strahler orders only are used because these are the ratios that most closely approximate to the established bifurcation ratio for a particular mode of growth. The overall bifurcation ratio exhibits too great a variability to reflect accurately the underlying growth process of the network (Hollingworth and Berry, 1975), and when networks of a similar size are being compared it is likely that the overall bifurcation ratio will be similar regardless of the mode of growth (see Table 7 and Figs. 14–16).

Connectivity of Networks

Network analysis defines exactly the manner in which individual segments join with one another and channel information to the root point of the tree (see Discussion above). This form of analysis is clearly applicable to the study of the role of branching in the integrative function of the dendritic tree, and it is perhaps surprising that this is the first time that a quantitative method can make this claim. The additional information about the lengths and diameters of individual segments and synaptic density can be incorporated readily into the analysis to define the system more accurately.

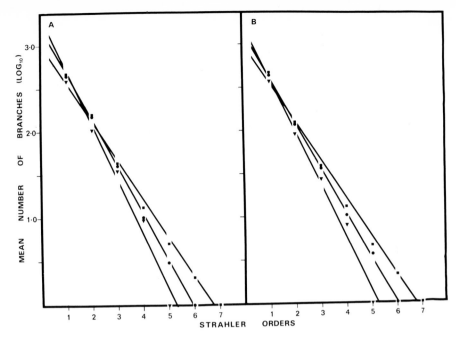

FIG. 15. Graph of the mean frequency of Strahler orders in 5th- (▼), 6th- (●), and 7th- (■) order networks. (A) Dichotomous branching on random arcs; (B) trichotomous branching on random pendant vertices. (A) 5th-order network: intercept, 3.34, slope −0.63, r, −1.0; 6th-order networks: intercept, 3.22, slope −0.54, r, −1.0; 7th-order networks: intercept, 3.05, slope −0.46, r, −1.0. (B) 5th-order networks: intercept, 3.23, slope −0.62, r, −0.99; 6th-order networks: intercept, 3.13, slope −0.52, r, −1.0; 7th-order networks: intercept, 2.99, slope −0.45, r, −1.0).

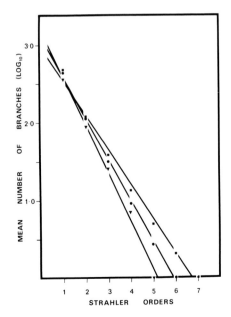

FIG. 16. Graph of the mean frequency of Strahler orders in 5th- (▼), 6th- (●), and 7th- (■) order networks produced by trichotomous branching on random arcs (5th-order network: intercept, 3.22, slope −0.62, r, −1.0; 6th-order networks: intercept, 3.13, slope −0.53, r, −1.0; 7th-order networks: intercept, 2.99, slope −0.45, r, −0.99).

SUMMARY

The technique of network analysis has been used to define the connectivity and growth of networks generated by monochotomous, dichotomous, and trichotomous branching.

The number of distinct topologic branching patterns exhibited by networks with a given number of pendant arcs is defined mathematically; when all types are represented, a complete pendant arc series is formed. The frequency of occurrence of topologic types in these series is unique for a given hypothesis of growth. The growth of the small dendritic arrays such as the basal dendritic fields of neocortical pyramids may be studied by comparing the actual frequency of topologic types with those computed according to given hypotheses. For larger dendritic networks such as those of Purkinje cells in the cerebellum it is only practicable to use the topologic types formed by the peripheral parts of the tree as a basis for comparison.

Individual dendritic segments can be ordered sequentially to define their hierarchical arrangement; the frequency of orders in a given network always forms an inverse geometric series. The ratio between orders is called the "bifurcation ratio," and the relationship in a given large series between adjacent orders becomes stabilized to a fixed or "established" bifurcation ratio at the periphery of the tree only. This "established ratio" characterizes the pattern of growth of the network. In the proximal part of the tree the ratio between adjacent orders is unstable and accounts for the variability of the overall bifurcation ratio exhibited by different networks with the same fundamental growth pattern and for the deviation of the overall from the established bifurcation ratio. For a given size of network the overall bifurcation ratio may be similar regardless of the mode of growth.

It is concluded that the precise definition of branching structures afforded by network analysis makes this technique well suited for the study of the connectivity, growth, and morphology of dendritic trees.

REFERENCES

Beresford, W. A. (1966): An evaluation of neuronatomical methods and their relation to neurophysiology. *Brain Res.,* 1:221–249.

Berge, C. (1958): *Théorie des graphes et ses applications.* Dunod, Paris. (English transl. by A. Doig, London, Methuen.)

Berry, M., Anderson, E. M., Hollingworth, T., and Flinn, R. M. (1972*a*): A computer technique for the estimation of the absolute three-dimensional array of basal dendritic fields using data from projected histological sections. *J. Microsc. (Oxf.),* 95:257–267.

Berry, M., Hollingworth, T., Flinn, R. M., and Anderson, E. M. (1972*b*): Dendritic field analysis—A reappraisal. *TIT J. Life Sci.,* 2:129–140.

Berry, M., Hollingworth, T., Flinn, R. M., and Anderson, E. M. (1973): Morphological correlates of functional activity in the nervous system. In: *Macromolecules and Behaviour,* edited by G. B. Ansell and P. B. Bradley. Macmillan, London.

Blackstad, T. W. (1970): Electron microscopy of Golgi preparations for the study of neuronal relations. In: *Contemporary Research Methods in Neuroanatomy,* edited by W. J. H. Nauter and S. O. E. Ebbesson. Springer-Verlag, Berlin, Heidelberg, and New York.

Busacker, R. G., and Saaty, T. L. (1965): *Finite Graphs and Networks.* McGraw-Hill, New York.

Coleman, P. D., and Riesen, A. H. (1968): Environmental effects on cortical dendritic fields. I. Rearing in the dark. *J. Anat.,* 102:363–374.

Etherington, I. M. H. (1937): Non-associate powers and a functional equation. *Math. Gaz.,* 21:36–39.

Eyles, R. J. (1968): Stream net ratios in the West Malaysia. *Bull. Geol. Soc. Am.,* 79:701–712.

Greenough, W. T., and Volkmar, F. R. (1973): Pattern of dendritic branching in occipital cortex of rats reared in complex environments. *Exp. Neurol.,* 40:491–504.

Gregory, K. J. (1966): Dry valleys and the composition of the drainage net. *J. Hydrol.,* 4: 327–340.

Haggett, P., and Chorley, R. J. (1969): *Network Analysis in Geography.* Arnold, London.

Hollingworth, T., and Berry, M. (1975): Network analysis of dendritic fields of pyramidal cells in neocortex and Purkinje cells in the cerebellum of the rat. *Phil. Trans. R. Soc. Lond. (Biol. Sci.),* 270:227–262.

Horton, R. E. (1945): Erosional development of streams and their drainage basins; hydrophysical approach to quantitative morphology. *Bull. Geol. Soc. Am.,* 56:275–370.

Liao, K. H., and Scheidegger, A. E. (1968): A computer model for some branching type phenomena in hydrology. *Bull. Int. Ass. Sci. Hydrol.,* 13:5–13.

Mitra, N. L. (1955): Quantitative analysis of cell types in the mammalian neocortex. *J. Anat.,* 89:467–483.

Nobach, C. R., and Purpura, D. P. (1961): Postnatal ontogenesis of neurons in cat neocortex. *J. Comp. Neurol.,* 117:291–308.

Ramon-Moliner, E. (1970): The Golgi–Cox technique. In: *Contemporary Research Methods in Neuroanatomy,* edited by W. J. H. Nauter and S. O. E. Ebbesson. Springer-Verlag, Berlin-Heidelberg-New York.

Schadé, J. P., and Caveness, W. F. (1968): Pathogenesis of x-irradiation effects in the monkey cerebral cortex. IV. Alteration in dendritic organization. *Brain. Res.,* 7:59–80.

Schadé, J. P., Van Backer, H., and Colon, E. (1964): Quantitative analysis of neuronal parameters in the maturing cerebral cortex. In: *Progress in Brain Research, Vol. 4: Growth and Maturation of the Brain,* edited by D. P. Purpura and J. P. Schadé. Elsevier, Amsterdam.

Scheidegger, A. E. (1966): Stochastic branching processes and the law of stream orders. *Water Res. Res.,* 2:199–203.

Scheidegger, A. E. (1967): On the topology of river nets. *Water Res. Res.,* 3:103–106.

Scheidegger, A. E. (1968a): Horton's Law of stream order numbers and a temperature-analog in river nets. *Water Res. Res.,* 3:103–106.

Scheidegger, A. E. (1968b): Horton's Law of stream numbers. *Water Res. Res.,* 4:655–658.

Shreve, R. L. (1963): Horton's "Law" of stream numbers for topologically random networks. *Trans. Am. Geophys. Un.,* 44:444–445.

Shreve, R. L. (1966): A comment on Horton's law of stream numbers. *Water Res. Res.,* 3: 773–776.

Smart, J. S., Surkan, A. J., and Considine, J. P. (1967): *Digital Simulation of Channel Networks,* pp. 87–98. Berne, IASH.

Smit, G. J., and Colon, E. J. (1969): Quantitative analysis of the cerebral cortex. I. Aselectivity of the Golgi–Cox staining technique. *Brain Res.,* 13:485–510.

Smit, G. J., Uylings, H. M. B., and Veldmaat-Wansink, L. (1972): The branching patterns in dendrites of cortical neurons. *Acta Morphol. Neerl. Scand.,* 9:253–274.

Stell, W. K. (1965): Correlation of retina cytoarchitecture and ultrastructure in Golgi preparations. *Anat. Rec.,* 153:389–397.

Strahler, A. N. (1953): Revisions of Horton's quantitative factors in erosional terrain. *Trans. Am. Geophys. Un.,* 34:345.

Van der Loos, H. (1965): Some notes on the properties of the Golgi-impregnation of vertebrate CNS. *Anat. Rec.,* 151:480.

Woldenberg, M. J. (1966): Horton's laws justified in terms of allometric growth and steady state in open systems. *Bull. Geol. Soc. Am.,* 77:431–434.

Advances in Neurology, Vol. 12, edited by
G. W. Kreutzberg, Raven Press, New York
© 1975.

Ordering Methods in Quantitative Analysis of Branching Structures of Dendritic Trees

H. B. M. Uylings, G. J. Smit, and W. A. M. Veltman

Central Institute for Brain Research, IJdijk 28, Amsterdam 1006, The Netherlands

Quantitative analysis of branching patterns in tree-like configurations, such as rivers, bronchial trees, arterial trees, wood trees, and neural dendritic trees, has been greatly enhanced by the method of ordering the segments or branches. In the literature, however, there exist several different methods of ordering the branching patterns. These can be grouped into two principal approaches, viz. the centripetal ordering system and the centrifugal ordering system.

The centripetal system starts with order numbering at the terminal segments of the tree, and numbers the segments progressively toward the stem. Different methods for centripetal ordering have been developed by Horton (1945), Strahler (1957), Scheidegger (1965), Horsfield and Cumming (1968), and Berry, Hollingworth, Anderson, and Flinn (1975).

In contrast, the centrifugal system starts with order numbering at the stem and then numbers upward toward the periphery (e.g., Rashevsky, 1960; Jones and Thomas, 1962; Weibel, 1963; Peters and Bademan, 1963; Coleman and Riesen, 1968).

The selection of the ordering method to be applied is of great importance because the different ordering methods may classify given segments into different groups. The main objective of ordering the segments is to group those which have similar definable structural and/or functional characteristics, for the purpose of correlating structure with function. Therefore, in view of this selection, this chapter compares certain properties of the centripetal ordering method that are most generally used, i.e., Strahler's method (e.g., Hollingworth and Berry, 1975) with properties of the centrifugal ordering method (e.g., Smit, Uylings, and Veldmaat-Wansink, 1972; Smit and Uylings, 1975), with respect to the analysis of neuronal dendritic trees. This chapter concludes with some preliminary criteria for selecting one of the two ordering systems.

DESCRIPTION OF THE TWO ORDERING METHODS

Strahler's Ordering Method

Using the Strahler method, we assign all terminal segments the order 1. The order is then raised by one wherever two segments of the same order

A   B

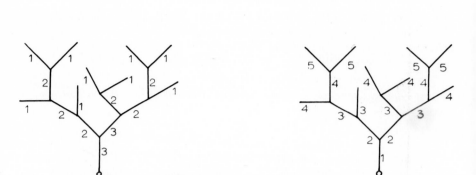

FIG. 1. (A) An example of the Strahler ordering method. (B) An example of the centrifugal ordering method.

meet. When two segments of unequal order meet, the highest-order number is retained (Fig. 1A). Thus it is possible that contiguous segments, before and beyond a bifurcation, have an identical order (Berry et al., 1975).

By applying Strahler's method, and by comparison with some growth hypotheses, Hollingworth and Berry (1975) have found in the cerebellar Purkinje cell dendrites of an adult rat that new dendritic segments arise mainly at the terminal segments. Furthermore, the Strahler method is suited for the study of connectivity of the dendritic segments within a dendrite (Berry et al., 1975).

Centrifugal Ordering Method

In the centrifugal system the proximal segment (i.e., the stem) is called the first-order segment. Beyond each bifurcation the order is raised by one, so that in each bifurcation the two daughter segments arising from a given mother segment always belong to the same order (Fig. 1B). Moreover, the mother segment is always one order lower than that of the two daughter segments.

By applying the centrifugal method, and by comparison with some growth hypotheses, Smit et al. (1972) have found in pyramidal cell dendrites in the visual cortex of an adult rabbit that new dendritic segments arise mainly at the terminal segments. Using the centrifugal method, it has been shown that the most peripheral part of the dendritic tree (i.e., segments of the higher orders) in several experimental studies undergoes the greatest change (e.g., Jones and Thomas, 1962; Greenough and Volkmar, 1973). Furthermore, the centrifugal method, too, is suited for the study of the connectivity of the dendritic segments within a dendrite.

SOME DIFFERENT PROPERTIES OF THE TWO ORDERING METHODS

It appears from the above discussion (see Description) that an analysis using one of the two ordering systems is more sensitive than the method of Sholl (1953). However, there are certain properties that differentiate these ordering methods, by virtue of which they cannot be used in the analysis of all kinds of branching patterns. The different properties are indicated below.

Applicability

1. In principle, the Strahler method is applicable to *all* types of branching patterns. It demands no special metrical and topologic characteristics of a branching pattern. The disadvantage of the Strahler method, viz. that contiguous segments can have the same order, can be overcome by noting, for instance, the number and order of the adjacent segments for a particular Strahler order (Hollingworth and Berry, 1975). 2. In a *metric* analysis, the centrifugal method can be applied only when the branching pattern is such that the two daughter segments of a bifurcation are metrically equivalent (i.e., have equal segment lengths and symmetric bifurcation angles). It is not necessary that a branching pattern be topologically symmetric, if in addition to the centrifugal order the segments are subdivided into terminal and intermediate segments (e.g., Peters and Bademan, 1963; Smit et al., 1972). A branching pattern is topologically symmetric when all the terminal segments have the same centrifugal order (i.e., the topologic distance from the stem to each terminal segment is equal, or the total number of segments at any order n is 2^{n-1}, if the stem is taken as the first order). Moreover, the bifurcation probability can be used as a parameter to describe the topologic asymmetry. The ith-order bifurcation probability is the quotient of the number of intermediate segments and the total number of segments of that order (Smit et al., 1972). When a branching pattern is completely symmetric in its topology, then the bifurcation probability for all the centrifugal orders is 1. Except for the highest order, the bifurcation probability is zero.

The more topologically asymmetric the branching pattern, the more will be the deviation of the above-mentioned relationship between bifurcation probability and order.

In the basal dendrites of cortical neurons, however, the daughter segments are equivalent with respect to segment lengths (Smit et al., 1972), and they generally have symmetric bifurcation angles (Smit and Uylings, 1975). Although apical dendrites do not have a completely symmetric branching pattern, it is possible to use the centrifugal method in the analysis of apical dendrites if the apical dendrites are subdivided into three sections: (a) the oblique dendrites, (b) the main shaft from soma until the so-called main bi-furcation point, and (c) the terminal tuft (Smit and Uylings, 1975).

Order of the Terminal Segments

1. When the Strahler method is used, all the terminal segments have the same Strahler order, whether they are near the soma or in the most distal part of the dendritic tree.

2. With the centrifugal method not all terminal segments need have the same centrifugal order, i.e., when the branching pattern is not topologically symmetric. The terminal segments near the soma will have in this case a lower order than the more distal terminal segments. Using the centrifugal method, Smit et al. (1972) found an overrepresentation of long segments in the highest-order terminal segments of basal dendrites in the visual cortex of an adult rabbit. Extrapolating from the segment lengths that had been found for the lower orders gave a specification of the growth potency assumed by Morest (1969) for dendrites in adult animals.

Effect of Missed Segments

1. In general, the Strahler method requires that no parts of the dendrites be missing, including the terminal portions, e.g., by cutting off a branch during sectioning. This is especially necessary for small topologically symmetric branching patterns. By missing a terminal segment (i.e., order 1 segment) in a topologically symmetric tree structure, the total ordering becomes altered.

The more a branching pattern is topologically asymetric, the less is the change in the Strahler ordering of the dendritic tree that is missing a terminal segment, and thus the less will be the change in the branching ratio (Barker, Cumming, and Horsfield, 1973). If a dendritic segment, or a part thereof, is missed, the Strahler ordering does not necessarily change.

2. If terminal parts of a dendrite are missed, e.g., in sectioning, the centrifugal ordering of the rest of the dendrite never changes. If a segment or segments within a given dendrite are missed, the ordering along the dendrite distal to the missed segment changes. The chance of missing a segment within a dendrite, however, is generally much smaller than that of missing the terminal parts.

Extensive Branching Patterns

1. The Strahler method seems to be very well suited for characterizing trees with a very extensive branching pattern, such as Purkinje cells of adult animals, because with this method the number of orders does not increase as much as the number of segments (see Fig. 1).

2. For characterizing entire trees having a very extensive branching pattern, the number of orders in the centrifugal method can be too unwieldy, especially if the analysis is intended to define the mode of growth of a full-grown branching pattern.

Bifurcation Angles

1. The Strahler method requires that the metric analysis of the spatial structure have at least some subordering. When the bifurcation angles are studied, the branching patterns have to be subordered in (a) bifurcations with a mother segment of a ith order and two daughter segments each of an $(i - 1)$th order, (b) bifurcations with a mother segment and a daughter segment of an ith order and a daughter segment of another order, separated into order $(i - 1)$, $(i - 2)$, etc. (See Fig. 2, the Strahler method, row C.)

In particular, the angle between successive, contiguous bifurcations (i.e., the torsion angle, Uylings and Smit, 1975) will be difficult to tabulate in relation to Strahler orders. It is possible to overcome this problem to a certain extent by tabulating the bifurcation in relation to the diameter of the mother segment (Horsfield, Dart, Olson, Filley, and Cumming, 1971). However, many segments of cortical neurons have a diameter at the limit of the resolving power of the light microscope.

2. Using the centrifugal method, we can tabulate the bifurcation angles in relation to the centrifugal order, and the torsion angles can be tabulated in relation to successive centrifugal orders.

Dendritic Outgrowth

1. The study of the dendritic outgrowth at different developmental stages necessitates an ordering method other than the centripetal method as the outgrowth is in a different direction (i.e., centrifugal). Berry et al. (1975) have therefore developed a *reversed Strahler method.* In this method the branching pattern is first ordered by the Strahler method, and then the sequence of the magnitude of the orders is reversed so that the branch of highest order becomes order 1, and a terminal segment is assigned the highest order (Fig. 2). Examining the consistency of the reversed Strahler order for already established branches during outgrowth, we have reversed the centripetal method of Horsfield-Cumming (1968), for comparing this with the reversed Strahler method (Fig. 2). It appears from Fig. 2 that with both of these reversed methods the orders of all established segments remains consistent, when new segments arise simultaneously at all terminal segments (see row D). It also appears that when the dendritic outgrowth is topologically more symmetric, the reversed Strahler order of many established segments changes, and that such changes are less with the reversed Horsfield-

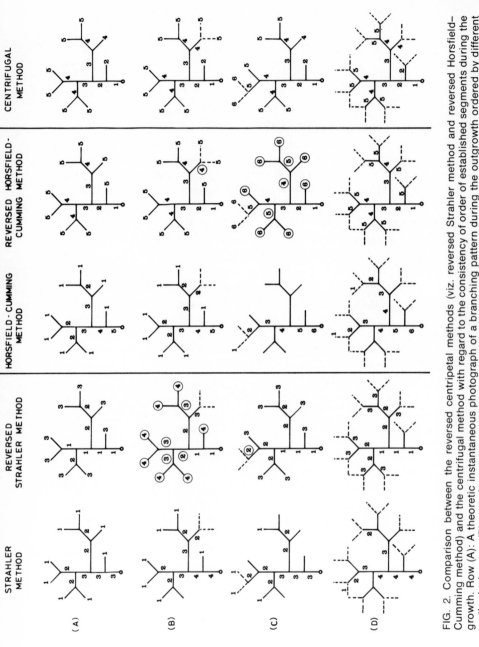

FIG. 2. Comparison between the reversed centripetal methods (viz. reversed Strahler method and reversed Horsfield–Cumming method) and the centrifugal method with regard to the consistency of order of established segments during the growth. Row (A): A theoretic instantaneous photograph of a branching pattern during the outgrowth ordered by different methods. In rows (B) and (C) one new segment has arisen, and in row (D) new segments have simultaneously arisen at all established terminal segments. The encircled numbers indicate those orders which are changed with respect to row (A). This was carried out only for the centrifugal method and the two reversed methods.

Cumming method (see row B). In contrast, it appears from Fig. 2 (row C) that, when the dendritic outgrowth is topologically totally asymmetric, the reversed Strahler order of the established segments practically does not change, unlike the reversed Horsfield-Cumming method.

2. The centrifugal order of established segments never changes during dendritic outgrowth (see Fig. 2).

CONCLUSION

In view of the different properties of the various methods described in the previous section, and in view of the main objective in ordering segments at all, viz. grouping together those which have similar characteristics, the following preliminary criteria are proposed.

When studying branching patterns that, when viewed metrically, are completely asymmetric, or when studying tree structures with a very extensive branching pattern such as the Purkinje cell dendrites, the application of the Strahler method is preferred.

When studying the outgrowth of dendrites, the reversed Strahler method is preferable only when the outgrowth is totally asymmetric (topologically and metrically). In all other cases, including that of full-grown apical dendrites of pyramidal neurons (see page 249), it appears that the centrifugal method is preferable.

In addition to the above-mentioned constellations, the following point is noteworthy with regard to research into the correlation between function and structure. So far as we know all of the models in the literature that describe physiologic phenomena in relation to the morphology of dendritic trees use the centrifugal ordering method (e.g., Rall and Rinzel, 1973).

SUMMARY

Two different ordering methods used in quantitative analysis of dendritic trees are compared with respect to the chief objective of doing the ordering, viz. grouping together those segments of a branching pattern which have similar characteristics.

After describing the different properties of these two ordering methods (i.e., Strahler method and centrifugal method), criteria are given for selecting one or the other of the two methods.

ACKNOWLEDGMENTS

We thank Mrs. S. W. Lust-Bosboom for typing the manuscript.

REFERENCES

Barker, S. B., Cumming, G., and Horsfield, K. (1973): Quantitative morphometry of the branching structure of trees. *J. Theor. Biol.*, 40:33–43.

Berry, M., Hollingworth, T., Anderson, E. M., and Flinn, R. M. (1975): This volume.

Coleman, P. D., and Riesen, A. H. (1968): Environmental effects on cortical dendritic fields. I. Rearing in the dark. *J. Anat.*, 102:363–374.

Greenough, W. T., and Volkmar, F. R. (1973): Pattern of dendritic branching in occipital cortex of rats reared in complex environments. *Exp. Neurol.*, 40:491–504.

Hollingworth, T., and Berry, M. (1975): Network analysis of dendritic fields of pyramidal cells in neocortex and Purkinje cells in the cerebellum of the rat. *Phil. Trans. R. Soc. Lond. (Biol. Sci.) (in press).*

Horsfield, K., and Cumming, G. (1968): Morphology of the bronchial tree in man. *J. Appl. Physiol.*, 24:373–383.

Horsfield, K., Dart, G. A., Olson, D. E., Filley, G. F., and Cumming, G. (1971): Models of the human bronchial tree. *J. Appl. Physiol.*, 31:207–217.

Horton, R. E. (1945): Erosional development of streams and their drainage basins; hydrophysical approach to quantitative morphology. *Bull. Geol. Soc. Am.*, 56:275–370.

Jones, W. H., and Thomas, D. B. (1962): Changes in the dendritic organization of neurons in the cerebral cortex following deafferentation. *J. Anat.*, 96:375–381.

Morest, D. K. (1969): The growth of dendrites in the mammalian brain. *Z. Anat. Entwicklungsgesch.*, 128:290–317.

Peters, H. G., and Bademan, H. (1963): The form and growth of Stellate cells in the cortex of the guinea pig. *J. Anat.*, 97:111–117.

Rall, W., and Rinzel, J. (1973): Branch input resistance and steady attenuation for input to one branch of a dendritic neuron model. *Biophys. J.*, 13:648–688.

Rashevsky, N. (1960): *Mathematical Biophysics. Physico Mathematical Foundations of Biology*, 3rd ed., Vol. II, Chapter 27, Dover, New York.

Scheidegger, A. E. (1965): The algebra of stream order numbers. *US Geol. Surv. Professional Pap.*, 525-B:187–189.

Sholl, D. A. (1953): Dendritic organization in the neurons of the visual and motor cortices of the cat. *J. Anat.*, 87:387–406.

Smit, G. J., and Uylings, H. B. M. (1975): The morphometry of the branching pattern in dendrites of the visual cortex pyramidal cells. *Brain Res.* 86.

Smit, G. J., Uylings, H. B. M., and Veldmaat-Wansink, L. (1972): The branching pattern in dendrites of cortical neurons. *Acta Morphol. Neerl. Scand.*, 9:253–274.

Strahler, A. N. (1957): Quantitative analysis of watershed geomorphology. *Trans. Am. Geophys. Un.*, 38:913–920.

Uylings, H. B. M., and Smit, G. J. (1975): Three-dimensional branching structure of pyramidal cell dendrites. *Brain Res.* 86.

Weibel, E. R. (1963): *Morphometry of the Human Lung.* Springer-Verlag, Berlin.

Advances in Neurology, Vol. 12, edited by
G. W. Kreutzberg, Raven Press, New York
© 1975.

Parameters of Dendritic Transport

Peter Schubert and Georg W. Kreutzberg

Max-Planck Institute for Psychiatry, D-8000 Munich 40, Federal Republic of Germany

The metabolic processes that take place in axons and dendrites require the presence of energy and of proteins acting as enzymes. Other proteins are used for the structural maintenance of the membranes, and it is postulated that specific macromolecules are released across the neuronal membranes to exert some influence on the microenvironment or on the metabolism of the target cells. Accordingly, the number of macromolecules needed in the neuronal processes is rather high; however, their capacity for local protein synthesis seems to be very low. No ribosomes are seen in axons, and the few ribosomes present in the peripheral dendrites are probably not sufficient to cover the demand for proteins. Therefore, most of the proteins needed in the neuronal processes have to be synthesized in the nerve cell soma, and must be transported into the periphery.

The transport within the axon has been thoroughly investigated (see recent review by Jeffrey and Austin, 1973), but less information has been obtained on the transport within dendrites. The existence of a dendritic transport system was demonstrated by the early experiments of Droz and Leblond (1963) and later by Young and Droz (1968). Its direct demonstration was possible with the aid of the single-cell injection technique developed in collaboration with Lux and Globus (Globus, Lux, and Schubert, 1968; Schubert, Lux, and Kreutzberg, 1971). It is the aim of this chapter to outline the parameters of dendritic transport as investigated with this technique, and to discuss its possible function and biologic significance.

MATERIALS AND METHODS

Dendritic transport of various macromolecules was studied in cat spinal motoneurons (total number about 600). Following intracellular application of radioactive precursors, their incorporation and the transport of the newly synthesized macromolecules within the individual neuron were made visible by autoradiography. The following substances have been injected: ^{3}H-glycine, ^{3}H-leucine, ^{3}H-proline, ^{3}H-histidine, ^{3}H-cystein as precursors for proteins; ^{3}H-fucose, ^{35}S-sulfate as precursors for glycoproteins and acid mucopolysaccharides; ^{3}H-choline as precursor for phospholipids; and ^{3}H-orotic acid, ^{3}H-uridine, ^{3}H-adenosine, ^{3}H-guanosine as precursors for RNA and other nucleoside derivatives.

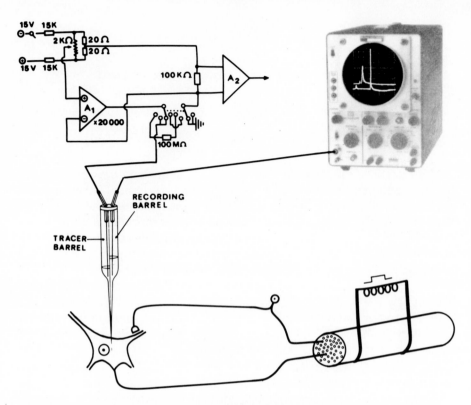

FIG. 1. Technique of intracellular tracer application. A double-barreled glass micropipette with a tip diameter of 1 to 2 μm is used. One barrel contains a highly concentrated acid or alkaline solution of the radioactive precursor to be applied. The other barrel serves as recording electrode and is connected to an oscilloscope. While the micropipette is advanced through the spinal cord, the peripheral sciatic and femoral nerves are stimulated by 1/sec current pulses. The elicited electrical potentials are continuously recorded and displayed on the oscilloscope screen. If the intracellular position of the pipette tip is indicated by the display of a stable resting and action potential, the precursor is applied by iontophoresis. The iontophoresis current is generated by a battery operated floating amplifier configuration. It can be switched as cross-barrel current from either barrel to ground. Usually, currents in the range of 20 to 40 nA were applied for 2 to 5 min (for technical details see Schubert et al., 1971; Neher, 1974; Schubert and Holländer, 1975).

   The technique of tracer application is demonstrated in Fig. 1. The intracellular position of the electrode and the effect of injection are electrophysiologically monitored by continuous recording of the nerve cell potentials. Only those neurons that showed normal resting potentials within minutes after injection and that responded to nerve stimulation were selected for further evaluation. The maintenance of normal electrical activity is probably a most sensitive indicator for the functional integrity of the neuron, ensuring that the transport is studied under physiologic conditions.

   This technique is found to be most suitable for studying fast transport ranging from minutes up to several hours. For longer survival times of up to 3 days, more complicated surgery and intensive postoperative care are required. At the end of the experiments the positions of the injection sites are marked, permitting the identification of the labeled neurons. The cats are killed by Formalin perfusion. The spinal cord is embedded in Paraplast, and 6-μm serial sections are prepared for autoradiography.

INTRADENDRITIC TRANSPORT OF PROTEINS

Within just 4 min after the intracellular application of radioactive amino acids, a distinct labeling is seen over the nerve cell soma indicating a rapid incorporation into proteins. The assumption that the autoradiographically demonstrable labeling represents almost exclusively incorporated proteins and peptides is generally accepted and is based on the quantitative investigations of Droz and Warshawsky (1963) as well as Peters and Ashley (1967). They showed that the free amino acids are almost completely removed from tissue during the Formalin perfusion and during the various steps of the subsequent histologic procedure.

Among the various amino acids tested, ^{3}H-glycine was found to be the most suitable precursor because it remains confined to the injected neuron (Fig. 2). This confinement and the high labeling of proteins obtained from bypassing the somal membrane uptake mechanism for amino acids make it possible to trace the transport of the newly synthesized proteins far into the

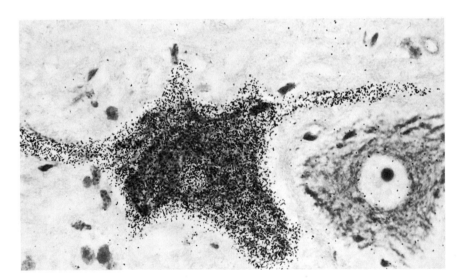

FIG. 2. Incorporation of ^{3}H-glycine, about 30 min after intracellular application. Labeling is confined to the soma and proximal dendrites of the injected neuron. No silver grains exceeding background level are seen over the neighboring glial and nerve cells. Autoradiography, stained by toluidine blue. (×670.)

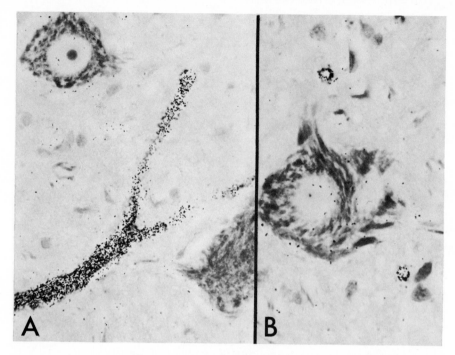

FIG. 3. (A) Transport of labeled proteins within peripheral dendrites, 30 min after injection of ³H-glycine into the cell soma. (×530.) (B) Ring-like appearance of labeling in a cross section of peripheral dendritic branches suggesting a replacement of membrane proteins by transported proteins. (×670.) Autoradiographs, counterstained by toluidine blue.

axon and dendrites (Fig. 3A). Within 15 min the entire dendritic tree is filled with radioactive material, and the labeling in the individual branches can be followed up to a distance of ~ 1000 μm from the soma.

It should be kept in mind that in addition to proteins free amino acids may also reach the dendritic periphery and may be incorporated locally. However, the minimal transport of RNA from the soma into dendrites (Kreutzberg and Schubert, 1973), the correspondingly small content of RNA determined biochemically in dendrites (Edstrom and Hydèn, 1954), and the few ribosomes seen in the peripheral branches suggest that their capacity to synthesize proteins is rather low compared to that of the cell soma. A considerable diffusion of free amino acids into the peripheral dendrites and local incorporation should also be excluded on the basis of the colchicine experiments described below. Therefore, the high labeling seen after short survival times within the peripheral dendritic branches primarily indicates a transport of proteins synthesized in the nerve cell soma.

In order to determine the velocity of dendritic transport, short-term experiments were performed (Schubert et al., 1971). Within 8 min after starting time and 4 min after the end of the iontophoretic tracer application, radioactive material is found transported up to a distance of 400 μm from the soma. The transport rate calculated from these data is at least 3 mm/hr.

The rapidly transported proteins often show a specific labeling pattern. Following the injection of glycine and especially of basic amino acids, many of the peripheral dendritic branches reveal in cross sections a ring-like formation of silver grains (Fig. 3B) (Kreutzberg, Schubert, Toth, and Rieske, 1973). This suggests an incorporation of the transported proteins into dendritic membranes, which are known to be particularly rich in basic proteins (Bloom 1970; Pfenninger 1971; Akert, Pfenninger, Sandri, and Moor, 1972). Therefore, the function of the rapid dendritic transport may be the same as shown for the fast axonal transport, i.e., to provide the synaptic membranes with proteins (Marko and Cuénod, 1973; Krygier-Brévart, Weiss, Mehl, Schubert, and Kreutzberg, 1974). This could also explain the distinct somatofugal gradient of the dendritic labeling observed after short survival times. In contrast to the labeling pattern seen in single axons, in which a wavefront of labeled material travels downward to reach the terminals (Lux, Schubert, Kreutzberg, and Globus, 1970), the grain density decreases in dendrites with further distance from soma. Because the synaptic membrane sites that must be supplied are situated along the entire length of the dendrites, the rapidly transported proteins should be used all along the way, and the amount transported must gradually decrease.

With time, the distribution of the radioactive proteins within the dendritic tree is equalized. Three days after injection of ^{3}H-glycine the peripheral branches reveal the same density of silver grains as the stem dendrites, and the overall intensity of labeling is considerably lower than at short survival times (Schubert et al., 1971). This may reflect that at this stage the export of radioactive proteins has ceased and that the radioactive proteins within the dendritic tree are continuously diluted by unlabeled proteins leading finally to the steady-state distribution observed. The homogeneous distribution might also be furthered by a retrograde transport of proteins as is shown to exist in dendrites, at least for exogenous material (Lynch, Smith, Browning, and Gall, 1975).

In addition to proteins, ^{3}H-choline-labeled phospholipids were found to be effectively transported within dendrites (Schubert et al., 1971; Kreutzberg and Schubert, 1973).

MECHANISM OF DENDRITIC TRANSPORT

The possibility that dendritic transport is operated by simple diffusion was tested by calculating the hypothetical diffusion coefficient of radioactive proteins from the experimental data. Within 15 min of tracer application, radioactive proteins reached the peripheral branches of the dendrites, 1,000 μm distant from the soma. The concentration at this locus was found to be ~ 10% of the concentration within the nerve cell soma determined by silver-grain counting.

Following intracellular injection, a surplus of radioactive amino acids is available for protein synthesis. Therefore, it is assumed that the amount of labeled proteins synthesized in the first minutes will be nearly constant. Under these conditions, the diffusion coefficient can be roughly calculated from the equation

$$c = c_0\left[1 - \phi\left(\frac{z}{2\sqrt{Dt}}\right)\right]$$

where D is the diffusion coefficient (cm^2/sec); c the concentration in peripheral dendrites (10%); c_0 the concentration in the cell soma (100%); t the time of diffusion (15 min); z the diffusion distance, i.e., distance of the peripheral dendrites from soma (1,000 μm). ϕ is the error function:

$$\phi\left(\frac{z}{2\sqrt{Dt}}\right) = \phi(x) = \frac{2}{\sqrt{\pi}}\int_0^x e^{-x^2}\,dx.$$

The diffusion coefficient calculated is 2.05×10^{-6} (cm^2/sec). This value is about 5 to 10 times higher than the known diffusion coefficients of most of the proteins determined in water (see tables in Altman and Dittmer, 1972). If, for example, globulin with a diffusion coefficient of 5.49×10^{-7} had to reach a 10% concentration in the peripheral dendrites by diffusion, it would need about 50 min instead of 15 min. Moreover, the data reported on the convection of procion yellow within dendrites point against diffusion (Llinás and Nicholson, 1971). Following local injection into the dendrites of alligator Purkinje cells, the dye was found to spread preferentially in a somatofugal direction from the injection site, which suggests a directed transport. Furthermore, the dendritic transport seems to be dependent upon the functional integrity of the neurons. In nerve cells that had been impaired during injection, as indicated by the loss of their resting potential, the spread of labeled material within the dendritic tree was found to be approximately 50% smaller than in control neurons.

In order to obtain more direct information on the possible mechanism of dendritic transport, the effect of colchicine, which is known to block the axonal transport (Kreutzberg, 1969) was tested (Schubert, Kreutzberg, and Lux, 1972). Three days after subdural colchicine application the affected neurons showed severe morphologic changes, as described by Wisniewski and Terry (1967). Large portions of the cell body and proximal dendrites were filled with filamentous material and the number of neurotubules was considerably reduced. The neurons were still able to synthesize proteins within the cell soma, but the dendritic transport of proteins was severely impaired (Fig. 4). This suggests that the transport within dendrites depends on the same mechanism as that of the axonal transport, and that it is linked to the integrity of the neurotubules.

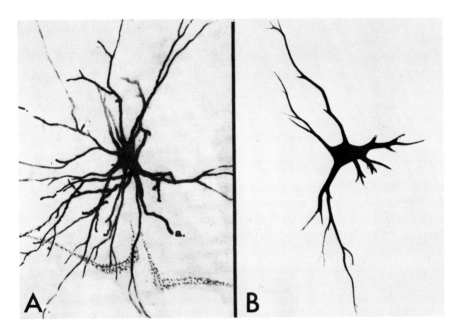

FIG. 4. Effect of colchicine on the dendritic transport of ³H-glycine-labeled proteins. The extension of the labeled dendritic tree is reconstructed from serial section autoradiographs. (A) Control neuron. All the dendrites with the individual branches can be followed throughout their entire length. (B) Colchicine treated neuron. The radioactive material is shown to be transported in some dendrites not further than 100 to 200 μm from the soma. Other dendrites are traceable up to 500 μm. But here also, the transport is stopped in some of the branches. (Schubert et al., 1972). (×80.)

No labeling is seen in the peripheral dendritic branches of the colchicine-treated neuron; therefore, even though the protein synthesis remains unaffected, it can be excluded that a considerable amount of free amino acids reaches the periphery of the dendritic tree by diffusion and is incorporated locally.

It is interesting to note that the colchicine-treated neurons show a normal excitability following antidromic stimulation. However, generally no action potentials could be elicited by orthodromic stimulation indicating an impairment of the synaptic transmission. This may be caused by a block of axonal transport in the afferent fibers (Perisic and Cuénod, 1972), or it may also result from a deficient supply of the dendritic membrane with substances involved in synaptic transmission.

REGULATION OF DENDRITIC TRANSPORT

If dendritic transport is an active process, it should be responsive to the functional requirements. This can be demonstrated in the regenerating neuron. Following nerve transection, the amount of proteins transported down the axon is increased considerably to cover the higher need for proteins in the axonal growth cone (Kreutzberg and Schubert, 1971). Simultaneously, the export of proteins into the dendrites is reduced (Schubert and Kreutzberg, 1975c). The amount exported is sufficient to supply the proximal dendrites but not the branches in the periphery of the dendritic tree. Such an impaired supply may lead to a kind of "dystrophy" of the peripheral branches. This could also explain the reduction of the dendritic tree and the loss of the peripheral dendrites observed after axotomy (cf. Sumner and Watson, 1971).

These findings suggest that the dendritic transport in the regenerating neuron is changed to compensate for the necessary increase of axonal transport material.

TRANSPORT OF GLYCOPROTEINS, ACID MUCOPOLYSACCHARIDES, AND RELEASE FROM DENDRITES

After the intracellular injection of ³H-fucose, the injected neuron shows a very typical labeling pattern (Kreutzberg et al., 1973). Although no incorporation is demonstrated in the cell nucleus, silver grains appear concentrated in several patches in the perikaryon (Fig. 5). This finding probably reflects an accumulation of the labeled material in the Golgi apparatus, where the glycoproteins are stored after glycosylation (Droz, 1967; Rambourg and Droz, 1969).

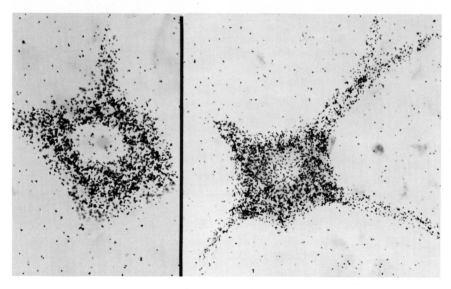

FIG. 5. Incorporation and dendritic transport of ³H-fucose-containing glycoproteins. The patchy labeling of the perikaryon indicates an accumulation of labeled material in the neuropil. Autoradiograph, counterstained with toluidine blue. (Left, ×650; right, ×550.)

Glycoproteins are transported from the perikaryon into the dendrites where they are found within 30 min after injection (Fig. 5). Dendritic labeling appears relatively weak and can be followed only up to 400 μm from the soma. This may be caused by the difficulties in injecting an uncharged molecule such as fucose into the neuron by iontophoresis or electro-osmosis. Thus the amount of precursor applied with fucose in our experiments might not be great enough to label intraneuronal glycoproteins to the extent that their transport can be traced throughout the entire dendritic tree.

In order to obtain a higher intracellular labeling, ^{35}S-sulfate has been used. It is considered to be a rather specific precursor of acid mucopoly-saccharides (Margolis, 1969). Again, the labeling pattern within the cell soma indicates an accumulation of the sulfate containing material in the Golgi complex. It is effectively transported within the dendrites even to the more peripheral branches (Fig. 6). In contrast to the transported proteins labeled by amino acids, however, the sulfate-containing material does not remain strictly confined to the dendrites of the injected neuron. Some of the transported material is able to pass the dendritic membrane, and apparently becomes bound to neuropil structures (Fig. 6). Such a release from dendrites is also seen after the injection of ^{3}H-fucose, but it is less prominent (Fig. 5). In an area of ~ 250 μm around the soma and around dendrites of the injected cell, radioactivity is distributed in a peculiar pattern. The silver

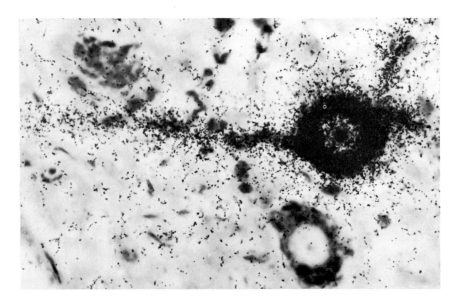

FIG. 6. Dendritic transport of sulfate-containing material, 2 hr after intracellular injection. Some of the radioactive material is released from dendrites and shows a peculiar distribution pattern within the neuropil (for details see text). Autoradiography, counterstained with toluidine blue. (×500.) (Schubert, 1974.)

grains appear slightly concentrated and are aggregated in strands. Other parts of the neuropil as well as the somata of neighboring nerve cells are nearly free of silver grains. This labeling pattern suggests a specific distribution.

It is well known that glycoproteins and acid mucopolysaccharides are important constituents of the extracellular space and of the outer membrane coat (see Schmitt and Samson, 1969). They are thought to contribute to the surface properties of the neuron, e.g., to the specificity of cell recognition (Barondes, 1970). It is conceivable that glycoproteins and acid mucopolysaccharides that had been released from the dendrites will move in the extracellular space and will become associated with the outer membranes of other cells. If this is true, such a release of substances could enable the neuron to exercise some influence or control on the composition of its microenvironment, which may be of functional significance.

DENDRITIC AND AXONAL TRANSPORT OF NUCLEOSIDE DERIVATIVES AND TRANSFER TO POSTSYNAPTIC NEURONS

Following intracellular injection of ^{3}H-adenosine and ^{3}H-guanosine, the cell nucleus and especially the nucleolus show the highest density of silver grains (Schubert and Kreutzberg, 1975b). A less but definite labeling is also seen in the perikaryon (Fig. 7A). The characteristic intracerebral distribution of the radioactive material suggests an incorporation into RNA. This is supported by the finding that the intensity of labeling is considerably reduced if the tissue sections have been incubated in a ribonuclease solution before the autoradiographs are prepared. Yet, in the tissue there remains a high proportion of radioactive material which is TCA-soluble (10 to 20%), indicating the presence of precursors which are incorporated into compounds other than RNA.

The nucleoside derivatives are effectively transported within the dendrites and within hours reach into the peripheral branches at about the same concentration as in the perikaryon (Fig. 7B). It is probably the nucleotides which are transported and which are obviously needed in the dendrites. They play a key role in the cell metabolism. Nucleotides supply the energy requirement of the neuron, and as constituents of a number of coenzymes they are involved in many metabolic processes. There is also a considerable release from dendrites. Many of the neighboring glial cells show an extremely high labeling of their nuclei, probably reflecting an incorporation of the released precursor into RNA or DNA. Some of the released radioactive compounds, probably the nucleosides, do also reach the neighboring vessels. This finding could be of some relevance for the local regulation of the intracerebral blood flow, since intracerebral application of adenosine was shown to result locally in an effective dilatation of the vessels (Berne et al., 1974).

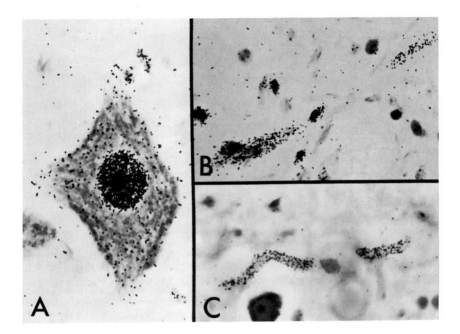

FIG. 7. (A) Incorporation of ³H-adenosine. Four hr after intracellular injection, the cell nucleus and nucleolus appear densely covered by silver grains. A less intensive but definite labeling is also seen over the perikaryon. (×600.) (B) Tritiated adenosine derivatives are effectively transported in dendrites. Some of the radioactive material obviously leaves the dendrites and is incorporated within the nuclei of some glial cells. (×400.) (C) Intra-axonal transport. Within just 4 hr a relatively high amount of ³H-adenosine derivatives has reached the level of root formation, i.e., a distance of ∼3 mm from the injected soma. Labeling remains rather confined to the axon. (×400.) Autoradiographs, counterstained with toluidine blue. (Schubert and Kreutzberg, 1975b).

In addition, a fast intraaxonal transport of nucleoside derivatives from the soma down to the periphery can be clearly demonstrated with the single-cell injection technique (Fig. 7C).

For further studies on the axonal transport of nucleoside derivatives into the terminal region, the extracellular application of nucleosides into a defined neuronal projection system seemed to be more advantageous (Schubert and Kreutzberg, 1974). One to 3 days following injection into the visual cortex, the transport of ³H-adenosine, ³H-uridine, and ³H-guanosine derivatives could be traced along the corticothalamic projection into the target area—the lateral geniculate nucleus (LGN). Here, the labeling does not remain confined to the neuropil where the axonal terminals are situated, but a high amount of radioactive material appears to accumulate in the neurons of the LGN (Fig. 8). Because contamination, spillover, and retrograde transport has been excluded, this finding suggests that nucleosides or nucleotides are transported into the terminals, are subsequently released, and are taken up by the postsynaptic neurons. Quantitative studies and

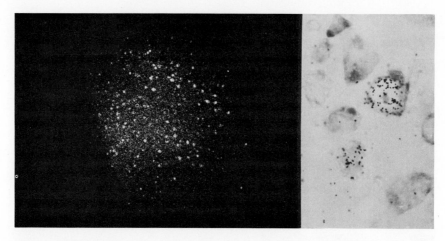

FIG. 8. (Left) Autoradiograph of the target area in the LGN 2 days after extracellular injection of ³H-adenosine into the ipsilateral striate cortex. Within the strictly confined
labeled area, silver grains are scattered over the neuropil and are highly accumulated over
the nerve cells. They appear as larger white dots. Dark-field illumination. (×50.) (Right)
Selective labeling of a few nerve cells located in the fifth layer of the contralateral non-
injected striate cortex, indicating a transcallosal projection to these neurons and a selective uptake of the transported ³H-adenosine derivatives. Autoradiograph, counterstained
with toluidine blue. (×500.) (Schubert and Kreutzberg, 1975a).

preliminary biochemical analyses revealed that surprisingly high quantities
of the TCA-soluble adenosine derivatives are transported, and that a
definite proportion is incorporated into cyclic AMP. Because of these
findings it is tempting to speculate that the well-known influence of a neuron
on the metabolism of its target cell may be mediated by the release and
transfer of nucleoside derivatives.

REFERENCES

Akert, K., Pfenninger, K., Sandri, C., and Moor, H. (1972): Freeze-etching and cytochemistry
    of vesicles and membranes in synapses of the central nervous system. In: *Structure and
    Function of Synapses,* edited by G. D. Pappas and D. P. Purpura, pp. 67–86. Raven Press,
    New York.
Altman, P., and Dittmer, D. S. (1972): Proteins: Physical properties. In: *Biology Data Book,*
    edited by P. Altman and D. S. Dittmer, pp. 370–385. Federation of American Societies
    for Experimental Biology, Bethesda, Maryland.
Barondes, S. H. (1970): Brain glycomacromolecules and interneuronal recognition. In: *The
    Neurosciences, Second Study Program,* edited by F. O. Schmitt, pp. 747–760. Rockefeller
    Univ. Press, New York.
Berne, R., Rubio, R., and Curnish, R. (1974): Release of adenosine from ischemic brain.
    Circ. Res., 35:262–272.
Bloom, F. E. (1970): Postsynaptic macromolecules. *Neurosci. Res. Program Bull.* 8:386–395.
Droz, B., and Leblond, C. P. (1963): Axonal migration of proteins in the central nervous
    system and peripheral nerves as shown by autoradiography. *J. Comp. Neurol.,* 121:325–345.

Droz, B., and Warshawsky, H. (1963): Reliability of the autoradiographic technique for the detection of newly synthesized protein. *J. Histochem. Cytochem.*, 11:426–435.

Droz, B. (1967): L'appareil de Golgi comme dite d'incorporation du galactose-³H dans les neurones ganglionnaires spinaux chez le rat. *J. Microsc. (Oxf.)*, 6:419–424.

Edström, J., and Hydèn, H. (1954): Ribonucleotide analysis of individual nerve cells. *Nature*, 174:128–129.

Globus, A., Lux, H. D., and Schubert, P. (1968): Somadendritic spread of intracellularly injected glycine in cat spinal motoneurons. *Brain Res.*, 11:440–445.

Jeffrey, P. L., and Austin, L. (1973): Axoplasmic transport. *Prog. Neurobiol.*, 2:207–255.

Kreutzberg, G. W. (1969): Neuronal dynamics and axonal flow. IV. Blockage of intra-axonal enzyme transport by colchicine. *Proc. Natl. Acad. Sci., USA*, 62:722–728.

Kreutzberg, G. W., and Schubert, P. (1971): Changes in axonal flow during regeneration of mammalian motor nerves. *Acta Neuropathol. (Suppl. V) (Berl.)*, 70–75.

Kreutzberg, G. W. and Schubert, P. (1973): Neuronal activity and axonal flow. In: *Central Nervous System—Studies on Metabolic Regulation and Function*, edited by E. Genazzani and H. Herken, pp. 84–93. Springer-Verlag, Berlin, Heidelberg, New York.

Kreutzberg, G. W., Schubert, P., Tóth, L., and Rieske, E. (1973): Intradendritic transport to postsynaptic sites. *Brain Res.*, 62:399–404.

Krygier-Brevart, V., Weiss, D. G., Mehl, E., Schubert, P., and Kreutzberg, G. W. (1974): Maintenance of synaptic membranes by the fast axonal flow. *Brain Res.*, 77:97–110.

Llinás, R., and Nicholson, C. (1971): Electrophysiological properties of dendrites and somata in alligator Purkinje cells. *J. Neurophysiol.*, 34:532–551.

Lux, H. D., Schubert, P., Kreutzberg, G. W., and Globus, A. (1970): Excitation and axonal flow. Autoradiographic study on motoneurons intracellularly injected with ³H-amino acid. *Exp. Brain. Res.*, 10:197–204.

Lynch, G., Smith, R. L., Browning, M., and Gall, Ch. (1975): This volume.

Margolis, R. W. (1969): Mucopolysaccharides. In: *Handbook of Neurochemistry*, edited by A. Lajtha, pp. 245–260. Plenum, New York.

Marko, P., and Cuénod, M. (1973): Contribution of the nerve cell body to renewal of axonal and synaptic glycoproteins in the pigeon visual system. *Brain Res.*, 62:419–423.

Neher, E. (1974): Elektronische Meßtechnik in der Physiologie. Springer-Verlag, Berlin, Heidelberg.

Peristic, M., and Cuénod, M. (1972): Synaptic transmission by colchicine blockade of axoplasmic flow. *Science*, 175:1140–1142.

Peters, T., and Ashley, C. A. (1967): An artefact in autoradiography due to binding of free amino acids to tissues by fixation. *J. Cell Biol.*, 33:53–60.

Pfenninger, K. (1971): The cytochemistry of synaptic densities. I. An analysis of the bismuth iodide impregnation. *J. Ultrastruct. Res.*, 34:103–122.

Rambourg, A., and Droz, B. (1969): Incorporation in vitro de la glucosamine-³H et du galactose-³H dans les cellules ganglionnaires spinales et les cellules hepatiques durrat. Etude radioautographie en microscopie électronique. *J. Microsc. (Oxf.)*, 8:79a.

Schmitt, F. O., and Samson, F. E. (1969): Brain cell microenvironment. *Neurosci. Res. Program Bull.*, 7:(4).

Schubert, P. (1974): Transport in Dendriten einzelner Motoneurone. *Bull. Schweiz, Akad. Med. Wiss.*, 30:56–65.

Schubert, P., and Holländer, H. (1975): Methods for the delivery of tracer to the central nervous system. In: *The Use of Axonal Transport for Studies of Neuronal Connectivity*, edited by M. W. Cowan and M. Cuénod. Elsevier, Amsterdam.

Schubert, P., and Kreutzberg, G. W. (1974): Axonal transport of adenosine and uridine derivatives and transfer to postsynaptic neurons. *Brain Res.*, 76:526–530.

Schubert, P., and Kreutzberg, G. W. (1975a): ³H-adenosine, a tracer for neuronal connectivity. *Brain Res.*, 85:317–319.

Schubert, P., and Kreutzberg, G. W. (1975b): Dendritic and axonal transport of ³H-nucleoside derivatives in single motoneurons and release from dendrites. *Brain Res. (In press.)*

Schubert, P., and Kreutzberg, G. W. (1975c): Changes in dendritic transport of regenerating motoneurons. *(In preparation.)*

Schubert, P., Kreutzberg, G. W., and Lux, H. D. (1972): Neuroplasmic transport in dendrites: Effect of colchicine on morphology and physiology of motoneurons in the cat. *Brain Res.*, 47:331–343.

Schubert, P., Lux, H. D., and Kreutzberg, G. W. (1971): Single cell isotope injection technique, a tool for studying axonal and dendritic transport. *Acta Neuropathol. (Berl.)*, 5:179–186.

Sumner, B. E. H., and Watson, W. E. (1971): Retraction and expansion of the dendritic tree of motor neurons of adult rats induced in vivo. *Nature,* 233:273–275.

Wisniewski, H., and Terry, R. D. (1967): Experimental colchicine encephalopathy. I. Induction of neurofibrillary degeneration. *Lab. Invest.,* 17:577–587.

Young, R. W., and Droz, B. (1968): The renewal of protein in retinal rods and cones. *J. Cell Biol.,* 39:169–184.

Advances in Neurology, Vol. 12, edited by
G. W. Kreutzberg, Raven Press, New York
© 1975.

Acetylcholinesterase as a Marker for Dendritic Transport and Dendritic Secretion

George W. Kreutzberg, L. Tóth, and H. Kaiya

Max-Planck Institute for Psychiatry, D-8000 Munich 40, Federal Republic of Germany

Acetylcholinesterase (EC 3.1.1.7; AChE) hydrolyzes and thereby inactivates the neurotransmitter acetylcholine after its release from presynaptic axon terminals. This function is performed by the enzyme at the postsynaptic dendritic membranes. Cytochemical studies have shown that the enzyme is synthesized in the perikaryon of the neuron and appears first in the cisternae of the granulated endoplasmic reticulum (ER) (Koelle, 1963). Its distribution from the cisternae to the postsynaptic membrane is the subject of this chapter.

MATERIALS AND METHODS

Our studies were performed in cats, guinea pigs, and Long-Evans hooded rats. Most of the investigations were carried out at the facial nucleus, which contains only motoneurons of a rather uniform multipolar isodendritic type. In one experimental series the facial nerve was cut unilaterally at the level of the stylomastoid foramen.

Experiments were performed by injecting diisopropyl fluorophosphate (DFP) intraperitoneally into rats and sacrificing the animals at 10 and 30 min, at 1, 3, 6, and 18 hr, and at 1, 2, 3, and 5 days postinjection. For light microscopy AChE activity was demonstrated in cryostat sections according to Gomori's (1952) modification of the Koelle and Friedenwald (1949) technique. For demonstration of AChE activity on the ultrastructural level, the animals were perfused with glutaraldehyde. Tissue blocks were rinsed in cacodylate buffer. Fifty-μm sections obtained by means of the Smith-Farquahr tissue chopper were incubated for 30 to 90 min in a medium containing acetylthiocholine iodide as substrate and ethopropazine as inhibitor of nonspecific cholinesterases. The procedure was carried out according to Karnovsky and Roots (1964) and according to Lewis and Shute (1969). The latter method is preferred because the reaction product allows a higher resolution. After osmication and block staining with uranyl acetate, the material was embedded in Araldite (Durcupan). Thin sections were viewed on a Zeiss EM 9. Thick sections measuring between 0.5 and 2 μm were investigated with a high-voltage electron microscope equipped with a scanning and a stereo device using the JSEM 200 of Jeol.[1]

OBSERVATIONS AND INTERPRETATIONS

Distribution of AChE in the Normal Facial Nucleus of Rats and Guinea Pigs

In the motoneurons the reaction product is visible in all cisternae of the rough endoplasmic reticulum (r-ER) and occasionally in tubular and vesicular parts of the Golgi complexes. It can also be demonstrated in the smooth endoplasmic reticulum (s-ER), in subsurface cisternae, occasionally in parts of the perinuclear cisternae, and finally in or on the plasmalemma (Fig. 1). In the dendrites, activity is demonstrated mainly in tubular and

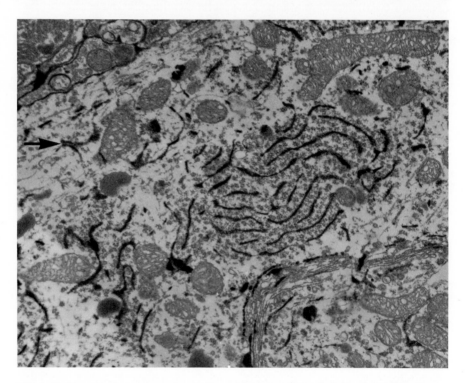

FIG. 1. Perikaryon of a motoneuron in the rat facial nucleus. Activity of AChE is demonstrated by electron-dense deposits in the cisternae of the r-ER, Golgi complex, the s-ER (*arrow*), and the plasma membrane. (×18,000.)

[1] We wish to thank the Kontron Company at München-Eching for offering the opportunity to work with this instrument. The technical help of Dr. Gensch is greatly appreciated.

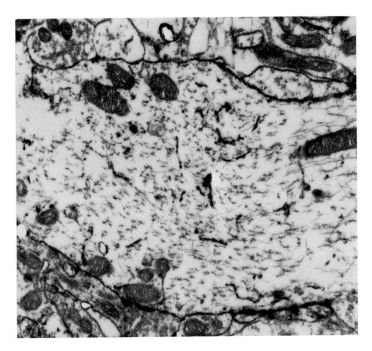

FIG. 2. Dendrites of facial motoneurons in guinea pig. AChE activity is located in tubular structures of the s-ER and in the dendritic membrane. (×18,000.)

vesicular structures of the s-ER and in subsurface cisternae (Fig. 2). If the r-ER is present, activity is also seen in the nissl bodies of the dendrites.

The plasmalemma of the dendrites show a high activity of AChE (Fig. 2). This is especially prominent at postsynaptic sites (Fig. 3). However, segments of the dendrites covered by astrocytotic processes also show enzyme activity. The quantitative difference of AChE activity in dendrites and axons of motoneurons is very striking. Over short stretches the axolemma shows occasional activity. AChE-containing structures are rarely seen inside the axon; if they are present, they appear to belong to the s-ER, as is the case in dendrites. Except in motoneurons, no AChE activity has been found inside other cellular elements of the facial nucleus such as incoming axons, glial cells, vascular cells. Yet there exist bundles of small neuronal fibers (diameter 0.1 to 0.3 μm), which are probably unmyelinated axons (C fibers) rather than dendritic bundles. In the extracellular space of these bundles AChE is often very prominent, although the fibers themselves do show some activity occasionally. If a capillary is seen in the vicinity of such bundles one might even detect continuous enzyme activity from the extracellular space to parts of the basement membrane of the endothelial cells. Such a distribution is frequently observed near the nucleus

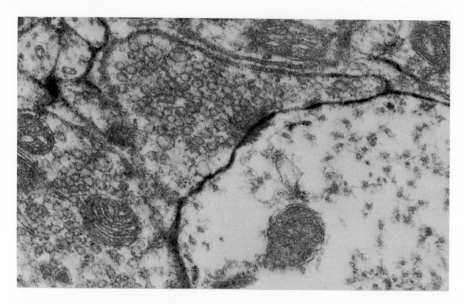

FIG. 3. Dense reaction product in the synaptic cleft indicates presence of AChE. Axodendritic synapse of guinea pig motoneuron. (×54,000.)

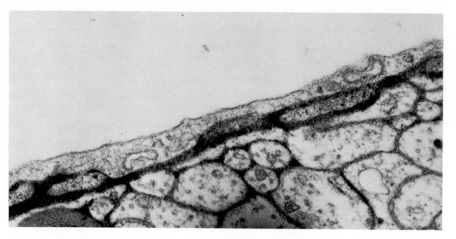

FIG. 4. Guinea pig, spinal tract of the trigeminal nerve. In certain areas of the brain, AChE activity is seen in the extracellular spaces between neuronal fiber bundles from which it reaches the basement membranes of brain capillaries. The vasculature appears AChE-positive, although endothelial cells cannot synthesize the enzyme. (×54,000.)

of the spinal tract of the trigeminal nerve at the level of the lower medulla oblongata (Fig. 4).

DFP EXPERIMENTS

Because the enzyme has been found in many different subcellular structures, it may be assumed that a transport process guides the enzyme from its site of synthesis in the ergastoplasm to its site of action at the synapse. The dynamics of such a process can be investigated by following the pathway of AChE through the cell with time. This is made possible through the use of DFP, which irreversibly inhibits all AChE activity. Accordingly, animals treated with DFP show no AChE activity in the nervous system. Yet, a few hours after the injection newly synthesized AChE again becomes visible in the neurons, and a reaction product first occurs in the cisternae of the nissl bodies (r-ER). In contrast to normal facial motoneurons, strong activity is also seen in the perinuclear cisternae, which are continuous with the r-ER cisternae (Fig. 5). Within 6 to 18 hr after DFP injection, AChE reappears in the dendrites. Activity is associated with tubulous and vesicular

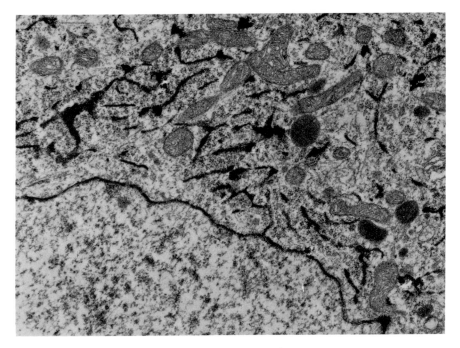

FIG. 5. Rat, facial motoneuron. Application of DFP leads to total and irreversible inhibition of AChE. Reappearance of strong enzyme activity is observed within hours in the r-ER and in the perinuclear cisternae. (×18,000.)

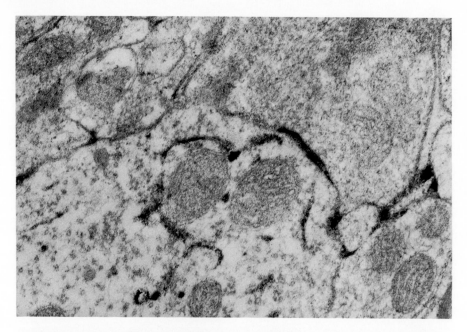

FIG. 6. Two days after DFP application AChE is seen again in the dendrites where it can be located in s-ER cisternae, in subsurface cisternae, and in synaptic clefts. The time sequence of enzyme appearance suggests a transport in s-ER structures and release from there to the postsynaptic membrane and the extracellular space. (×54,000.)

structures of the s-ER. These structures very often show an impressive length of several microns and can also be observed to branch. Although very often oriented along the longitudinal axis of the dendrites, we also see these cisternae oriented in a transverse direction, forming subsurface cisternae (Fig. 6). There seems to be a certain reciprocity of the activity of the subsurface cisternae and the overlying dendritic membrane. If activity in the cisternae is low, activity in the dendritic membrane seems to be high. In our opinion this is caused by a release of the enzyme to the dendritic membrane.

The observation in normal and DFP-treated neurons suggests compartmentalization of AChE in the s-ER of dendrites and probably also in the axons. It is interesting that this is essentially in agreement with the general concept of s-ER, which is involved in transportation and maturation of membrane constituents (Morré, Keenan, and Huang, 1974). AChE at its final destination is indeed a membrane enzyme performing its tasks predominately on the outer surface of dendritic, axonal, and cellular envelopes.

The fact that AChE is compartmentalized and transported in s-ER does not necessarily imply that this is the system for dendritic transport. It could very well be envisaged that the microtubular transport mechanism also drives transport in s-ER compartments.

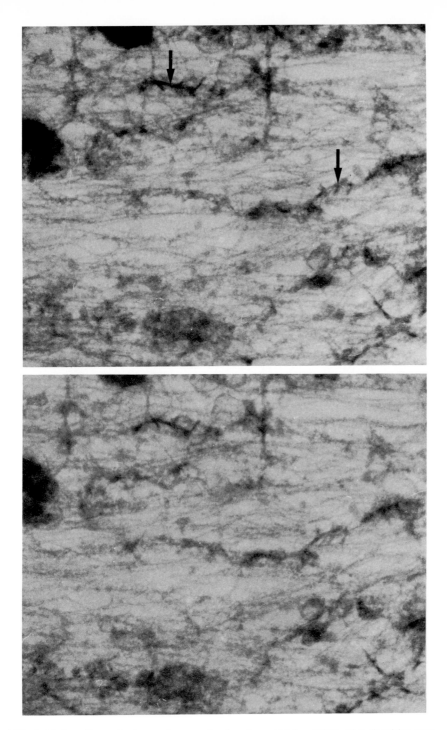

FIG. 7. High-voltage electron micrograph of a 1-μm-thick section of a dendrite, two-dimensional image of a stereoscopic figure. AChE-containing s-ER structures (*arrow*) are recognized as a tubulous system branching at regular angles with continuity over remarkably long distances. (×35,000.)

An interesting aspect to this problem is supplied by high-voltage electron microscopy of 0.5 to 2-μm-thick sections. Owing to the deposits of electron-dense reaction product in the AChE preparation, s-ER can be stained in dendrites. By tilting the object in the microscope for 5° or 10°, it is possible to prepare stereoscopic pictures. Analysis of such stereo-electron micrographs taken with transmission or scanning transmission instruments (TEM or STEM) will probably lead to a revised concept of the s-ER. It appears that the s-ER system consists of branching tubules of considerable length. The possibility of having continuous tubes from the perikaryon into the peripheral sites of the axon has been considered (Droz, 1975).

In our material, the tubular cisternae are most frequently oriented along the longitudinal axis of the dendrites. They give rise to tubular branches that run perpendicular to the main tubule. The impression is that branching occurs in regular distances and at certain angles. Figure 7 shows such a system, although most of the impressive appearance in stereoscopy is lost by the two-dimensional representation.

CHANGES IN AChE SYNTHESIS AND DISTRIBUTION DURING CHROMATOLYSIS OF MOTONEURONS

Changes in AChE activity in chromatolytic neurons and in regenerating nerves have been described for a number of years (e.g., Schwarzacher, 1958; Lewis et al., 1971; Frizell and Sjöstrand, 1974; literature reviewed by Silver, 1974). It is most interesting to see that species differences in this experimental situation offer further evidence for somatofugal dendritic transport of AChE. In the rat, as in most other animals, chromatolytic neurons diminish or even give up synthesis of AChE during the first 2 weeks after axotomy. In the facial nucleus, which is uniformly populated by motoneurons, activity totally disappears, confirming the cytochemical finding that the only source for AChE in this region is indeed the motoneurons.

In the guinea pig the change is very different. Light-microscopic histochemistry shows an unchanged or even increased AChE activity in the cell bodies of the motoneurons. Yet, distribution of activity decreases dramatically in the neuropil. This is because there is less activity in the dendrites and especially in the dendritic membrane (Fig. 8). Rather than in these normally positive structures, the enzyme accumulates in the basement membrane of the capillaries (Fig. 9) (Kreutzberg and Tóth, 1974; Kreutzberg, Tóth, Weikert, and Schubert, 1974). It appears that the dendritic membrane becomes leaky to AChE or that the enzyme can no longer be fixed on the outer surface of the membrane, and is therefore released into the extracellular spaces. From here, it reaches the basement membranes (basal lamina) of the capillaries, which are known to form a spe-

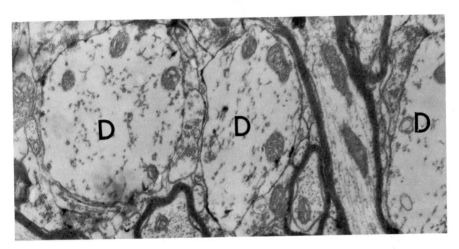

FIG. 8. Dendritic profiles, D, of chromatolytic facial motoneurons of guinea pig, 2 weeks after axotomy. AChE activity, can be seen in a few intradendritic structures, but it has been lost from most of the dendritic membrane. (×18,000.)

cialized part of the extracellular space. By some yet-unknown mechanism, basement membrane material seems to be able to concentrate AChE. This has also been demonstrated after injection of exogenous AChE into rat brain (Kreutzberg and Kaiya, 1974).

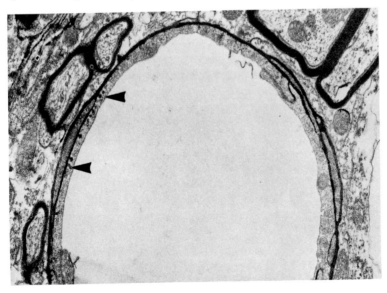

FIG. 9. Chromatolytic facial motoneuron of the guinea pig, showing loss of AChE to the extracellular space by "dendritic secretion." Within days enzyme activity is accumulating in the basement membranes of the local capillaries. AChE-containing pinocytotic vesicles can be observed near the basement membranes (*arrow*). On other occasions cytopempsis of such vesicles has been seen. (×12,000.)

"DENDRITIC SECRETION" AND TRANSNEURONAL
TRANSPORT OF MATERIAL

The most interesting aspect of the changes in AChE location in the guinea pig experiments is certainly the demonstration of a pathway for macromolecules from the neuron to other cells — in this case to the vasculature. It may be demonstrated that such a transfer occurs not only under the conditions of chromatolysis, but it is also observed under normal conditions in a number of brain regions (Flumerfelt, Lewis, and Gwyn, 1973), very prominently, for instance, in the spinal nucleus of the trigeminal tract (see Fig. 4). It also occurs in the recovery phase 3 or more days after DFP treatment of rats (Kreutzberg and Schubert, 1975).

Obviously, there is a release of macromolecules from the neuronal or dendritic membrane to the extracellular space, which we would like to term "dendritic secretion" (Kreutzberg and Tóth, 1974).

Distribution of AChE at motoneuron synapses also suggests a transsynaptic transfer of the enzyme. In a number of axodendritic and axosomatic synapses primarily resembling the L type as described by Bodian (1970) AChE activity can be detected very strongly in the synaptic cleft and in synaptic vesicles at the presynaptic membrane (Fig. 10). Very rarely an AChE-activity-containing free vesicle can also be seen within the presynaptic terminals. The pictures are almost identical to those obtained with horseradish peroxidase (Ceccarelli, Hurlbut, and Mauro, 1972) at the motor end plate, and the interpretation is similar. Apparently synaptic vesicles do open toward the synaptic cleft, most probably releasing the neurotransmitter. After this exocytotic process, material from the cleft can reach the open empty vesicle to become enclosed in an endocytotic process.

It is possible that AChE is not the only substance that is secreted from the neuron and taken up by other cells, thereby influencing the general metabolism or specific functions such as barrier and carrier functions in the endothelium, regulatory functions in glial cells, and trophic functions of neurons. Another substance that is transferred from presynaptic to postsynaptic sites is adenosine or adenosine derivatives (Schubert and Kreutzberg, 1974, 1975). The assumption that these nucleosides or nucleotides have a trophic function is reasonable because cyclase activity is abundant at the postsynaptic site and can easily transform nucleosides into cyclic forms. These could influence the metabolism of the postsynaptic cell.

Finally, we have evidence from our single-cell injection experiments with radioactive glycine that transfer of material occurs selectively between interconnected motoneurons. When spinal motoneurons of the cat are injected electrophoretically with radioactive amino acids (^{3}H-glycine) by means of double-barreled microelectrodes, it occurs frequently that not only the injected cell but also 1 to 3 cells in the environment show radioactivity. However, after careful checking electrode tracks, sites of injection, direction of

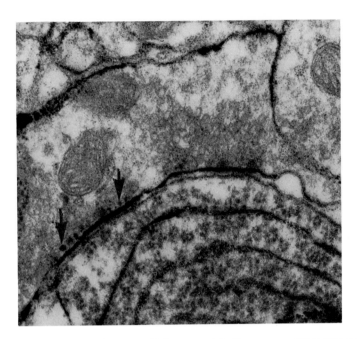

FIG. 10. AChE uptake from the extracellular space into the presynaptic terminal by endocytosis is seen frequently at dendritic or somatic synapses of facial motoneurons in both rats and guinea pigs. Electron micrograph showing a L-type Bodian synapse with a nissl body and a subsurface cisterna at the postsynaptic site. High activity in the cisternae and in the synaptic cleft. Synaptic vesicles some pinched off some in contact with the presynaptic membrane show AChE activity (*arrows*). (×54,000.)

cutting, possibility of leaks and diffusion, we concluded that there must exist a specific transfer for this material for a very distinct number of cells. It is not clear from the experiments whether there is a transfer of the amino acids or of macromolecules such as peptides or proteins (Globus, Lux, and Schubert, 1968; Kreutzberg, Schubert, and Lux, 1975; Schubert, Kreutzberg, Puzich, and Lux, *in preparation*).

CONCLUSION

After a period of intensive study of intraneuronal transport initiated by the discovery of axonal flow by Paul Weiss, it seems that transneuronal and intercellular transport phenomena are gaining in significance. Functionally, they seem to be closely related to dendritic and axonal transportation.

As demonstrated for AChE this enzyme is transported in axons and dendrites and becomes built into neuronal plasmalemma. It can be released from this site and may be taken up from the extracellular space by presynaptic terminals. It also can travel along extracellular pathways and reach basement membranes of brain capillaries. The enzyme will be concentrated in these structures, and it can be taken up by endothelial cells in an endocytotic process. Therefore, AChE cytochemistry has demonstrated (for one enzyme) several complex transport pathways including intraneuronal, transmembraneous, extracellular, and endocytotic mechanisms.

REFERENCES

Bodian, D. (1970): An electron microscopic characterization of classes of synaptic vesicles by means of controlled aldehyde fixation. *J. Cell Biol.*, 44:115–124.

Ceccarelli, B., Hurlbut, W. P., and Mauro, A. (1972): Depletion of vesicles from frog neuromuscular junctions by prolonged tetanic stimulation. *J. Cell Biol.*, 54:30–38.

Droz, B. (1975): Radioautography as a tool for visualizing neurons and neuronal processes. In: *The Use of Axonal Transport for Studies of Neuronal Connectivity*, edited by W. M. Cowan and M. Cuénod. Elsevier, Amsterdam. (Also, *personal communication.*)

Flumerfelt, B. A., Lewis, P. R., and Gwyn, D. G. (1973): Cholinesterase activity of capillaries in the rat brain: A light and electron microscopic study. *Histochem. J.*, 5:67–77.

Frizell, M., and Sjöstrand, J. (1974): Transport of proteins, glycoproteins and cholinergic enzymes in regenerating hypoglossal neurons. *J. Neurochem.*, 22:845–850.

Globus, A., Lux, H. D., and Schubert, P. (1968): Somadendritic spread of intracellularly injected tritiated glycine in cat spinal motoneurons. *Brain Res.*, 11:440–445.

Gomori, G. (1952): *Microscopic Histochemistry.* Univ. of Chicago Press, Chicago, Illinois.

Karnovsky, M. J., and Roots, L. (1964): A direct-coloring thiocholine method for cholinesterase. *J. Histochem. Cytochem.*, 12:219–221.

Koelle, G. B. (1963): Cytological distributions and physiological functions of cholinesterases. In: *Handbuch der experimentellen Pharmakologie, Erg.* XV, edited by O. Eichler and A. Farah. Springer-Verlag, Berlin.

Koelle, G. B., and Friedenwald, J. S. (1949): A histochemical method for localizing cholinesterase activity. *Proc. Soc. Exp. Biol. Med.*, 70:617–622.

Kreutzberg, G. W., and Tóth, L. (1974): Dendritic secretion: a way for the neuron to communicate with the vasculature. *Naturwissenshaften*, 61:37.

Kreutzberg, G. W., and Kaiya, H. (1974): Exogeneous acetylcholinesterase as tracer for extracellular pathways in the brain. *Histochemie*, 42:233–237.

Kreutzberg, G. W., and Schubert, P. (1975): The cellular dynamics of intracellular transport. In: *The Use of Axonal Transport for Studies of Neuronal Connectivity*, edited by M. W. Cowan and M. Cuénod. Elsevier, Amsterdam.

Kreutzberg, G. W., Schubert, P., and Lux, H. D. (1975): Neuroplasmic transport in axons and dendrites. In: *Proceedings of the Golgi Centennial Symposium*, edited by M. Santini, pp. 315–320. Raven Press, New York.

Kreutzberg, G. W., Tóth, L., Weikert, M., and Schubert, P. (1974): Changes in perineuronal capillaries accompanying chromatolysis of motoneurons. In: *Pathology of Microcirculation*, edited by J. Cervos-Navarro, pp. 282–288. de Gruyter, Berlin, New York.

Lewis, P. R., Flumerfelt, B. A., and Shute, C. C. D. (1971): The use of cholinesterase techniques to study topographical localization in the hypoglossal nucleus of the rat. *J. Anat.*, 110:203–213.

Lewis, P. R., and Shute, C. C. (1969): An electron microscopic study of cholinesterase in the rat adrenal medulla. *J. Microsc. (Oxf.)*, 89:181–193.

Morré, D. J., Keenan, T. W., and Huang, C. M. (1974): Membrane flow and differentiation: Origin of Golgi apparatus membranes from endoplasmic reticulum. In: *Advances in Cytopharmacology, Vol 2: Cytopharmacology of Secretion*, edited by B. Ceccarelli, F. Clementi, and J. Meldolesi. Raven Press, New York.

Schubert, P., and Kreutzberg, G. W. (1974): Axonal transport of adenosine and uridine derivatives and transfer to postsynaptic neurons. *Brain Res.*, 76:526–530.

Schubert, P., and Kreutzberg, G. W. (1975): [³H]-adenosine, a tracer for neuronal connectivity. *Brain Res.*, 78:317–319.

Schubert, P., Kreutzberg, G. W., Puzich, R., and Lux, H. D. (1975): Neuro-neuronal transfer of radioactivity following intracellular injection of [³H]-glycine. (*In preparation.*)

Schwarzacher, H. G. (1958): Der Cholinesterasegehalt motorischer Nervenzellen während der axonalen Reaktion. *Acta Anat. (Basel)*, 32:51–65.

Silver, A. (1974): *The Biology of Cholinesterases. Frontiers of Biology*, Vol. 36. North-Holland Publ. Corp., Amsterdam and New York.

Advances in Neurology, Vol. 12, edited by
G. W. Kreutzberg, Raven Press, New York
© 1975.

The Microstream Concept of Axoplasmic and Dendritic Transport

Guenter W. Gross

Max-Planck Institute for Psychiatry, D-8000 Munich 40, Federal Republic of Germany

EVIDENCE SUGGESTING CHROMATOGRAPHIC TRANSPORT PROCESSES

The investigation of isotope concentration distributions established by the transport system in axons and dendrites has provided a direct and accurate method of measuring transport velocities (Ochs, 1972; Edström and Hanson, 1973; Gross, 1973; Gross and Beidler, 1973). It now appears that these distributions may also be a valuable source of information on the utilization of molecules along dendrites and axons as well as on certain aspects of the transport mechanism.

A quantitative profile analysis of protein transport in the long and homogeneous garfish olfactory nerve has produced evidence for an asymmetric peak broadening and an exponential peak amplitude decrease with distance from the cell bodies. The material lost by the peak is found deposited along the axon behind the peak (Figs. 1–3). Furthermore, movement of some material in the deposited plateau region is still possible because the label accumulates at both sides of nerve transections or local cold blocks (Fig. 4). In this particular nerve the salient profile variations cannot be produced by hypothetical velocity differences in different axons (Gross and Beidler, 1975), and it must be assumed that profile variations with distance along the nerve are caused primarily by intraaxonal redistributions of transported material. The mass fluxes required to explain the observed redistribution of label are depicted in Fig. 5. Loss of material from the rapid transport system must be possible along the entire axon. Once deposited in what has been called a "deposition phase," the macromolecules may be picked up by organelles, by the membrane, by a retrograde transport process, or they may desorb and reenter the rapid orthograde transport system. Evidence also exists for a loss from the axon of rapidly transported macromolecular material (Gross and Beidler, 1975).

A simple physical process that could account for the profile variations demonstrated is a chromatographic process. In such a case, transported material alternates between a carrier medium and a stationary phase. Transport velocities are determined by the time spent by the substance

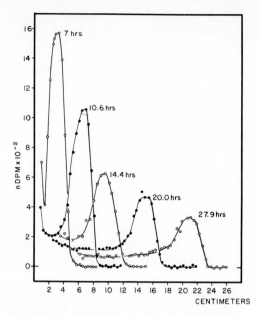

FIG. 1. Normalized isotope concentration distributions obtained at various times after application of labeled leucine and plotted as functions of distance from the olfactory mucosa. Nerves were cut behind the olfactory mucosa 6 hr after isotope application (see also Fig. 7). The macromolecule-bound isotope distributions display characteristic changes with distance from the olfactory mucosa. Peak heights decrease exponentially, peaks broaden, and wavefronts become more shallow. Plateau regions are established behind the peaks reflecting a deposition of material along the axons. Upon arrival at the synaptic region, the peak contains only 20% of the total activity in the nerve. (Gross and Beidler, 1975).

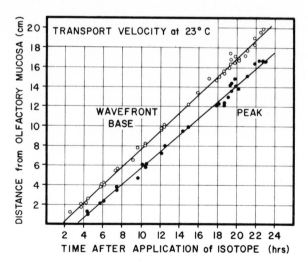

FIG. 2. Transport velocities of two profile loci at 23°C. The velocity of the wavefront base locus is 221 ± 2 mm/day, whereas that of the peak apex locus is 201 ± 6 mm/day. Therefore, the two loci separate at 20 mm/day reflecting a peak dispersion process. (Gross and Beidler, 1975).

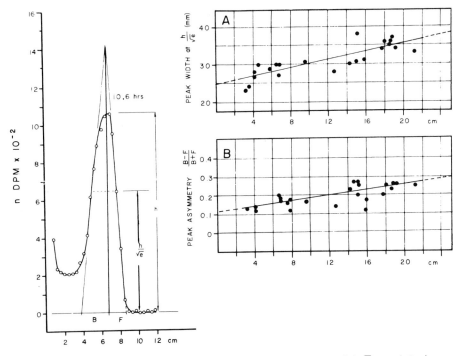

FIG. 3. Analysis of peak broadening in cut nerves. Peak widths at $h/\sqrt{e}$ are plotted as a function of peak apex position in (A). At 23°C the peak width increases at a constant rate of 0.51 mm for every 1-cm-peak displacement. This peak dispersion is asymmetric (B). The base of the peak is divided into front, F, and back, B, segments by a perpendicular line through the intersection of leading and trailing edge tangents. The asymmetry ratio is defined as $B - F/B + F$. (Gross and Beidler, 1975).

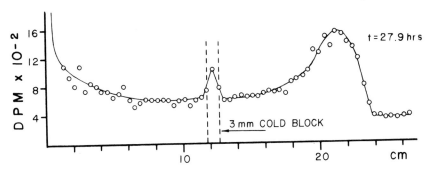

FIG. 4. Isotope accumulation in the plateau region of a cut nerve at a 3-mm nerve segment that was lowered to 5°C for 6.7 hr after the trailing edge of the peak had passed that location. The accumulation suggests that movement of some material in the plateau region is possible.

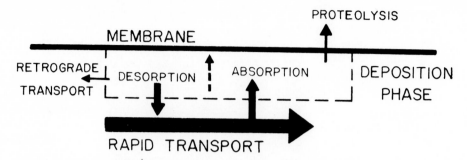

FIG. 5. Mass fluxes required to explain profile variations if they reflect primarily intra-axonal redistributions and if only one rapid transport system exists in these fibers. A deposition phase (stationary and slowly moving axonal constituents) sorbs material from the rapid transport system. The material may then become part of the membrane and organelles, undergo retrograde transport, or reenter the orthograde transport system. Labeled macromolecules may also be subjected to some proteolysis and are lost from the axon. (Gross and Beidler, 1975).

in each of the two phases; peak broadening is caused by simple molecular diffusion, convective dispersion, and the mass transfer kinetics of sorption and desorption. Peak tailing can be explained in theoretical terms by creating tail-producing sites with slow desorption rates; even level plateaus can be produced by high affinity sites (Giddings, 1965, Chapter 2). Such a chromatographic process would be relatively nonspecific and would carry a great variety of material. Instead of moving in a transport package through a viscous, stationary axoplasm, material would be carried within a streaming medium.

THE MICROSTREAM HYPOTHESES

A model has been developed that adapts the concepts of chromatography to solving the problem of dendritic and axoplasmic transport. It is based on the following five hypotheses:

1. Material is not transported through a stationary medium but is moved by carrier streams that will be called microstreams.
2. The microstreams are located in annular regions around the micro-tubules.
3. The streaming velocity is highest in the vicinity of the microtubule surface and decreases with distance from the tubule.
4. The force-generating mechanism is situated at the microtubule surface and exerts a shear force on the adjacent fluid.
5. The shear force is generated by a vectorial enzyme reaction at an ATPase situated on the surface of the microtubule. The vectorial properties result from the association of this enzyme with the oriented microtubule

structure and from the directional release of the electrostatic energy of repulsion residing in the ATP side chain.

THE ROLE OF THE MICROTUBULE IN THE MICROSTREAM CONCEPT

The microstream hypotheses utilize the microtubules as the seat of the force-generation process. Although direct evidence is still lacking, the data linking microtubules with the transport phenomenon in different types of cells are substantial. The mitotic apparatus of dividing cells is constructed of microtubules along which chromosomes move and in the vicinity of which the movement of particles increases (Taylor, 1965). Saltation (i.e., discontinuous but directional movement of particles) is frequently observed in cellular regions where microtubules are found, but is absent in areas displaying only microfilaments (Wohlfarth-Botterman, 1964; Freed and Lebowitz, 1970). In cultured fibroblast-like cells the microtubules are implicated in bidirectional saltatory mitochondrial movements, oriented dispersion of filaments, and cell translocation (Goldman, 1971). In the protozoan *Tokophrya,* two-directional particle movement occurs during feeding in tubes containing 49 microtubules arranged in clusters (Rudzinska, 1965). Finally, a statistical association between microtubules and pigment granules in melanophores has been established recently (Murphy and Tilney, 1974).

In the realm of neuronal transport the mitotic inhibitors colchicine and vinblastine, which are known to interact with tubulin (Wilson and Meza, 1973), have long been observed to inhibit this process (Dahlström, 1968; Kreutzberg, 1969; James, Bray, Morgan, and Austin, 1970; Hinckley and Green, 1971). Axoplasmic transport also ceases at temperatures at which microtubules dissociate (Fernandez, Huneeus, and Davison, 1970). In axons in which separate regions of microtubules and microfilaments often occur, labeled transported material is seen primarily in the microtubule regions (Lentz, 1972; Droz, Koenig, and Di Giamberardino, 1973), and associations of vesicles or granules with microtubules have been demonstrated in synaptic regions (Smith, Järlfors, and Beránek, 1970), as well as along axons (Banks, Mayor, and Tomlinson, 1971). In spinal root fibers mitochondrial movement is observed to occur more frequently in axons with higher microtubule density, and a microtubule–mitochondrion association has been considered necessary for such movement (Smith, 1973).

The microtubule is a comparatively high-inertia, rigid structure that has been appropriately assigned a skeletal function (Porter, 1966). It is also an oriented structure as it grows only in one direction from a site of nucleation (Borisy and Olmsted, 1972; Dentler, Granett, Witman, and Rosenbaum, 1974). The tubule is therefore a logical support for a force-generating mechanism because it can absorb the recoil resulting from such a process and can also serve to orient this process along the longitudinal axis of the microtubule. Membranes such as the axolemma or smooth endoplasmic reticulum do not appear to have these properties. Also, the latter structure sometimes forms transverse cisternae lying perpendicular to the axonal axis (Lieberman, 1971). These cisternae are fenestrated by microtubules which represent the only continuous structures in the axoplasm. Furthermore, a membrane-free region up to 1,500 Å in diameter surrounds the microtubules at the point of penetration through the transverse membranes. These regions could be the direct result of microstream activity.

THE GENERATION OF AN UNSPECIFIC SHEAR FORCE

The rapid movement of large macromolecules or particles through axoplasm of substantial viscosity has always been energetically unattractive and has led to Weiss' proposal of low-viscosity channels in axons (Weiss, 1967, page 380). The more specific microstream concept proposed here suggests that material is moved with neuroplasm and not through it. The directional release of energy at the tubule surface should automatically lower the viscosity of the adjacent neuroplasm as a result of molecular orientation and the continuous breaking of ionic and hydrogen bonds. This assumes that axoplasm is a thixotropic medium with non-Newtonian viscosity characteristics as has been demonstrated for the cytoplasm of *Nitella* (Kamiya and Kuroda, 1965). Forces are exerted on the fluid and not on a specific transport particle or vesicle within that fluid. Transport is a fluid-carrier phenomenon and is, within certain limits, nonspecific.

It is evident from the literature that the material transported in neurons is very heterogeneous. A vast variety of molecules, from amino acids (Csanyi, Gervai, and Lajtha, 1973) and nucleosides (Schubert and Kreutzberg, 1974) to large proteins and glycoproteins (Ochs, 1972; Jeffrey and Austin, 1973) are known to be a part of neuronal transport. In addition, molecular aggregates and a variety of organelles are also moved (Lubinska, 1964; Dahlström, 1971; Jeffrey and Austin, 1973). Of special interest are the observations of exogenous particle transport such as horseradish peroxidase (Kristensson and Olsson, 1971; LaVail and LaVail, 1972), viruses (Bodian and Howe, 1941; Constantine, Emmons, and Woodie, 1972), ferritin, and colloidal gold (De Lorenzo, 1970). Because many of these particles do not appear to be located in vesicles, it is difficult to visualize how a specific mechanism could move such foreign particulate substances.

If we take into consideration that neuroplasmic transport and protoplasmic streaming phenomena probably result from contiguous processes, further arguments for the existence of nonspecific shear forces in axons can be made. Stationary lipid droplets pushed with microneedles into the vicinity of an active streaming region at the mitotic spindle participate subsequently in the streaming (Chambers, 1917). Rotating fibril loops that are presumably bundles of microtubules have been observed in the isolated protoplasm of *Chara foetida* by Jarosch (1957; see also Kamiya, 1959, pages 150–155). Particles in the path of the rotating fibrils are suddenly accelerated in the direction opposite to the motion of the fibril without contacting the latter. Also, chloroplasts shaken loose from the cortical gel display rotatory movement. If such movement is prevented by touching a chloroplast with a microneedle, a local streaming of endoplasm takes place around the chloroplast in a direction opposite to that of the original rotation (Kuroda, 1964). These examples suggest the existence of shear forces that have a general effect on the surrounding medium. A specific protein–protein interaction may not be necessary to generate such shear forces.

THE VECTORIAL ENZYME REACTION

The force-generation hypothesis is highly speculative and a specific mechanism is premature. However, it is well established that axoplasmic transport is ATP dependent (Ochs and Hollingsworth, 1971) and that the primary energy-supply molecule for other streaming processes is also ATP (Kamiya, 1959, pages 74–81). Therefore, the need to create movement in a particular direction necessitates the conceptualization of a vectorial ATP hydrolysis. The usual thermodynamic treatment of this reaction ignores the structure of the molecule and its unique vectorial properties. At pH 7 the ATP phosphate chain has one of the highest charge densities in the realm of biologic molecules (Lehninger, 1965). Regardless of the exact configuration of the side chain in solution, a repulsive force between the chain's center of charge and the terminal phosphate group should always exist. According to Segal (1967) the electrostatic repulsion contributes about 2 kcal/mole to the free energy of hydrolysis of ATP to ADP. This energy release could be vectorial, and the aligning of numerous ATP molecules may result in the generation of a transport force. This can be accomplished by orienting all transport ATPases along the longitudinal axis of the axon or dendrite. As discussed previously, the microtubules are the best candidates for such a task.

Upon energy release, there are two general ways in which a directional fluid movement may be produced. A conformational change of a section of the ATPase could have a microciliary effect, or an electro-osmotic flow could result from directional charge fluctuations. To support streaming, ATP molecules must continually condense on the tubule structure and are hydrolyzed randomly. No coordination process is required. Only a tubule, its ATPase, a sufficiently high ATP concentration, and a proper ionic medium should be essential for an initiation of streaming. It is of interest that a dynein-like protein with possible ATPase activity has recently been found associated with microtubules isolated from mammalian brain (Gaskin, Kramer, Cantor, Adelstein, and Shelanski, 1974).

Preliminary calculations have revealed that a steady state, laminar Newtonian flow of a 1.3-cP fluid moving with a maximum velocity of 220 mm/day through an annulus with inner and outer radii of 125 and 475 Å, respectively, requires about 1.4×10^{-12} ergs of energy per micrometer (approximately 3.6 ergs/sec). It can also be inferred that approximately 650 ATP molecules could be hydrolized per tubule, per 1 μm length, per second. If only the 2 kcal/mole of electrostatic repulsion residing in the ATP side chain are utilized, the available energy per second would be about 90×10^{-12} ergs. Consequently, further and substantial inefficiencies can be introduced before one is confronted with an energy shortage.

MICROSTREAM DYNAMICS

The location of the microstream defined by hypothesis 2 is depicted for a C-fiber cross section in Fig. 6. The concentric rings around the microtubule represent the low viscosity regions in which movement occurs. The velocity profile of the streaming medium around the microtubule has been assumed to decrease exponentially from a maximum, close to the tubule surface, to zero a few hundred angstroms away from the tubule (Fig. 6B). Cooperative effects between tubules in close proximity are possible, and streaming rates may be enhanced in these regions. The mitochondria should also be affected by the microstreams. However, the large frictional forces produced by their enormous size should preclude anything but a very slow average transport velocity. According to the Bernoulli principle, pressure is lower in the higher kinetic energy regions, and microtubules would be inclined to arrange themselves around mitochondria, which has indeed been observed (Raine, Ghetti, and Shelanski, 1971). The resulting cooperative effect could induce a more rapid mitochondrial movement over short distances. Considering the elastic nature of these organelles, a discontinuous but oriented movement can be easily visualized. It is also reasonable to suspect that the frictional forces to which mitochondria are subjected may be a function of fiber diameter, whereas the microstreams are essentially independent of this parameter.

The microtubules should also be affected by the Bernoulli principle and would tend to aggregate unless this is prevented through space-preserving arms or anchoring filaments extending from the tubule surface. Such structures have been observed (Smith, 1971; McIntosh, 1974), but have not been interpreted in this manner. The aggregation tendency of intact tubules predicted by the microstream concept suggests that the position of microtubules may be stabilized in the neuroplasm, although repeated mitochondrial disruption of the stabilizing system should be expected.

According to the hypotheses presented, the transport velocity of a molecule or particle is determined by its position in the microstream velocity profile. This position may be a complicated function of time since movement

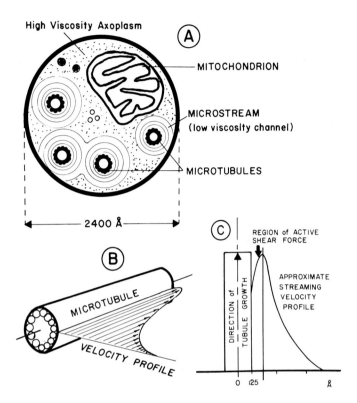

FIG. 6. Schematic representation of postulated microstreams within C fibers. A cross section of a C fiber containing one mitochondrion and four microtubules is shown in (A). The movement of molecules known as rapid axoplasmic transport is thought to occur within low viscosity channels surrounding the microtubules. These regions are thought to be induced by a shear force generating mechanism based on a vectorial ATPase reaction occurring at enzymes attached to the surface of the microtubules. A hypothetical streaming velocity profile is depicted in (B) and (C) which show that the streaming velocity decreases with distance from the microtubule. Average transport velocities are determined by the time a particle or molecule spends in different regions of this profile. All orthograde transport, including that of mitochondria, is assumed to depend on microstreams.

perpendicular to the surface of the tubule is probable. Such lateral movement is under the influence of several physical factors, such as the size of the particle, the shape of the particle, and its affinity for stationary or slowly moving axonal components. In addition, local obstructions to the microstream as well as other medium inhomogeneities will probably produce a turbulent flow, disrupting the laminar velocity profile depicted in Fig. 6B. Consequently, one should expect a considerable convective dispersion within microstreams, resulting in peak broadening of the isotope distribution profile, in direct analogy to peak broadening in chromatographic columns.

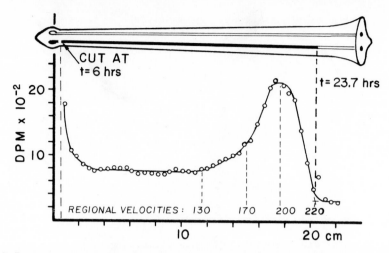

FIG. 7. Regional velocities demonstrated with a 23.7-hr cut nerve profile. In the exponential tailing region of the peak, material is transported at approximately 130 mm/day. Slower velocities cannot be shown because of the level plateau created by the deposition phenomenon. It is apparent that, at least in the peak region, a velocity spectrum is produced by the transport system. The garfish rostrum containing the two olfactory nerves is depicted above the profile for reference. In all profile depictions, the olfactory mucosa from which the C fibers of the olfactory nerve originate is placed at the origin, with the nerve extending along the abscissa.

The microstream may produce a continuum of transport velocities if there is a continuum of the physical factors mentioned above. The cut nerve profile depicted in Fig. 7 reveals a velocity range from 221 ± 2 mm/day at the wavefront base to approximately 170 mm/day in the trailing edge of the peak, and 130 mm/day at the point at which a level plateau is established. A velocity continuum appears to exist in this range. Slower transport rates probably also occur but cannot be demonstrated with a simple isotope profile. The plateau region is thought to result from a deposition of labeled material onto the stationary structures (membranes and microtubules), onto slowly moving organelles such as mitochondria, and into stationary regions of axoplasm. Moreover, desorbed material may also be moving at higher velocities in this region.

Although the dimensions of a particle or molecule should have some influence on its average transport velocity, the influence may not be a simple one. The hydrodynamic properties of a microstream are complex and cannot yet be visualized in detail. For example, particle spin, induced by the nonhomogeneous velocity profile may serve to stabilize a particle in the microstream, and its large size may make a penetration into the more viscous and stationary regions of the axoplasm difficult. In contrast, a smaller molecule would have greater lateral freedom in the microstream and a higher probability of penetrating into viscous regions. In such a case, some of the smaller molecules may display a slower average transport velocity than do vesicles or granules. In fact, it may be incorrect to assume that a specific molecular species is transported at a specific velocity because many molecular species may themselves contribute to the observed velocity continuum. However, it is reasonable to expect that a certain maximum velocity is not exceeded and that this velocity begins to become a function of particle size in the range of macromolecular aggregates and organelles. Consequently the rapid transport peak should contain a great variety of labeled material, including particulate material. Such a variety has been demonstrated in mammalian sciatic nerves (Sabri and Ochs, 1972). Nevertheless, as the size of the transported moiety increases, some separation should occur and should be experimentally demonstrable.

CONCLUSIONS

The vesicle transport hypothesis (Schmitt, 1968), the transport filament hypothesis (Ochs, 1971), and the mechanochemical hypothesis (Samson, 1971) represent the primary models established to explain the rapid transport phenomenon. They may be classified as impulse models because they suggest the application of a force to a specific transport moiety over a specific instant of time. Because the variety of material found to be transported has been steadily increasing and includes observations of exogenous particle movement, the need for a highly specific transport system is now more open to question. In addition, an investigation of isotope distributions has suggested the existence of relatively nonspecific carrier processes. The emergence of a streaming model is therefore the result of certain incompatibilities between proposed mechanisms and new transport data. The microstream concept presented here brings the field of axoplasmic transport closer to the realm of protoplasmic streaming, as the latter has given rise to several nonspecific streaming hypotheses (Kamiya, 1959; Tazawa, 1968; Donaldson, 1972), and represents a return to the earlier general concepts of cytoplasmic streaming in neurons proposed by Lubinska in 1964.

The microstream concept suggests the possibility that in a neuron one mechanism can induce a great variety of transport velocities, from the very slow to the maximum streaming velocity that the system can generate. From this point of view, it is no longer obvious that a separate slow transport mechanism is necessary. Although some experimental findings have suggested that after subcellular fractionation the specific activity of the particulate fraction is higher for the rapidly transported material than for the slowly transported axonal constituents, the deposition phenomenon associated with the rapid transport makes identification of material in transit extremely difficult.

In a closed system, the forward pumping of fluid results also in a backward pressure flow. Although the axon is not a closed system, as material is lost across the axolemma as well as from the synaptic region, it cannot be considered an open system. Therefore, a retrograde flow is a consequence of orthograde transport. The microstreams arriving at the synaptic region will exert a pressure on the surrounding membrane. Indeed, this may contribute to the driving force behind axonal sprouting and growth-cone activity. However, this pressure cannot be expected to produce a retrograde movement of axoplasm over more than a few hundred micrometers. It is more likely that local eddy currents or vortices result along the entire axon, creating a backward flow of axoplasm. Neither can an active transport along the membrane or along tubules oriented toward the cell body be excluded as a possibility. Retrograde transport is therefore an important area of investigation that will make essential contributions to the unraveling of the transport phenomenon.

It is a direct consequence of the microstream model that any microtubule to which transport ATPases are attached has the potential of producing microstreams. Therefore many perikaryal tubules may transport material to specific regions and represent a supply network with which the cell body achieves its high degree of compartmentalization. The different proteins observed to migrate into the different branches of bifurcating axons (Anderson and McClure, 1973) may therefore not be an example of transport mechanism specificity, but rather a reflection of a difference in tubule origin and subsequent pathway.

The question as to whether material is moving through or with a medium is important because it influences the experimental approaches designed to elucidate the transport mechanism. The data presently available are not sufficiently specific to allow a clear decision in favor of one of these two alternatives. An experimental emphasis on the transport of exogenous particles, on water transport in axons, on the characterization of labeled material in the different regions of the rapid transport profile, and on a correlation of transport velocities with particle or molecular dimensions would probably allow such a decision in the near future. Thereafter, the path to an understanding of the molecular mechanism underlying the longitudinal transport phenomena in neurons should appear less difficult.

REFERENCES

Anderson, L. E., and McClure, W. O. (1973): Differential transport of protein in axons: Comparison between the sciatic nerve and dorsal columns of cats. *Proc. Natl. Acad. Sci. USA,* 70:1521–1525.

Banks, P., Mayor, D., and Tomlinson, D. R. (1971): Further evidence for the involvement of microtubules in the intra-axonal movement of noradrenaline storage granules. *J. Physiol. (Lond.),* 219:755–761.

Bodian, D., and Howe, H. A. (1941): Experimental studies on intraneuronal spread of poliomyelitis virus. *Johns Hopkins Med. J.,* 68:148–167.

Borisy, G. G., and Olmsted, J. B. (1972): Nucleated assembly of microtubules in porcine brain extracts. *Science,* 177:1196–1197.

Chambers, R., Jr. (1917): Microdisection studies. *J. Exp. Zool.,* 23:483–487.

Constantine, D. G., Emmons, R. W., and Woodie, J. D. (1972): Rabies virus in nasal mucosa of naturally infected bats. *Science,* 175:1255–1256.

Csanyi, V., Gervai, J., and Lajtha, A. (1973): Axoplasmic transport of free amino acids. *Brain Res.* 56:271–284.

Dahlström, A. (1968): Effects of colchicine on transport of amine storage granules in sympathetic nerves of rat. *Eur. J. Pharmacol.,* 5:111–113.

Dahlström, A. (1971): Axoplasmic transport (with particular respect to adrenergic neurons). *Phil. Trans. R. Soc. Lond. B,* 261:235–358.

De Lorenzo, A. J. D. (1970): The olfactory neuron and the blood-brain barrier. In: *Taste and Smell in Vertebrates,* edited by G. E. W. Wolstenhome and J. Knight. Churchill, London.

Dentler, W. L., Granett, S., Witman, G. B., and Rosenbaum, J. L. (1974): Directionality of brain microtubule assembly in vitro. *Proc. Natl. Acad. Sci. USA,* 71:1710–1714.

Donaldson, I. G. (1972): The estimation of the motive force for protoplasmic streaming in *Nitella. Protoplasma,* 74:329–344.

Droz, B., Koenig, H. L., and Di Giamberardino, L. (1973): Axonal migration of protein and glycoprotein to nerve endings. I. Radioautographic analysis of the renewal of protein in nerve endings of chicken ciliary ganglion after intracerebral injection of ^{3}H-lysine. *Brain Res.,* 60:93–127.

Edström, A., and Hanson, M. (1973): Temperature effects on fast axonal transport of proteins in vitro in frog sciatic nerves. *Brain Res.,* 58:345–354.

Fernandez, H. L., Huneeus, F. C., and Davison, P. F. (1970): Studies on the mechanism of axoplasmic transport in the crayfish cord. *J. Neurobiol.,* 1:395–409.

Freed, J. J., and Lebowitz, M. M. (1970): The association of a class of saltatory movements with microtubules in cultured cells. *J. Cell Biol.,* 45:334–354.

Gaskin, F., Kramer, S. B., Cantor, C. R., Adelstein, R., and Shelanski, M. L. (1974): A dynein-like protein associated with neurotubules. *FEBS Lett.,* 40:281–286.

Giddings, J. C. (1965): *Dynamics of Chromatography, Part 1: Principles and Theory,* Chapter 2. Dekker, New York.

Goldman, R. (1971): The role of three cytoplasmic fibers in BHK-21 cell motility. *J. Cell Biol.,* 51:752–762.

Gross, G. W. (1973): The effect of temperature on the rapid axoplasmic transport in C-fibers. *Brain Res.,* 56:359–363.

Gross, G. W., and Beidler, L. M. (1973): Fast axonal transport in the C-fibers of the garfish olfactory nerve. *J. Neurobiol.,* 4:413–428.

Gross, G. W., and Beidler, L. M. (1975): A quantitative analysis of isotope concentration profiles and rapid transport velocities in the C-fibers of the garfish olfactory nerve. *J. Neurobiol.* 6. (*In press.*)

Hinckley, R. E., and Green, L. S. (1971): The effects of colchicine and halothane on microtubules and electrical activity of rabbit vagus nerves. *J. Neurobiol.,* 2:97–106.

James, K. A. C., Bray, J. J., Morgan, I. G., and Austin, L. (1970): The effect of colchicine on the transport of axonal proteins in the chicken. *Biochem. J.,* 117:767–771.

Jarosch, R. (1957): Zur Mechanik der Protoplasmafibrillenbewegung. *Biochim. Biophys. Acta,* 25:204–205.

Jeffrey, P., and Austin, L. (1973): Axoplasmic transport. *Prog. Neurobiol.,* 2/3:205–255.

Kamiya, N. (1959): Protoplasmic streaming. *Protoplasma tologia,* 8(3a).

Kamiya, N., and Kuroda, K. (1965): Rotational protoplasmic streaming in *Nitella* and some physical properties of the endoplasm. In: *Proceedings of the Fourth International Congress on Rheology,* Part 4, edited by E. H. Lee and A. L. Copley. Wiley, New York.

Kreutzberg, G. W. (1969): Neuronal dynamics and axonal flow. IV. Blockage of intra-axonal enzyme transport by colchicine. *Proc. Natl. Acad. Sci. USA,* 62:722–728.

Kristensson, J. H., and Olsson, Y. (1971): Uptake and retrograde axonal transport of peroxidase in hypoglossal neurons. *Acta Neuropathol.,* 19:1–7.

Kuroda, K. (1964): Behavior of naked cytoplasmic drops isolated from plant cells. In: *Primitive Motile Systems in Cell Biology,* edited by R. D. Allen and N. Kamiya. Academic Press, New York.

LaVail, J. H., and LaVail, M. M. (1972): Retrograde axonal transport in the central nervous system. *Science,* 176:1416–1417.

Lehninger, A. L. (1965): *Bioenergetics.* Benjamin, New York.

Lentz, T. L. (1972): Distribution of leucine-³H during axoplasmic transport within regenerating neurons as determined by electron microscope radioautography. *J. Cell Biol.,* 52:719–732.

Lieberman, A. R. (1971): Microtubule-associated smooth endoplasmic reticulum in the frog's brain. *Z. Zellforsch. Mikrosk. Anat.,* 116:564–577.

Lubinska, L. (1964): Axoplasmic streaming in regenerating and normal nerve fibers. *Prog. Brain Res.,* 13:1–66.

McIntosh, J. R. (1974): Bridges between microtubules. *J. Cell Biol.,* 61:166–187.

Murphy, D. B., and Tilney, L. G. (1974): The role of microtubules in the movement of pigment granules in teleost melanophores. *J. Cell Biol.,* 61:757–779.

Ochs, S. (1971): Characteristics and a model for the fast axoplasmic transport in nerve. *J. Neurobiol.,* 2:331–345.

Ochs, S. (1972): Fast transport of materials in mammalian nerve fibers. *Science,* 176:252–260.

Ochs, S., and Hollingsworth, D. J. (1971): Dependence of fast axoplasmic transport in nerve on oxidative metabolism. *J. Neurochem.,* 18:107–114.

Porter, K. R. (1966): Cytoplasmic microtubules and their function. In: *Ciba Foundation Symposium on Principles of Biomolecular Organization,* edited by G. E. W. Wolstenholme and J. O'Connor. Little, Brown, Boston, Massachusetts.

Raine, C. S., Ghetti, B., and Shelanski, M. L. (1971): On the association between microtubules and mitochondria within axons. *Brain Res.,* 34:389–393.

Rudzinska, M. A. (1965): The fine structure and function of the tentacle in *Tokophrya infusionum. J. Cell Biol.,* 25:459–477.

Sabri, M. I., and Ochs, S. (1972): Characterization of fast and slow transported proteins in dorsal root and sciatic nerve of cat. *J. Neurobiol.,* 4:145–165.

Samson, F. E., Jr. (1971): Mechanism of axoplasmic transport. *J. Neurobiol.,* 2:347–360.

Schmitt, F. O. (1968): Fibrous proteins – neuronal organelles. *Proc. Natl. Acad. Sci. USA,* 60:1092–1101.

Schubert, P., and Kreutzberg, G. W. (1974): Axonal transport of adenosine and uridine derivatives and transfer to postsynaptic neurons. *Brain Res.,* 76:526–530.

Segal, I. (1967): Phosphate bond energies. In: *Encyclopedia of Biochemistry,* edited by R. Williams and E. Lansford, Jr. Reinhold, New York.

Smith, D. S. (1971): On the significance of cross-bridges between microtubules and synaptic vesicles. *Phil. Trans. R. Soc. Lond. (Biol. Sci.),* 261:395–405.

Smith, D. S., Järlfors, U., and Beránek, R. (1970): The organization of synaptic axoplasm in the lamprey (*Petromyzon marinus*) central nervous system. *J. Cell Biol.,* 46:199–219.

Smith, R. S. (1973): Microtubule and neurofilament densities in amphibian spinal root nerve fibers: Relationship to axoplasmic transport. *Can. J. Physiol. Pharmacol.,* 51:798–806.

Taylor, E. W. (1965): Brownian and saltatory movements of cytoplasmic granules and the movement of anaphase chromosomes. In: *Symposium on Biorheology, Proceedings of the Fourth International Congress on Biorheology.* Wiley (Interscience), New York.

Tazawa, M. (1968): The motive force of the cytoplasmic streaming in *Nitella. Protoplasma,* 65:207–222.

Weiss, P. (1967): Neuronal dynamics. In: *Axoplasmic Transport Neurosci. Res. Program Bull.,* 5:371–400.

Wilson, L., and Meza, I. (1973): The mechanism of action of colchicine. *J. Cell Biol.,* 58:709–719.

Wohlfarth-Botterman, K. E. (1964): Cell structures and their significance for ameboid movement. *Int. Rev. Cytol.,* 16:61–73.

Advances in Neurology, Vol. 12, edited by
G. W. Kreutzberg, Raven Press, New York
© 1975.

Evidence for Bidirectional Dendritic Transport of Horseradish Peroxidase

Gary Lynch, Rebekah L. Smith, Michael D. Browning,
and Sam Deadwyler

Department of Psychobiology, University of California, Irvine, Irvine, California 92664

The study of the transport of materials within the neuron has become a prominent subfield of modern neurobiology. Until recently, attention has been focused exclusively on the movement of proteins and other macromolecules from the cell body to the axon terminal. A number of important characteristics of axoplasmic flow have been established from such studies. In particular, it appears that the cell may use more than one transport mechanism, as evidenced by the variety of flow rates (e.g., McEwen and Grafstein, 1968; Lasek, 1970; Karlsson and Sjöstrand, 1971; Ochs, 1972*b*), and their differential content and susceptibility to drug treatment (Kidwai and Ochs, 1969; Sabri and Ochs, 1972; Fernandez and Samson, 1973).

An exciting development in this field has been the experimental demonstration that axoplasmic transport is a bidirectional process (Lubinská, 1964; Dahlström, 1965; Lasek, 1967; Kristensson, 1970; LaVail and LaVail, 1972). This finding suggests that neurons may have mechanisms for reciprocal communication between soma and terminal fields, and thus would be important to theories of the trophic functions of neurons (Rosenbluth and Wissig, 1964; Guth, 1969; Harris, 1974). That is, somatopetal axonal transport, in conjunction with uptake of materials at the terminal fields, may provide feedback monitoring of the extracellular environment by the metabolic center of the cell.

It has long been suspected that comparable transport phenomena occur in dendrites, but until very recently this field has remained neglected. This is understandable in view of the technical difficulties created by the short length of dendrites. Clearly, the material used as a marker would have to be placed very discretely; even moderately sized injections would cover both soma and dendritic ramifications, making it impossible to separate local uptake from dendritic transport. Kreutzberg, Schubert, and their associates (Globus, Lux, and Schubert, 1968; Schubert, Lux, and Kreutzberg, 1971; Schubert, Kreutzberg, and Lux, 1972; Kreutzberg, Schubert, Tóth, and Rieske, 1973) have recently used neurophysiologic techniques to obviate this difficulty. In a series of elegant experiments they have studied the movement of radioactive amino acids from extremely small and accurately placed injections. By iontophoresing labeled glycine inside the somata of spinal motoneurons and processing the tissue autoradiographically, they were able to follow the movement of label (presumably as proteins) throughout the dendritic trees of these cells. Beyond this, they were able to provide preliminary evidence that dendritic transport, like its axonal counterpart, may involve the microtubule system of the cell (Schubert et al., 1972).

In our laboratory we have used a different approach to the problem of the transport of materials within dendrites. The following sections summarize the results of our efforts to date. First, we review the evidence that the enzyme horseradish peroxidase is accumulated by neurons and moved bidirectionally through the dendritic tree. We then discuss in some detail a technique that we feel will ultimately permit an analysis of the mechanisms subserving this dendritic "transport."

EVIDENCE FOR DENDRITIC TRANSPORT OF HORSERADISH PEROXIDASE *IN VIVO*

Horseradish peroxidase (HRP) is an enzyme that cytologists have used for years to study pinocytosis and the intracellular fate of exogenously applied compounds (see Holtzman, 1971). Kristensson and Olsson (1971) were the first to use this enzyme to study axonal transport. They concluded that HRP taken up at the gastrocnemius muscle moved from the neuromuscular junction in a somatopetal direction to the parent cell bodies in the spinal cord. These findings were replicated in hypoglossal neurons (Kristensson, Olsson, and Sjöstrand, 1971; Kristensson and Olsson, 1973; Kuypers, Kievit, and Groen-Klevant, 1974), and extended by LaVail and LaVail (1972), who followed somatopetal flow of HRP from the chick optic tectum to cell bodies in the retina. LaVail, Winston, and Tish (1973) also documented several cases of somatopetal axonal transport entirely within the brain and have demonstrated the value of the procedure as a neuroanatomic tracing technique. In addition, the somatopetal transport of HRP in the brain has now been replicated by several laboratories (Jones and Leavitt, 1973; Ralston and Sharp, 1973; Kuypers et al., 1974; Nauta, Pritz, and Lasek, 1974). Work in our laboratory has shown that HRP will also travel in a somatofugal direction in axons (Lynch, Smith, Mensah, and Cotman, 1973; Lynch, Gall, Mensah, and Cotman, 1974), and in some, but certainly not all cases, HRP can be used to follow an entire anatomical system from cell bodies to axon terminals. Kuypers and his associates (1974) have also reported the existence of such transport in axons.

Further studies in our laboratory have revealed that HRP can be ejected from recording micropipettes by electrophoresis (Lynch, Deadwyler, and Gall, 1974). This suggested that the enzyme might be used to study dendritic as well as axonal transport in the central nervous system. That is, by combining high impedance recording with electrophoresis, we felt it would be possible to place very discrete ejections near somata or at some point along their dendrites and to follow the subsequent movement of the enzyme. This would also provide a means of labeling the elements recorded by extracellular microelectrodes, a technique not previously available to neurophysiologists.

To date we have performed the majority of our experiments in the hippocampal formation of the rat. There are several reasons for choosing this system. First, the cell bodies of this region form two compact layers with long, outwardly radiating dendrites (Fig. 1). Furthermore, these cells and their processes are oriented roughly perpendicular to the septotemporal axis of the hippocampus. Together these features make it possible to place ejections at various points along the length of the dendrites and compare these results with those obtained after ejections in the cell layers. In addition, the afferents to the dendritic zones separate themselves into discrete layers, and electrical stimulation of these afferents produces monosynaptic negative potentials localized to the terminal field of that afferent. Therefore,

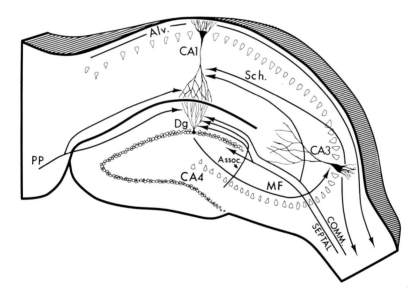

FIG. 1. Diagram of the cellular arrangement of the hippocampal formation. This schematic represents a typical *in vitro* tissue section cut perpendicular to the septo-temporal axis of the hippocampal formation. *Abbreviations:* Alv, alveus, containing axons of CA1 cells exiting the hippocampus; Assoc, ipsilateral associational axons arising from CA3 cells and terminating in middle molecular layer of the dentate gyrus and CA1; CA1, CA3, and CA4, subfields of pyramidal cells; Comm., hippocampal commissural axons from contralateral CA3 cells, terminating in same dendritic fields as Assoc.; Dg, dentate gyrus (granule cell layer); MF, mossy fiber axons of the granule cells innervating the inner molecular layer of CA3 cells; PP, perforant path, containing axons originating in cells of the entorhinal cortex and terminating in dentate gyrus and CA1 outer molecular layers; Sch, Schaeffer collaterals of CA3 axons, terminating in middle dendritic zone of CA1 cells; Septal, septal axons terminating in the inner molecular layer of the dentate gyrus.

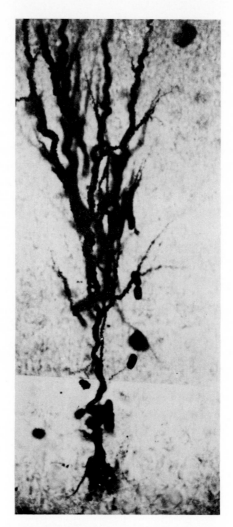

FIG. 2. *In vivo* labeling of single hippocampal pyramidal cell by somatofugal transport of HRP. Montage of photomicrographs of a subicular cell recorded from and labeled with HRP with an ejection current of 500 nA for 10 sec. (From Lynch, Deadwyler, and Gall, 1974a.)

by using stimulation and recording techniques, it is possible to place ejections in the dendrites at specific distances from the cell body.

All *in vivo* experiments were performed on adult rats anesthetized with urethane. Glass microelectrodes filled with 2% HRP (Sigma, type II) in 2 M NaCl were lowered into the hippocampus until the pyramidal cell layer was identified by spontaneous electrical activity. A positive current of up to 2 μA was then applied to the electrolyte for 10 to 15 sec. Following the ejection, the electrode was raised, moved several hundred micrometers, and lowered into the apical dendrites, about 300 to 350 μm below the CA1 pyramidal cell layer. This process was repeated several times per animal. In a few animals, ejections were also made in the dorsal thalamus immediately below the hippocampal formation, in the caudate nucleus, and in the cerebellum. Survival times after the last ejection varied from 2 min (immediate sacrifice) to several hours. The animals were perfused with 10% Formalin and the brains removed and postfixed in cold (4°C) Formalin for 12 to 24 hr. The brains were then sectioned at 50 μm on a freezing microtome, and relevant sections processed for the demonstration of HRP (Strauss, 1964; Lynch et al, 1973, 1974*b*).

Figure 2 shows the result of an early experiment in which a subicular cell was isolated by electrophysiologic criteria and 500 nA of current was briefly applied to the HRP-filled recording electrode. Notice that the enzyme has traveled from the region of the soma outward through the apical shafts of the neurons for a total distance of over 400 μm. Figure 3 indicates that transport in the reverse direction also takes place. In this case, the electrode was localized in the dendrites of the hilus just ventral to the dorsal leaf of the dentate gyrus. A single polymorph cell is labeled. It is

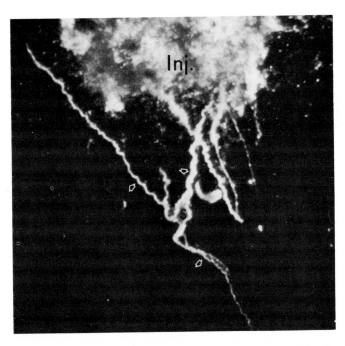

FIG. 3. Bidirectional dendritic movement of HRP through a single cell *in vivo*. Dark-field photomicrograph of a single neuron labeled with HRP following passage of a small current into the hilar region of the dentate gyrus (at Inj). HRP has traveled somatopetally to the soma, S, then somatofugally through other dendrites. Probable direction of movement of the enzyme through the dendrites is indicated by arrows.

evident that the HRP has traveled in a somatopetal direction to the cell body, at which point it was transported in a somatofugal fashion into other dendrites of the cell. It appears, then, that HRP is taken up by somata or by dendrites and transported rapidly in both somatofugal and somatopetal directions.

These experiments provide evidence that bidirectional dendritic transport of HRP takes place in the brain and lead naturally to questions about the time course and mechanisms underlying this effect. It would be useful to know, for instance, whether active cellular processes such as underlie axonal transport, or whether passive diffusion may underlie this dendritic movement of protein. It appears from our studies that the total time of uptake and transport in hippocampal neurons is extremely rapid. Measurements taken from those experiments in which animals were sacrificed within 2 min of the beginning of the current ejection indicate that the enzyme was transported approximately 100 to 150 μm into the dendrites after ejection into the pyramidal cell layer. This suggests that the somatofugal movement must take place at a rate of at least 50 μm/min (including uptake), a value comparable to that reported for spinal cord cells (Globus et al., 1968; Schubert et al., 1971).

The precise measurement of the time of transport cannot be accurately accomplished in the brain because the dendrites are short and critical time is lost with ordinary perfusion methods. A further complication is that we have no data on the rate of uptake of HRP into neuronal perikarya or dendrites. Holtzman and Peterson (1969) have presented evidence that uptake into dorsal root ganglion neurons is rapid, but unfortunately they did not test this at times shorter than 15 min. In addition, although a variety of drugs have been used to manipulate axonal transport in peripheral nerves (Dahlström, 1968; Kreutzberg, 1969; Sjöstrand, Frizell, and Hasselgren, 1970; England, Kadin, and Goldstein, 1973; and many others), such manipulations are less convenient in subcortical brain structures such as the hippocampus.

IN VITRO STUDIES OF THE HIPPOCAMPUS

In order to pursue the mechanistic questions mentioned above with regard to dendritic transport in neurons of the central nervous system, we have begun using a procedure and apparatus similar to that described by Yamamoto (1972) for his *in vitro* studies of the mossy fiber system of the hippocampus. Slices of the hippocampal formation are prepared and maintained in the following way. Animals are stunned by a sharp blow to the back of the neck, then decapitated. The brains are quickly removed and one hippocampal formation from each animal is sectioned perpendicular to the septotemporal axis, at 400 μm, using a Sorvall tissue sectioner. Sections are immediately placed into a recording chamber (Fig. 4) containing a glucose–

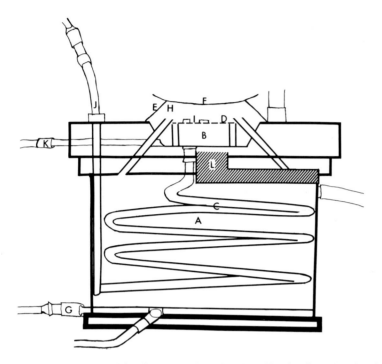

FIG. 4. Schematic diagram of *in vitro* recording chamber. The *in vitro* chamber is constructed of clear Plexiglas, and consists of a water bath, A, on which a well, B, is placed. A glass tube containing the bathing medium, C, coils through the warm (37°C) water bath and inserts into the bottom of the well. The well is covered by a 50-μm mesh nylon net, D, which is surrounded by a plastic cone, E, on which rests a watch glass, F. A gas containing 95% O_2–5% CO_2 is bubbled, G, through the water bath, creating a heated, high-humidity atmosphere in the area immediately above the net, H. The tissue slices, 1, are placed on this net. Oxygenated medium (glucose–Ringer's) is dripped into the glass coil, J, and flows into the net-covered well and exits through plastic tubing, K. Illumination is provided by a light, L, located immediately below the well.

Ringer's solution (Yamamoto, 1972). The medium is maintained at 35 to 37°C, pH 7.0 to 7.4, and is continually aerated with 5% CO_2–95% O_2.

We have found through electrophysiologic analyses that the hippocampal explants thus prepared exhibit neurophysiologic behavior similar to that recorded in the intact rat. Both spontaneous and evoked activity can be recorded from all subdivisions of the hippocampal explant. We have tested the response characteristics of a number of intrinsic and extrinsic pathways and have shown that each exhibits field potentials, extracellular unit driving, and in some cases synaptic potentials, which are all comparable to those widely reported from intact preparations (e.g., Andersen and Lømo, 1970).

Figure 5 shows the response characteristics of a single hippocampal explant in which we found three separate fiber systems (perforant path, mossy fibers, and Schaeffer collaterals) to be operative. Note that both the dentate gyrus and CA1 field potentials show reversals of the extracellular

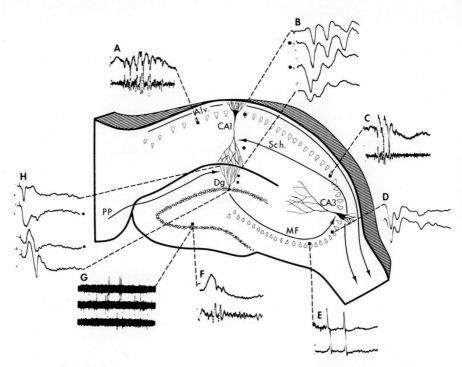

FIG. 5. Extracellular potentials recorded during stimulation of three separate fiber systems of a single hippocampal explant. Abbreviations as in Fig. 1. (A) Unitary discharges from CA1 cell layer to stimulation of Schaeffer collaterals; upper trace is unfiltered record, lower is after high pass (500 Hz–10 kHz) filtering. Stimulus at onset of trace. Amplitude of units is 500 μV; sweep duration 50 msec. In this and all other traces, negativity is down, positivity is up. (B) Field-potential profile from CA1 region to Schaeffer collateral stimulation. Dotted lines indicate potentials recorded from tip of apical and basilar dendrites. Filled dots represent maximal negative (synaptic) potential (lower) and cell-layer responses (upper). Note series of three distinct "population spikes" within the cell layer, which increase in latency when recorded in the alveus (top trace). Largest peak negativity is 4.0 mV, sweep duration is 20 msec. (C) Driven unitary activity recorded from the CA3 region from stimulation of the mossy fiber pathway. Calibration same as in (A). (D) Higher-intensity stimulation of mossy fibers elicits short-latency negative potentials in CA3. Calibration same as in (B). (E) Spontaneously firing CA3 unit well isolated by microelectrode (unfiltered recording). Amplitude 2 mV, sweep duration 20 msec. (F) Driven dentate granule cell unitary discharge (lower trace) and field potential (upper trace) from low intensity stimulation of perforant path axons. Calibration same as in (A) and (C). (G) Spontaneous activity of dentate units. Spike amplitude 100 μV; sweep duration 500 msec. (H) Field-potential profile from dentate molecular and cell layers. Dotted lines indicate potentials recorded at the obliterated hippocampal fissure (upper) and within the dentate cell layer (lower). Note "population spike" negativity on cell-layer response. Dotted traces indicate maximal extracellular synaptic potential (upper) and reversal point of negativity at positions from which recordings were obtained in the molecular layer. Calibration, peak negativity 2.5 mV; sweep duration 20 msec. (From Deadwyler, Rose, Stanford, Lynch, and Cotman, *in preparation*).

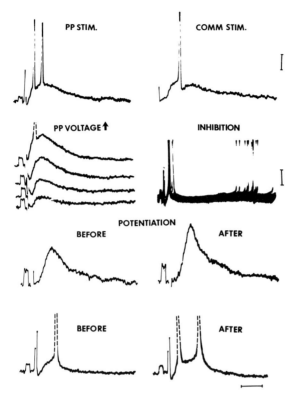

FIG. 6. Intracellular responses of dentate granule cells recorded from *in vitro* hippocampal explants. PP stim, Response of a granule cell to stimulation of perforant path axons. Note double discharge. Calibration pulse is 4 mV followed by stimulus artifact. Spike amplitude approximately 55 mV, EPSP 12 mV, total sweep duration 50 msec. Comm stim, Response of a different granule cell to stimulation of commissural axons. Spike amplitude 60 mV; EPSP 15 mV. Calibration 15 mV; sweep duration 40 msec. PP voltage, Response of another granule cell to increases in stimulus voltages; bottom to top stimulus voltages were 15, 25, 40, and 70 V applied to perforant path axons. Calibration pulse 4.0 mV, sweep duration 50 msec. Inhibition, Inhibitory period (60 msec) following initial excitation by perforant path stimulation. This cell was depolarized by positive current injection through the microelectrode in order to elicit spontaneous activity. Sweep duration approximately 125 msec; calibration 15 mV; spike amplitude 50 mV. Seventeen superimposed sweeps. Potentiation, Sub- and suprathreshold responses of two granule cells (upper and lower traces) to 1.5/sec perforant path stimulation before and after a 15-sec train of 15/sec pulses. The top set of traces utilized a stimulus intensity that was insufficient to elicit an action potential and only effected an increase in the amplitude of the EPSP (compare before and after), which lasted for at least 1.0 min. The bottom set of traces shows another cell in which the stimulus intensity was sufficient to elicit a single discharge (before potentiation, left trace). After potentiation the stimulus elicited two action potentials. Calibration pulse is 2.0 mV in the upper traces and 5.0 mV in the lower traces; total sweep is 50 msec in all cases. Note that spike in lower traces has been clipped because of high amplification. Calibration bar is 10 msec (same cell as shown for "inhibition" above). (From Deadwyler, Dudek, Lynch, and Cotman, *in preparation*).

dendritic negativity in the respective cell layers, and that each positive-going field potential has the "population spike" superimposed (at arrows). All three cellular subdivisions (granule cells, CA1 and CA3 pyramidal cells) were also spontaneously active. The activation of CA3 neurons through stimulation of the mossy fiber axons is similar to that previously reported by Yamamoto (1972) in hippocampal explants from the guinea pig. In all three fiber systems stimulated, bursts of individual unitary potentials were easily obtained with relatively low current levels (delivered through 62-μm bipolar electrodes).

Figure 6 shows the results of intracellular recordings from granule cells in the dentate gyrus. These cells are exceedingly small and are normally difficult to impale *in vivo* (Andersen, Holmquist, and Voorhoeve, 1966; Lømo, 1971a). We have succeeded in recording for up to 1 hr from impaled dentate granule cells that exhibited stable resting potentials and synaptic driving through known input pathways. Spontaneously firing as well as synaptically driven granule cells often exhibited action potentials of 60 to 80 mV. Frequently these cells could be depolarized to firing level by injection of positive current, or hyperpolarized by the injection of negative currents through the recording electrode. In addition, both single- and multiple-action potential discharges arising from 5 to 15 mV and long duration excitatory postsynaptic potentials (EPSP's) were often observed following stimulation of the perforant path axons. Measurement of conductance changes indicated that the EPSP's were probably sodium-mediated. EPSP's were enhanced following brief trains of 15/sec stimuli delivered to the perforant path, but such potentiation was difficult to obtain in a number of neurons, and appeared to be dependent upon stimulus intensity to a large extent (Lømo, 1971*b*; Kuno and Weakly, 1972). Impalement of CA3 and CA1 neurons has also been obtained; however, because the intracellular response characteristics of these neurons has been extensively reported elsewhere (Spencer and Kandel, 1968), pyramidal cell activity will not be reiterated here.

Effects of this sort are obtained in the explants for up to 8 to 10 hr after their preparation. Recently, we have modified the bathing medium to include amino acids and vitamins (Eagle's minimal essential medium), and found that the survival time can be greatly extended.

From the above-described physiologic analyses it is evident that the explants exhibit many of the characteristics of the hippocampus *in vivo* and are therefore appropriate as a model system in which to study basic neurobiologic phenomena, including dendritic transport.

IN VITRO STUDIES OF DENDRITIC TRANSPORT

We have found that dendritic transport is readily obtained *in vitro*. We regularly use 3 to 5-MΩ glass micropipettes filled with 1% HRP in 1 M

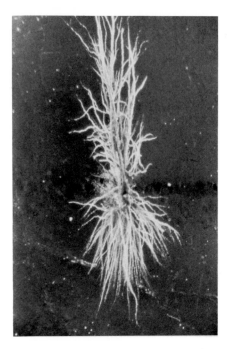

FIG. 7. Distribution of HRP after a small ejection into the CA1 pyramidal cell layer of the hippocampus. In this *in vitro* experiment, the enzyme is accumulated by two to four somata then transported throughout their extensive apical and basal dendritic trees. Two fine axons are also visible for a considerable distance from the cells.

NaCl, buffered at pH 6.2 with 0.2 M phosphate (Strauss, 1958). Ejection currents range from 500 nA to 5 μA for 10 to 30 sec. Immediately after the last ejection, the explants are fixed in a cold, cacodylate-buffered (pH 7.4) solution of 3% glutaraldehyde, 10% formaldehyde, and 15% sucrose for 2 hr. The tissue is then transferred to buffered sucrose and kept at 4°C for an additional 2 to 24 hr before it is sectioned and stained as in the *in vivo* preparations.

In Fig. 7, a small ejection was made into the pyramidal cell layer of the subfield CA1 and the enzyme was incorporated by a very small population of cells. As is evident from the micrograph, HRP was transported throughout both apical and basal dendritic ramifications. In this experiment we were also able to follow the axons for a short distance. Figure 8 is an example in which the enzyme was ejected onto a neuron isolated by neurophysiologic criteria and was transported into the dendritic fields. Note, as pointed out by Kuypers et al. (1974), that dark-field microscopy reveals more detail than does bright-field. It should be emphasized that only a portion of the dendritic field is contained on the 50-μm-thick section from which this micrograph was taken. Retrograde transport is also common, as indicated by the cells labeled in Fig. 9. In this case the enzyme was ejected

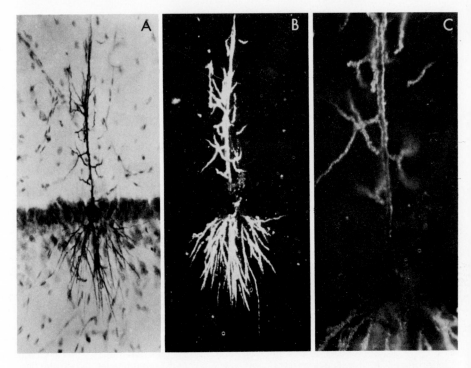

FIG. 8. Localization of HRP after ejection near electrophysiologically isolated pyramidal cell. Another example of the somatofugal movement of HRP following a very discrete ejection onto one or possibly two pyramidal cells *in vitro*. Note the greater detail revealed by dark-field microscopy (B) than found in bright-field photographs of the same material (A). (C) High-power detail of the dendritic arborization.

under visual control into the pyramidal cell dendritic tree. Again note the relative advantages of dark- and bright-field photography with regard to HRP.

Use of the *in vitro* preparations has allowed for a more precise measurement of flow rates than is possible in intact animals, because flow can be terminated more quickly and reliably by immediate cold fixation. Initial measurements on those ejections that were placed in the middle of the dendritic tree of the pyramidal cells suggest that up to 200 μm may be labeled in either the somatopetal or somatofugal direction in 1 min. The rate ranged between 140 and 200 μm/min (including uptake) among the 16 ejections measured to date. This represents a considerably faster rate than the 50 μm/min reported in the intact spinal cord (see above). Further experiments directed at obtaining a more precise measurement of dendritic flow rates are currently in progress.

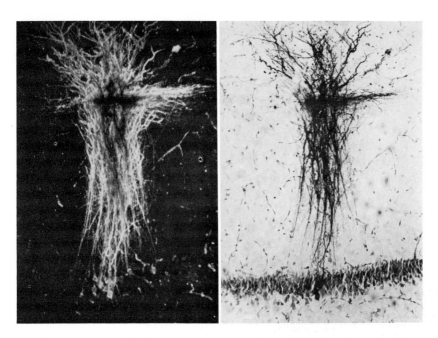

FIG. 9. Distribution of HRP following an ejection in the dendritic field of the zone CA1. In this *in vitro* experiment, HRP was applied to the hippocampal explant approximately 300 μm from the pyramidal cell bodies. (Right) Bright-field photomicrograph; whereas (left) is the same material photographed with a dark-field condensor. The enzyme has traveled somatopetally to reach the cell bodies and somatofugally through the dendritic ramifications above the ejection. Note that in this case there appears to be some labeling of axons passing through the ejection site.

DISCUSSION

These experiments indicate that HRP histochemistry is a valuable tool for the study of intradendritic movement of macromolecules. A chief advantage of the procedure is that the enzyme can be ejected extracellularly, thereby obviating the great difficulties associated with intracellular neurophysiology. Several workers using a variety of test systems have shown that HRP is accumulated by neurons, and our results are certainly in accord with this. However, it should be noted that our procedures may have produced some damage to the cells under study, and that this may have facilitated the "loading" of the cells with enzyme. In most cases we were able to record from the same cell before and after application of current to the microelectrode, and we found that after a short period of depression the cell would show apparently normal spontaneous activity. In these cases it would seem that any immediate damage caused by the presence of the electrode or the ejection of electrolytes and enzyme would have to be relatively minor.

A second advantage of HRP histochemistry is that by using electrophoresis, extremely discrete ejections can be made. After carefully isolating a cell according to neurophysiologic criteria, we have been able on many occasions to label single neurons. Finally, although we have not exploited this feature, the reaction product can easily be made electron dense, making HRP histochemistry appropriate for ultrastructural studies (Graham and Karnovsky, 1966). This is an invaluable feature, as electron microscopic studies will be required in order to elucidate the cellular machinery responsible for the transport-like effects we have obtained.

Our findings with HRP indicate that very rapid movement of materials takes place within dendrites. Following ejections at the cell body, enzyme was distributed throughout both apical and basal dendrites, including, in our best preparations, secondary and tertiary branches. When ejections were made in dendritic fields a similar rapid distribution of enzyme was observed, indicating that dendritic flow is bidirectional. A curious feature of this retrograde movement was that in some regions it did not appear to move effectively past the soma, whereas in others it clearly did. This failure may have been due to an insufficient quantity of enzyme reaching the soma because of its dilution by distribution into very extensive dendritic ramifications; but other mechanisms are possible. Ochs (1972a) has suggested in his studies of axonal transport that there exists a "gate" at the point of transfer of transported substances from cell cytoplasm into the axons; it is possible that a comparable transport "gate" also operates for materials entering dendrites from the cell body.

It is tempting to hypothesize that this movement of HRP in the dendrites is mediated by mechanisms similar to those underlying bidirectional axoplasmic transport, rather than by simple diffusion. A necessary first step in testing this possibility will involve an electron-microscopic analysis of the ultrastructural localization of the enzyme. As mentioned, HRP histochemistry is readily adaptable to electron-microscopic studies and we are currently pursuing this line of investigation. Beyond this, it would be particularly useful to measure the response of the dendritic "transport" to treatments known to interrupt axoplasmic flow by means of microtubule disruption or metabolic inhibition. We have recently begun studies of this type using the explant techniques described above. To date we have found that the transport of HRP is unimpaired (although possibly slowed) by temperatures as low as 22°C. In addition, we have obtained preliminary evidence that 10^{-3} M colchicine in the bathing medium appears to interfere with transport, and possibly uptake, of HRP. We have also used colchicine (10^{-2} M in 2 M NaCl) in glass micropipettes to make discrete ejections of the chemical at known distances from HRP ejections. Pilot studies using this method indicate that when colchicine is ejected into the middle of the dendritic layer somatofugal HRP transport may be blocked within 20 min. This effect occurs even though the cells at the area of HRP ejection remain spontaneously active throughout the experiment. Although these findings are fragmentary, they do support the conclusions of Schubert et al. (1972) that dendritic transport is retarded by colchicine, and may therefore involve the microtubule system of the cell.

If the movement of HRP described above is caused by processes normally active in neurons, it would appear that a very rapid bidirectional exchange of materials takes place between the soma and its dendritic ramifications. Presumably this could serve functions comparable to those proposed for axoplasmic flow. Materials synthesized in the cell body would be transported by the somatofugal mechanisms throughout the dendritic tree, whereas the reverse flow might serve to provide a means for events taking place in distal synaptic zones to influence the basic biochemistry of the entire neuron. The suggestion has been made that axons exert long-term or trophic influences on the cells they innervate (cf. Guth, 1969), and it seems plausible that interactions of this type would involve a retrograde dendritic transport mechanism.

ACKNOWLEDGMENTS

We are pleased to acknowledge the helpful suggestions and assistance of Dr. Timothy J. Teyler, of Harvard University, in the design of the in vitro recording chamber. We would also like to thank Dr. F. E. Dudek, Greg Rose, and Edward Stanford for their valuable contributions to the in vitro hippocampal neurophysiology, and Valentine Gribkoff for his assistance in preparing the figures. Research supported by grants NS 11589–01 (NIH) and BMS 7702237–2 (NSF).

REFERENCES

Andersen, P., Holmquist, B., and Voorhoeve, P. E. (1966): Entorhinal activation of dentate granule cells. Acta Physiol. Scand., 66:448–460.

Andersen, P., and Lømo, T. (1970): Mode of control of hippocampal pyramidal cell discharges. In: The Neural Control of Behavior, edited by R. E. Whalen, R. F. Thompson, M. Verzeano, and N. M. Weinberger. Academic Press, New York.

Dahlström, A. (1965): Observations on the accumulation of noradrenalin in the proximal and distal parts of peripheral adrenergic nerves after compression. J. Anat., 99:677–689.

Dahlström, A. (1968): Effect of colchicine on transport of amine storage granules in sympathetic nerves of rat. Eur. J. Pharmacol., 5:111–113.

England, J. M., Kadin, M. E., and Goldstein, M. N. (1973): The effect of vincristine sulphate on the axoplasmic flow of proteins in cultures of sympathetic neurons. J. Cell Sci., 12:549–565.

Fernandez, H. L., and Samson, F. E. (1973): Axoplasmic transport: Differential inhibition by cytochalasin-B. J. Neurobiol., 4:201–206.

Globus, G., Lux, H. D., and Schubert, P. (1968): Somadendritic spread of intracellularly injected tritiated glycine in cat spinal motoneurons. Brain Res., 11:440–445.

Graham, R. C., and Karnovsky, M. J. (1966): The early stages of absorption of injected horseradish peroxidase in the proximal tubules of mouse kidney: Ultrastructural cytochemistry by a new technique. J. Histochem. Cytochem., 14:291–302.

Guth, L., editor (1969): "Trophic" effects of vertebrate neurons. In: *Neurosciences Research Program Bulletin*, Vol. 7, pp. 1–73. MIT Press, Cambridge, Massachusetts.

Harris, A. J. (1974): Inductive functions of the nervous system. *Annu. Rev. Physiol.* 36:251–305.

Holtzman, E. (1971): Cytochemical studies of protein transport in the nervous system. *Phil. Trans. Soc. Lond. (Biol. Sci.)*, 261:407–421.

Holtzman, E., and Peterson, E. R. (1969): Uptake of protein by mammalian neurons. *J. Cell Biol.*, 40:863–868.

Jones, E. G., and Leavitt, R. Y. (1973): Demonstration of thalamo-cortical connectivity in the cat somato-sensory system by retrograde axonal transport of horseradish peroxidase. *Brain Res.*, 63:414–418.

Karlsson, J., and Sjöstrand, O. (1971): Synthesis, migration and turnover of proteins in retinal ganglion cells. *J. Neurochem.*, 18:749–767.

Kidwai, A. M., and Ochs, S. (1969): Components of fast and slow phases of axoplasmic flow. *J. Neurochem.*, 16:1105–1112.

Kreutzberg, G. W. (1969): Neuronal dynamics and axonal flow. IV. Blockage of intraaxonal enzyme transport by colchicine. *Proc. Natl. Acad. Sci., USA*, 62:722–728.

Kreutzberg, G. W., Schubert, P., Tóth, L., and Rieske, E. (1973): Intradendritic transport to postsynaptic sites. *Brain Res.*, 62:399–404.

Kristensson, K. (1970): Transport of fluorescent protein tracer in peripheral nerves. *Acta Neuropathol. (Berl.)*, 16:293–300.

Kristensson, K., and Olsson, Y. (1971): Retrograde axonal transport of protein. *Brain Res.*, 29:363–365.

Kristensson, K., and Olsson, Y. (1973): Uptake and retrograde axonal transport of protein tracers in hypoglossal neurons. *Acta Neuropathol. (Berl.)*, 23:43–47.

Kristensson, K., Olsson, Y., and Sjöstrand, J. (1971): Axonal uptake and retrograde transport of exogenous proteins in the hypoglossal nerve. *Brain Res.*, 32:399–406.

Kuno, M., and Weakly, J. N. (1972): Facilitation of monosynaptic facilatory synaptic potentials in spinal motorneurons evoked by internuncial impulses. *J. Physiol. (Lond.)*, 224:271–286.

Kuypers, H. G. J. M., Kievit, J., and Groen-Klevant, A. C. (1974): Retrograde axonal transport of horseradish peroxidase in rat's forebrain. *Brain Res.*, 67:211–218.

Lasek, J. (1967): Bidirectional transport of radioactivity-labelled axoplasmic components. *Nature*, 216:1212–1214.

Lasek, R. J. (1970): Protein transport in neurons. *Int. Rev. Neurobiol.*, 13:289–324.

LaVail, J. H., and LaVail, M. K. (1972): Retrograde axonal transport in the central nervous system. *Science*, 176:1416–1417.

LaVail, J. H., Winston, K. R., and Tish, A. (1973): A method based on retrograde intraaxonal transport of protein for the identification of cell bodies of origin of axons terminating within the CNS. *Brain Res.*, 58:470–477.

Lømo, T. (1971a): Patterns of activation in a monosynaptic cortical pathway: The perforant path input to the dentate area of the hippocampal formation. *Exp. Brain Res.*, 12:18–45.

Lømo, T. (1971b): Potentiation of monosynaptic EPSP's in the perforant path–dentate granule cell synapse. *Exp. Brain Res.*, 12:46–63.

Lubinská, L. (1964): Axoplasmic streaming in regenerating and in normal nerve fibers. In: *Progress in Brain Research, Vol. 13: Mechanisms of Neural Regeneration*, edited by M. Singer and J. P. Schade, pp. 56–66. Elsevier, Amsterdam.

Lynch, G., Deadwyler, S., and Gall, C. (1974a): Labeling of central nervous system neurons with extracellular recording microelectrodes. *Brain Res.*, 66:337–341.

Lynch, G., Gall, C., Mensah, P., and Cotman, C. W. (1974b): Horseradish peroxidase histochemistry: A new method for tracing efferent projections in the central nervous system. *Brain Res.*, 65:373–380.

Lynch, G. S., Smith, R. L., Mensah, P., and Cotman, C. W. (1973): Tracing the dentate gyrus mossy fiber system with horseradish peroxidase histochemistry. *Exp. Neurol.*, 40:516–524.

McEwen, B. S., and Grafstein, B. (1968): Fast and slow components in axonal transport of protein. *J. Cell Biol.*, 38:494–508.

Nauta, H. J. W., Pritz, M. B., and Lasek, R. J. (1974): Afferents to the rat caudoputamen studied with horseradish peroxidase. An evaluation of a retrograde neuroanatomical research method. *Brain Res.,* 67:219–238.

Ochs, S. (1972a): Fast transport of materials in mammalian nerve fibers. *Science,* 176:252–260.

Ochs, S. (1972b): Rate of fast axoplasmic transport in mammalian nerve fibres. *J. Physiol. (Lond.),* 227:627–645.

Ralston, H. J. III, and Sharp, P. V. (1973): The identification of thalamocortical relay cells in the adult cat by means of retrograde axonal transport of horseradish peroxidase. *Brain Res.,* 62:273–278.

Rosenbluth, J., and Wissig, S. L. (1964): The distribution of exogenous ferritin in toad spinal ganglia and the mechanism of its uptake by neurons. *J. Cell Biol.,* 23:307–325.

Sabri, M. I., and Ochs, S. (1972): Characterization of fast and slow transported proteins in dorsal root and sciatic nerve of cats. *J. Neurobiol.,* 4:145–165.

Schubert, P., Kreutzberg, G. W., and Lux, H. D. (1972): Neuroplasmic transport in dendrites: Effect of colchicine on morphology and physiology of motoneurones in the cat. *Brain Res.,* 47:331–343.

Schubert, P., Lux, H. D., and Kreutzberg, G. W. (1971): Single cell isotope injection technique, a tool for studying axonal and dendritic transport. *Acta Neuropathol. (Berl.),* 5:179–186.

Sjostrand, J., Frizell, M., and Hasselgren, P.-O. (1970): Effects of colchicine on axonal transport in peripheral nerves. *J. Neurochem.,* 17:1563–1570.

Spencer, W. A., and Kandel, E. R. (1968): Cellular and integrative properties of the hippocampal pyramidal cell and the comparative physiology of cortical neurons. *Int. J. Neurol.,* 6:266–297.

Strauss, W. (1958): Colorimetric analysis with *N,N*-dimethyl-*p*-phenylenediamine of the uptake of intravenously injected horseradish peroxidase by various tissues of the rat. *J. Biophys. Biochem. Cytol.,* 4:541–549.

Strauss, W. (1964): Factors affecting the cytochemical reaction of peroxidase with benzidine and the stability of the blue reaction product. *J. Histochem. Cytochem.,* 12:462–469.

Yamamoto, C. (1972): Activation of hippocampal neurons by mossy fiber stimulation in thin brain sections *in vitro. Exp. Brain Res.,* 14:423–435.

Advances in Neurology, Vol. 12, edited by
G. W. Kreutzberg, Raven Press, New York
© 1975.

Observations on Cortical Neurons Retrogradely Labeled with Horseradish Peroxidase

Horstmar Holländer

Neuroanatomical Laboratory, Max Planck Institute for Psychiatry, D-8000, Munich 40, Federal Republic of Germany

Cell bodies originating in the central nervous pathways may be identified after injections of horseradish peroxidase (HRP) into the region of axonal terminations. The enzyme is transported retrogradely through the axons and accumulates in the parent cells where it can be shown histochemically (LaVail, Winston, and Tish, 1973; Nauta, Pritz, and Lasek, 1974). In studies on corticotectal projections in the cat (Holländer, 1974) cortical neurons projecting to the superior colliculus were demonstrated by this technique. This chapter describes light microscopical aspects of tracer storage and distribution in the labeled cells.

In four adult cats 150 μg HRP dissolved in 0.5 μl of water was stereotaxically injected into the left superior colliculus. The times of postinjection survival were 17 hr, 3 days, and 8 days (two experiments). In deep Nembutal narcosis the animals were perfused transcardially with a mixture of 0.5% paraformaldehyde and 2.5% glutaraldehyde in cacodylate buffer at pH 7.2 preceded by washing with Macrodex to remove erythrocytes from the capillaries (Jacobson and Trojanowski, 1974). Tissue blocks were sampled from various cortical regions of the ipsilateral hemisphere immersed overnight in a 30% sucrose solution and were cut serially at a section thickness of 40 μm. The sections were collected in buffer and for histochemical reaction were transferred into the incubating medium 0.05% 3.3'-diaminobenzidine tetrahydrochloride and 1% H_2O_2 in tris buffer at pH 7.6 (Graham and Karnovsky, 1966). After 30 min the sections were rinsed in distilled water and mounted with alcoholic gelatin.

Most of the labeled cells were found in the Clare-Bishop area, which is a strip of cortex situated in the depth of the suprasylvian sulcus and in area 17, and virtually all were layer V pyramids. The labeled cells could be easily identified by dark-brown HRP-positive granules occurring in the cytoplasm of the perikaryon and the dendrites (Fig. 1A,B,C). The size of the granules was not uniform. Some cells contained exclusively fine granules (Fig. 1B), whereas others contained also coarser granules (Fig. 1C). The type of granulation was not dependent on the time of postinjection survival. However, fine granulation was more frequently observed in the large cells of the

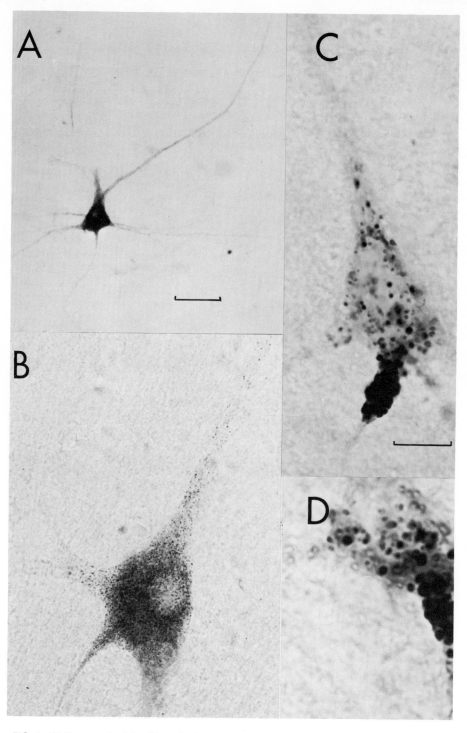

FIG. 1. (A) Nerve cell of the Clare-Bishop area. Scale: 50 μm. (B) Nerve cell of the Clare-Bishop area. Scale: 25 μm. (C) Nerve cell of area 19. Scale 10 μm. (D) Stuffing of the axon hillock with HRP-positive granules. Scale: 5 μm.

Clare-Bishop area, and coarse granulation more often in the small pyramids of the medial regions. In all four experiments most of the HRP-positive cells were only weakly labeled.

The percentage of heavily labeled cells was lowest in the 17-hr animal (19%) highest in the 3-day animal (43%) and intermediate in the 8-day animals (27%, 28%). The weakest labeled cells contained only a few HRP-positive granules, which were always found near the nucleus of the cell. With increased labeling, granules were also found aggregated in the axon hillock region and in the stem dendrites. In all of the labeled cells a distinct gradient was observed from the perikaryon with the highest concentration of granules to the dendritic periphery with lower concentrations. In the 8-day cases a diffuse light-brown labeling of the cytoplasm was frequently observed. The axon was in most instances free of any granulation. Only occasionally were fine granules observed beyond the hillock region. Coarse granules were never observed in axons. In some of the cells that contained coarse granules the axon hillock was swollen and stuffed with granules (Fig. 1C,D). In the 3-day experiment, 13% of all labeled cells showed this phenomenon. In dendrites, however, the stuffing phenomenon was never observed. Even in fine dendritic branches coarse granules were frequently seen.

In the axons the tracer was presumably transported in organelles too small to be resolved by the light microscope, such as small membrane-bound vesicles or multivesicular bodies (LaVail and LaVail, 1972; Turner and Harris, 1974). In the perikaryon, however, larger granules are known to occur with a diameter of up to 0.5 μm (Ralston and Sharp, 1973). In the present material many of the granules seemed to be even larger. Although HRP granules may be found in great number in cell bodies and dendrites, no sign of a cytotoxic effect was hitherto observed (Kristensson and Olsson, 1973). In rats and mice it was shown that the HRP labeling disappeared from labeled cells 6 to 11 days postoperatively (Kristensson and Olsson, 1973). The process of tracer removal is not yet understood. In the present material it is presumably reflected by the decrease of heavily labeled cells in the 8-day cases. The stuffing phenomenon that was observed in axon hillocks indicates a gating mechanism in corticotectal nerve cells that prevents the axonal export of HRP granules.

REFERENCES

Graham, R. C., and Karnovsky, M. J. (1966): The early stages of absorption of injected horse-radish peroxidase in the proximal tubules of mouse kidney: Ultrastructural cytochemistry by a new technique. *J. Histochem. Cytochem.*, 14:291–302.

Holländer, H. (1974): On the origin of the corticotectal projections in the cat. *Exp. Brain Res.*, 21:433–439.

Jacobson, S., and Trojanowski, J. Q. (1974): The cells of origin of the corpus callosum in rat, cat and rhesus monkey. *Brain Res.*, 74:149–155.

Kristensson, K., and Olsson, Y. (1973): Uptake and retrograde axonal transport of protein tracers in hypoglossal neurons fate of the tracer and reaction of the nerve cell bodies. *Acta Neuropathol. (Berl.)*, 23:43–47.

LaVail, J. H., and LaVail, M. M. (1972): Retrograde axonal transport in the central nervous system. *Science*, 176:1416–1417.

LaVail, J. H., Winston, K. P., and Tish, A. (1973): A method based on retrograde intraaxonal transport of protein for identification of cell bodies of origin of axons terminating within the CNS. *Brain Res.*, 58:470–477.

Nauta, H. J. W., Pritz, M. B., and Lasek, R. J. (1974): Afferents to the rat caudoputamen studied with horseradish peroxidase. An evaluation of a retrograde neuroanatomical research method. *Brain Res.*, 67:219–238.

Ralston, H. J., and Sharp, P. V. (1973): The identification of thalamus cortical relay cells in the adult cat by means of retrograde axonal transport of horseradish peroxidase. *Brain Res.*, 62:273–278.

Turner, P. T., and Harris, A. B. (1974): Ultrastructure of exogenous peroxidase in cerebral cortex. *Brain Res.*, 74:305–326.

Advances in Neurology, Vol. 12, edited by
G. W. Kreutzberg, Raven Press, New York
© 1975.

The Appearance of Dendrites of Callosal and Corticothalamic Neurons in Somatosensory Cortex of Immature Rats Demonstrated by Horseradish Peroxidase

Stanley Jacobson and John Q. Trojanowski

Anatomy Department, Erasmus University, Rotterdam, The Netherlands and Anatomy Department, Tufts University School of Medicine, Boston, Massachusetts 02111

The morphology of neurons at light-microscopic levels has most commonly been demonstrated with the Golgi neuronal method as in the studies of Lorente de Nó (1949), Morest (1969), and Scheibel and Scheibel (1970). This method is excellent for demonstrating neurons as well as their full compliment of processes throughout the entire central nervous system (CNS). Despite the remarkable details of neuronal morphology revealed by this technique, it suffers from the severe limitation of being nonselective in staining specific neuronal populations.

Recently developed techniques employing tracer substances applied intracellularly and extracellularly permit somewhat greater selectivity (Kreutzberg, Schubert, Tóth, and Rieske, 1973; Lynch, Deadwyler and Gall, 1974). However, for neuroanatomic studies of neuronal connectivity, as well as morphology of the neuronal projections, even these techniques as currently applied are not completely adequate. The ideal technique would combine certain characteristics of both the classic Golgi method and a retrograde neuroanatomic method such as the horseradish peroxidase (HRP) technique. More specifically, such a technique would entail a tracer that, after injection into an area under investigation, would be (1) limited closely to the injection site; (2) picked up primarily by synaptic endings of axons terminating in or close to the injection site and not by the axons themselves; (3) thereafter transported retrogradely to the neuronal cell bodies giving rise to the axons; and (4) render not only the soma of the neuron opaque but also its processes such that the morphology of these cells could be studied in as much detail as neurons stained by the Golgi method. In the CNS of the adult mammal the HRP technique effectively labels the neurons —though possibly not all of them—that project to the injected area (LaVail, Winston, and Tish, 1973; Jacobson and Trojanowski, 1975; Kuypers, Kievit, and Groen-Klevant, 1974; Nauta, Pritz, and Lasek, 1974). However, only a limited portion of the morphologic details of these neurons can be visualized, i.e., the soma and the immediately adjacent portions of the apical and basilar dendritic tree. Nevertheless, in a recent study of the cells of origin of the corpus callosum in adult mammals, we were able to visualize enough of the neuronal processes to be able to classify the labeled neurons as pyramidal, stellate, or fusiform, using HRP (Jacobson and Trojanowski, 1975). In an attempt to better visualize the dendritic field of the neurons that form callosal and corticothalamic connections we have carried out experiments on the CNS of maturing albino rats with the HRP technique. We have confined this experiment to rats from birth to 22 days postnatal, a span of time during which the cerebrum progresses from a relatively undifferentiated state to one in which the cortex becomes six-layered with all the appearances of the adult cortex (Eayrs and Goodhead, 1959; Purpura, Shofer, Housepean, and Noback, 1963; Schadé, Van Backer, and Colon, 1963; Altman, 1967; Caley and Maxwell, 1968*a,b*). Reference is made, however, to earlier experiments in adult rats, and some of this material is presented for comparison with the immature material.

MATERIALS AND METHODS

Young rats were injected with HRP using a 10-μl Hamilton syringe with a 30-gauge needle. The syringe was mounted on a stereotactic apparatus, and the needle was introduced into motor or sensory cortex or into the thalamus. The concentration of the HRP was in all instances 10% (Sigma VI) in distilled water. The animals were anesthetized for all procedures.

The rats were injected at birth (5 animals), 3 days (5 animals), 7 days (5 animals), 10 days (19 animals), 14 days (5 animals), 15 days (19 animals) and 20 days (15 animals). The rats at birth and 3, 7, and 14 days postnatal received injections of 0.1 μl, while the rats in the remaining age groups received injections of either 0.1, 0.2 or 0.4 μl with at least five animals in each group receiving injections of these amounts. The rats injected at birth and 3 days postnatal survived 1 day, whereas the remaining rats survived 1 to 2 days; consequently, the animals were sacrificed on the following postnatal days: 1, 4, 8, 9, 11, 12, 15, 16, 17, 21, 22. The observations will be presented with the rats referred to according to the age at which they were sacrificed.

At the time of sacrifice, the rats were deeply anesthetized and perfused with 25 to 50 ml of 6% dextran in a 0.9% aqueous solution of NaCl followed by 50 to 100 ml of 0.5% paraformaldehyde and 2.5% glutaraldehyde buffered with sodium cacodylate at pH 7.2. After removal, the brains were left in the concentrated fix for at least 1 hr at which time they were transferred to a mixture of one part fixative to one part sodium cacodylate with 30% sucrose added to reduce freezing artifact. After 12 hr in this solution, the brains were transferred to a solution of sodium cacodylate–30% sucrose until they sank. Thereafter the brains were cut at 80 μm on a freezing microtome, and every third section was collected in the sucrose–cacodylate mixture and later incubated, usually on the same day, in 3,3'-diaminobenzidine tetrahydrochloride in tris buffer at pH 7.6 to which was added 1% hydrogen peroxide. After 30 min the reaction was stopped by transferring the sections to distilled water, and the sections were then mounted from alcoholic gelatin. The sections were examined, unstained, with both light- and dark-field illumination. After the HRP-labeled neurons were identified and localized, in many instances the coverslips were removed and the sections were counterstained with cresyl violet to permit identification of the area and layer in which the neurons were found. In order to permit a clearer identification of the HRP reaction in the 11-, 12-, 16-, 17-, 21-, and 22-day-old rats, incubated sections cut at 80 μm containing HRP-positive callosal and corticothalamic neurons were osmicated (2% buffered) for 2 hr dehydrated, and embedded in Epon, and 1 to 7 μm thick sections were cut on a ultramicrotome and examined with the light microscope. The identification of rat sensorimotor cortex is after Krieg (1946).

OBSERVATIONS

Previous investigators have reported that two different reactions are observed with the HRP technique (Jacobson and Trojanowski, 1974; Lynch et al., 1974; Nauta et al., 1974; Turner and Harris, 1974). At the injection site or in the vicinity of the injection site one finds an even, brown agranular reaction; the cells resemble neuronal perikarya stained by the Golgi method. This phenomenon apparently results from direct injury to the neuron, while usually at some distance from the injection site—i.e., the thalamus, contralateral hemisphere, or ipsilateral areas projecting into the injection site—one finds the granular reaction, which the typical appearance of HRP in neurons labeled retrogradely with the tracer. Throughout this study we refer to both types of reactions—the agranular reaction, which is useful for determining the stage of development of the cells in and around the injection site, and the granular reaction, which not only labels those neurons with afferents to the injection site, but also visualizes many details of the dendritic trees of such labeled neurons.

One Day Postnatal

The cortical mantle at this stage of development is very immature (Fig. 1A). Differentiation of the layers has just begun, but the only layer actually identifiable is layer i. The neurons also are only just beginning to differentiate, and they are very tightly packed. By this time the majority of macroneurons have reached the cortex with only a few microneurons yet to migrate toward the cortex (Angevine and Sidman, 1961; Berry and Rogers, 1965; Altman, 1967). After injections of HRP into cortex, no evi-

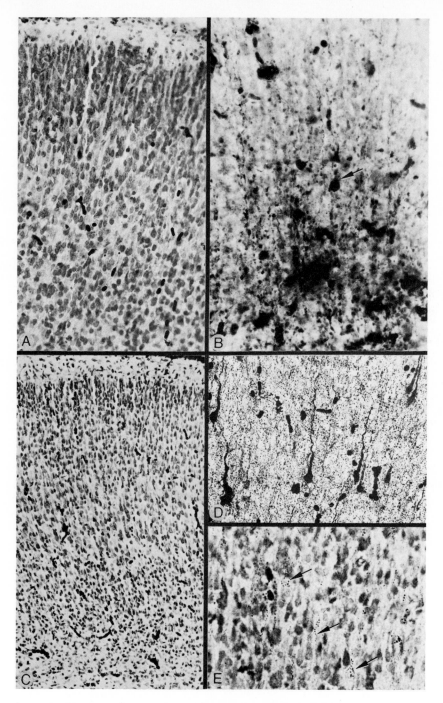

FIG. 1.(A,B) One day postnatal. (A) Undifferentiated cortex, nissl stain. (×33.) (B) Cortical injection site shows agranular reaction. (×55.) (C,D,E) Four days postnatal. (C) Sensory cortex starting to show a six-layered cortex. (×33.) (D) Injection site in sensory cortex with the neuroblasts having a prominent apical dendrite and a few basilar dendrites. (×110.) (E) HRP-positive callosal cells in layers ii and iii of sensory cortex, counterstained with cresyl violet. (×110.)

dence of the granular reaction was noted in cortex or thalamus. However, there was evidence of the agranular reaction at the injection site. Here HRP was noted in cells that had profiles of an immature neuronal cell body with a vertically oriented apical dendrite (Fig. 1B).

Four Days Postnatal

At this stage of cortical development it is possible to identify the various cortical regions in the cerebrum, as the cortical mantle has begun to differentiate and the nerve cells appear less densely packed; in some instances they are seen to have apical and basilar dendrites (Fig. 1C).

Injection of HRP into cortex results in agranularly labeled HRP-positive neurons at the injection site; the granular-type HRP reaction was noted at a distance from the injection site in the same and opposite hemisphere, as well as the ipsilateral thalamus-labeled neurons. At the injection site the cells have an even brown stain with the cells having a pyramidal shape and a prominent but immature apical dendrite and some basilar dendrites (Fig. 1D). Callosal and corticothalamic neurons are labeled with the granular-type HRP reaction. They have a prominent but immature apical dendrite; however, far less of the apical dendrite is visualized by the granular reaction than with the agranular reaction, and no basilar dendrites could be seen (Fig. 1E). Therefore, although retrograde transport is sufficiently mature at this stage to reveal the cell bodies with afferents to the injection site, the morphology of the immature dendritic trees of these neurons is poorly visualized, as is the case in adult rats (Fig. 3K,L). To verify that the cells labeled with the granular reaction were actually neurons and not glia cells, pericytes, or macrophages, sections were counterstained with cresyl violet; the granules of HRP were noted in the neuronal perikarya and apical dendrites of these counterstained neurons. In the callosal system the labeled cells were found primarily in layers iii and v, whereas in the thalamus they were noted primarily in the ventrobasal complex and in the ventrolateral nucleus.

Eight and Nine Days Postnatal

At this stage of development the nissl-stained material at both postnatal days reveals that the cortical lamination is more distinctly apparent than at 4 days, and that the neurons are more widely spaced (Fig. 2A). At the injection site neurons stained with the agranular reaction are seen to have a much more developed but still immature dendritic tree (Fig. 2B). The callosal neurons labeled with the granular HRP reaction in the opposite hemisphere are more obvious than was the case at 4 days postnatal, and the fact that the granules are found in neurons is verified by the cresyl violet-stained sections (Fig. 2C). The callosal and corticothalamic neurons contain

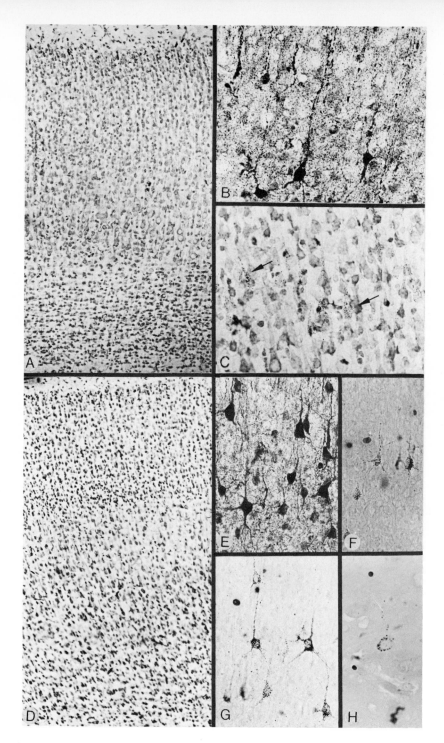

FIG. 2.(A–C) Eight days postnatal. (A) Sensory cortex shows a nearly complete six-layered cortex with prominent pyramidal cells. (×33.) (B) Injection site in motor cortex with the pyramidal cells having an apparently more mature dendritic tree. (×110.) (C) HRP-positive callosal neurons in layer iii of sensory cortex shows cells more mature than at 4 days. (×110.) (D–H) Eleven and 12 days postnatal. (D) Sensory cortex appears nearly mature. (×33.) (E) Injection site in sensory cortex showing numerous mature appearing neurons. (×110.) (F,G) Callosal neurons in layers iii and v of sensory cortex. (×110.) (H) Five-μm section reveals the dense bodies that form the most visible portion of the reaction in light-microscopic preparations. (×110.)

more granules at this stage than at 4 days postnatal making the cells stand out more prominently. The granules reveal the profile of the soma, but they also reveal adjacent portions of the apical and occasionally the basilar dendrites. Still, at this stage the agranular reaction seems far more effective in revealing details of dendritic morphology than the granular reaction. The retrogradely labeled neuronal elements still appear to be pyramidal in shape, although it is difficult to be certain of the identity of each cell, probably because of the immaturity of the cells.

Eleven and Twelve Days Postnatal

The animals sacrificed at these 2 days are discussed together because the material appears essentially the same. The cortex at this stage has progressed further toward maturity but still shows evidence of not being quite fully developed (Fig. 2D). Compared with the HRP-stained neurons seen at 8 days postnatal those observed at 11 and 12 days are dramatically different, especially with regard to the cells stained with the granular reaction. The neurons, whether stained with the agranular reaction at the injection site (Fig. 2E) or by the granular reaction in the opposite hemisphere (Fig. 2F and G), seem to have many characteristics of mature neurons with a much more elaborate-appearing dendritic field. The HRP granules are distributed for a considerable distance into the apical and basilar dendrites, and there is also the appearance of some staining of the cell neuroplasm, making the identification and classification of the neurons as pyramidal, stellate, or fusiform more simple. The granular reaction noted in these rats also differs rather considerably from that seen in neurons retrogradely labeled in adult rats (Fig. 3K,L) and, as will be seen subsequently, it also differs from the reaction seen in similar neurons in rats at the 21- and 22-day postnatal stage (Fig. 3G,H,I,J). The difference between the granular reaction at this stage and the later stages mentioned is that the granules now are not confined to the soma and immediately adjacent dendrites only, but for some reason are visible for a considerable distance away from the cell body in these processes. Although the neurons are still immature at this stage, they have developed sufficiently so that a more positive identification of the cell type may be made.

By far the most common cell type found among the retrogradely labeled neurons in the callosal and corticothalamic system is the pyramidal neuron. However, we have also noted fusiform cells, large stellate neurons, and stellate pyramids (Fig. 2G) following the classification system of Lorente de Nó (1949). In the callosal system the HRP-positive neurons are seen in layers ii to vi with the heaviest concentration of labeled neurons being found in layers iii and v (Fig. 4A) as is the case in adult rat, whereas the corticothalamic neurons are found only in infragranular layers (Fig. 4B) as is also the case in adult rats. The neuron labeled retrogradely with HRP

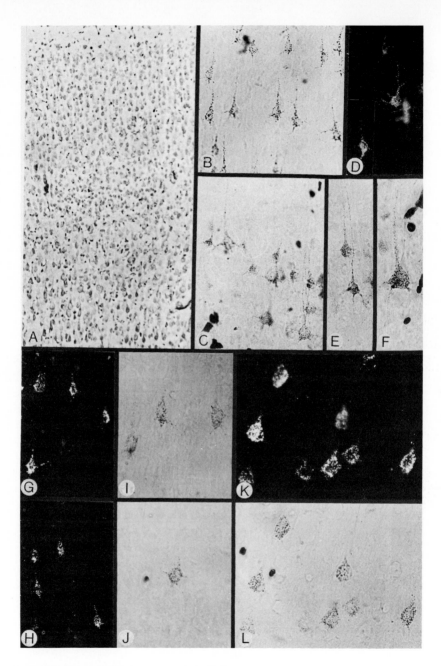

FIG. 3.(A–F) Fifteen to 17 days postnatal. (A) Sensory cortex appears mature. (×33.) (B–F) Neurons shows the maximal response of HRP-positive cells. (B) Pyramidal callosal cells in layers ii and iii. (C) Pyramidal thalamocortical neurons in layer v. (×110.) (D) Callosal neurons in layer iii. Inset shows fusiform cell, dark field. (×110.) (E,F) Pyramidal corticothalamic cells in layer v. (E) (×110.) (F) (×220.) (G–J) Twenty-one and 22 days postnatal. Callosal neurons show that less of the neuron is visible than at 15–17 days (cf. Fig. 3A–F) and that the reaction is similar to the adult neurons shown in K and L. (G,H) (×110.) (I,J) (×220.) (K,L) Adult callosal neurons. (K,L) Same fields but (K) is dark field and (L) is light field. (×220.)

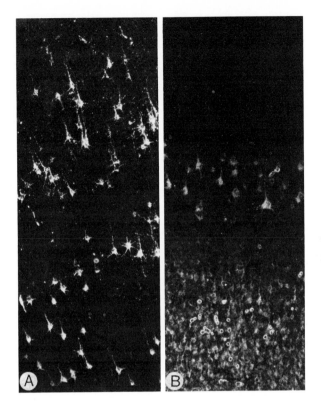

FIG. 4.(A) Distribution of callosal cells in sensory cortex of 15-day postnatal animal; note that the cells are in layers ii–vi, whereas in (B), also 15 days, where the corticothalamic neurons are shown, the cells are only in layers v and vi. (×66.)

granules in Fig. 2H is a photomicrograph taken from a 5-μm epoxy section showing in greater detail the appearance of the HRP granules in the soma and dendrites of a neuron. Figure 2 is a series of photomicrographs, which show slightly less of the dendritic field than is actually labeled by the granular reaction; nevertheless, it is clear that although more of the dendritic tree is visualized at this stage than at the later stages mentioned, far less is visualized than can be demonstrated by the Golgi method.

Fifteen to Seventeen Days Postnatal

These rats are also discussed as a group, as the material is essentially the same. The nissl-stained material shows an apparently mature cortex at this stage with the neurons more dispersed than in previous stages (Fig. 3A). The neurons stained with both types of HRP reaction at this stage are similar to those observed in the 11- and 12-day postnatal rats and are therefore dramatically different from the neurons observed at earlier stages. Again, this is particularly true for the granular reaction seen in retrogradely labeled neurons in that far more morphologic details of the dendritic fields of these neurons are shown than at earlier stages of cortical development or in older rats (see Fig. 3; compare B–F with G–L). The cells that form callosal connections labeled with the granular HRP reaction are prominent in layers ii–vi (Fig. 4A).

In the supragranular layers the pyramidal cells are smaller; nearly the entire dendritic field of the labeled neurons was visualized, whereas in the infragranular layers, where cells are larger, slightly less of the dendritic field could be seen. The cells that form the corticothalamic system also are more extensively visualized than in the earlier developmental stages examined, and again the cells are found in layers v and vi. The most common neuronal profile seen at this stage is the pyramidal neuron with the largest in the callosal system being found in layer iii and the largest in the corticothalamic system being found in layer v. This material has also been examined in the identification of labeled neurons giving rise to associational projections. Surrounding the injection site one can see evidence of the retrograde granular reaction in all cell types distributed throughout all cell layers; however, at distances more removed from the injection site only a few retrogradely labeled cells are apparent, and these are pyramidal and found primarily in layer v.

Although it is obvious that more of the dendritic field of the neurons retrogradely labeled with the granular reaction is seen at this stage of cortical development than is visualized at earlier or later stages, it is also obvious that less of the morphology of the neuron can be demonstrated with this technique than with the classic Golgi method. However, the advantage of the HRP technique over the Golgi method at this stage of development is that the morphology of the visualized dendritic fields is that of a select group of neurons with projections into the area in which the HRP has been injected.

Twenty-One and Twenty-Two Days Postnatal

The material from these animals is similar and is therefore presented together. At this stage of development one is dealing with apparently fully mature cortex. At the injection site neurons labeled with the agranular reaction are very much similar to those found in adult animals and are not remarkably different in appearance from similarly stained neurons about 15 days postnatal and older. The agranular HRP reaction reveals not only the neuronal profile but also apical and basilar dendrites in great detail as noted by others (Lynch et al., 1974), but it does not reveal as much of the morphologic detail of neurons as does the Golgi technique. It is in the retrogradely labeled neurons that a change is noted compared with the rats at 11 to 12 and 16 to 17 days. Callosal and corticothalamic neurons so labeled with the granular reaction greatly resemble similarly labeled neurons in adult rats (Fig. 3 G–L) and are quite unlike the granularly labeled neurons noted in the two developmental periods that were previously examined (Fig. 3B–F). Much as in the adult, the HRP granules are confined to the neuronal somata and the immediately adjacent dendritic processes, which makes classification of the neurons according to cell type less certain. Nevertheless, the pattern of distribution of the retrogradely labeled callosal and corticothalamic neurons remains the same as that seen previously in earlier developmental periods and as is found in adult rats.

In addition to the differences between immature and adult rats with regard to the HRP technique, it should be noted that some of the results obtained using these young animals differed in yet another striking way from those obtained using adult rats. In the immature rats it was noted that when injections of HRP involved all layers of the cortex but did not involve the medullary center, retrogradely labeled neurons were seen in only the same area of the contralateral hemisphere. However, in several instances the injection was partially or completely restricted to fibers in the medullary center. In such cases a far greater number of retrogradely labeled neurons were seen in both hemispheres laterally from the dorsal rim of the rhinal sulcus to the longitudinal fissure medially. Such cells were concentrated in the same cell layers as are the cells of origin of the corpus callosum and were restricted only to those areas that are interconnected by fibers crossing in the corpus callosum. This suggested a significant uptake of HRP by callosal axons and subsequent retrograde transport in these immature rats. In adult animals the evidence indicates that significant uptake by axons does not occur (Nauta et al., 1974; Turner and Harris, 1974).

DISCUSSION

The criteria for classifying neurons according to cell type have been based upon studies using the classic Golgi method in which the total appearance of the neuronal perikaryon with all its processes is determined by making camera lucida drawings of thick sections. Although an excellent technique for studying individual neurons and some aspects of local anatomy, the Golgi method stains nerve cells in a nonselective manner and is of only very limited use in investigations of neuronal connectivity. The classic silver techniques used for investigating neuronal connectivity have depended either on the destruction of the neurons giving rise to the projections being studied or on the disappearance or pathologic changes in the neurons projecting to a previously ablated distant area. More recently developed neuroanatomic methods that take advantage of anterograde and retrograde transport leave the cells of origin of the projections under investigation intact, and to a limited extent they reveal some of the morphologic details of these cells. However, as was mentioned earlier, neither these techniques nor the Golgi method possesses all of the characteristics that a neuroanatomic technique should if both neuronal connectivity and neuronal morphology are to be studied simultaneously.

The HRP technique as currently used in adult animals comes closest to such a neuroanatomic method in its visualization of the soma of neurons and the immediately adjacent parts of the dendritic field. However, as we noted in our earlier study of the callosal system, many neurons are so poorly visualized that classification according to cell type is impossible. The results derived from a similar study of the callosal and corticothalamic system in immature animals reported in this chapter indicate that there are dramatic differences in the way HRP behaves in young and adult animals. With regard to the agranular HRP reaction, differences between the cells visualized in young animals compared to those seen in adult animals are largely dependent upon the morphology of the neurons themselves at the different maturational stages rather than upon differences in the ability with which HRP stains such neurons in and around the injection site. This is not true of the retrograde granular reaction, for which, aside from the differences in the morphology of the neurons, there are distinct differences in the extent of the dendritic field that can be stained retrogradely with the HRP at different maturational stages.

At earlier stages of development examined, 1 day postnatal, a time at which nerve cells are undifferentiated (Caley and Maxwell, 1968a,b) we could detect no evidence at the light-microscopic level of retrograde transport of HRP and subsequent labeling of neurons with HRP granules. The first evidence of this phenomenon came at 4 days postnatal. However, from this time until 8 days, a time at which the dendritic fields of neuroblasts are rapidly developing (Eayrs and Goodhead, 1959; Caley and Maxwell, 1968a,b), visualization of the retrogradely labeled neurons is very poor. The soma was noted to contain HRP granules and in a few cases apical dendrites, but only occasionally were other processes noted to have sufficient quantities of these granules so as to be well visualized. At some point between 8 and 10 days postnatal dramatic changes occur in the way in which the retrogradely transported HRP is handled by the labeled neurons for at 11 days—not only are the neuronal soma and immediately adjacent portions of the dendritic fields visualized, but the more distal parts of dendritic processes are now seen to contain granules rendering them visible in the light microscope. Apical and basilar dendrites as well as axons are visualized at this point in development. Some processes, especially apical dendrites, can be traced for several hundred microns. The ability to visualize a large part of the dendritic field of neurons retrogradely labeled with HRP persists in increasingly older animals to at least 17 days postnatal, and perhaps somewhere between 15 to 16 days postnatal the amount of the dendritic field stained with the HRP granules reaches a maximum.

Even as late as 17 days postnatal, the neurons in rat neocortex are clearly not mature; however, they very closely resemble neurons of adult rats in morphology, and development has progressed far enough to allow classification of these neurons according to cell type. Certainly far less of the dendritic field is seen of the retrogradely labeled HRP-positive neurons than can be demonstrated by the Golgi method. With the Golgi method the complete apical and basilar dendritic fields including spines can be demonstrated. The retrogradely stained HRP material visualizes the apical and basilar dendrites including dendritic branches, but to a lesser extent, and no dendritic spines can be seen. Nevertheless, a sufficiently larger extent of the dendritic field can be seen in nearly all labeled neurons so as to permit a more satisfactory determination of cell type than is possible in adult material.

After 17 days postnatal, less of the dendritic field is visualized by the HRP granules in retrogradely labeled neurons. At 22 and 23 days postnatal, labeled cells appear very much like HRP-positive neurons in adult rats, i.e., only the soma and immediately adjacent portions of neuronal processes are labeled; although this is sufficient labeling to localize cells with afferents to the injection site, the classification of neurons according to cell type is more difficult. That the labeled neurons resemble adult labeled neurons at this stage of development is consistent with the observations of Caley and Maxwell (1968*a,b*) that by 21 days of age in the rat the organelles, neuropil, and the neuron itself have all the properties of the adult. Also in the rat Eayrs and Goodhead (1959) have reported that by 18 days of age the cells in the cortex have the appearance of mature neurons and that changes after this time are quantitative rather than qualitative. Moreover, by 14 days the electrocorticogram of the rat has been shown to be similar to that of the adult (Crain, 1952). In the kitten a similar developmental pattern has been shown, and by 21 days of age the cortex is similar to that seen in the adult cat (Purpura et al., 1963). It is therefore not surprising that at about 21 days postnatal the granular reaction in retrogradely labeled neurons very much resembles that seen in adult cortical neurons. The intriguing question that remains to be answered is why a much greater extent of the dendritic field is visualized by the retrograde HRP reaction between 11 and 17 days postnatal.

The difference in the way HRP is handled by these younger animals compared to older ones may well reflect changes in the metabolism of neurons as they mature. Although the reason for this difference is not clear, it is known that different precursors injected intracellularly into adult neurons are differentially transported intradentritically, and thus label the soma and neuronal processes to a greater or lesser extent (Kreutzberg et al., 1973). In contrast, a study similar to that of Turner and Harris (1974) or LaVail (1974) carried out on immature animals may reveal a difference in the distribution of the lysosomal bodies labeled with HRP, particularly in dendrites of immature versus mature neurons. A second significant difference between the response to HRP injections in the immature and mature CNS is the far greater number of retrogradely labeled cells distributed over a wider area that results from injections in young animals, which involve the medullary center. This suggests that in immature rats significant uptake of HRP may occur along the axon with the subsequent occurrence of a widespread labeling of callosal neurons in the opposite hemisphere. If this is in fact the case, it may well be a result of the incomplete myelination of these axons in the medullary center at this time (Jacobson, 1963). An investigation at the electron-microscopic level should resolve this question.

Although inferior to the classic Golgi method in demonstrating the details of dendritic morphology, the HRP technique as used in this investigation in immature rats does enable the investigator to locate those neurons that project into the region of the injection site. Between 11 and 17 days postnatal not only is the soma of such neurons visualized by the HRP granules, but so is a large portion of the dendritic field, making it possible to analyze the morphology of these neurons in more satisfactory detail than in adult animals. Thus, the morphology of a select group of neurons as well as their efferent projections can be studied. It is precisely this selective quality, so important to the neuroanatomist, which is lacking in the classic Golgi method.

ACKNOWLEDGMENTS

The authors wish to thank E. Dalm and Mrs. M. Heung for their expert technical assistance, W. van den Oudenalder and Miss P. Delfos for their help with the figures and photography, and Mrs. E. Jongbloed for typing the manuscript. This investigation was supported by USPHS Grant NS 07666 and the Charlton Fund of Tufts University.

REFERENCES

Altman, J. (1967): Postnatal growth and differentiation of the mammalian brain, with implications for a morphological theory of memory. In: *The Neuroscience: A study program*, edited by G. Quarton, T. Melnechuk, and F. O. Schmitt, pp. 723–743. Rockefeller University Press, New York.

Angevine, J. B., and Sidman, R. L. (1961): Autoradiographic study of cell migration during histogenesis of cerebral cortex in the mouse. *Nature*, 192:766–768.

Berry, M., and Rogers, A. W. (1965): The migration of neuroblasts in the developing cerebral cortex. *J. Anat.*, 99:691–709.

Caley, D., and Maxwell, D. S. (1968a): An electron microscopic study of neurons during postnatal development of the rat cerebral cortex. *J. Comp. Neurol.*, 133:17–44.

Caley, D. W., and Maxwell, D. S. (1968b): Development of the blood vessels and extra cellular spaces during postnatal maturation of rat cerebral cortex. *J. Comp. Neurol.*, 138:31–48.

Crain, S. M. (1952): Development of electrical activity in the cerebral cortex of the albino rat. *Proc. Soc. Exp. Biol. Med. N.Y.*, 81:49–51.

Eayrs, J. T., and Goodhead, B. (1959): Postnatal development of the cerebral cortex in the rat. *J. Anat.*, 93:385–402.

Jacobson, S. (1963): Sequence of myelinization in the brain of the albino rat. *J. Comp. Neurol.*, 121:5–29.

Jacobson, S., and Trojanowski, J. Q. (1974): The cells of origin of the corpus callosum in rat, cat and rhesus monkey. *Brain Res.,* 74:149–155.

Jacobson, S., and Trojanowski, J. Q. (1975): Corticothalamic neurons and thalamocortical terminal fields: An investigation in rat using horseradish peroxidase, autoradiography and the Fink-Heimer method. *Brain Res.,* 85:385–401.

Kreutzberg, G. W., Schubert, P., Toth, L., and Rieske, E. (1973): Intradendritic transport to postsynaptic sites. *Brain Res.,* 62:399–404.

Krieg, W. J. S. (1946): Connections of the cerebral cortex. I. The albino rat. (b) Structure of the cortical areas. *J. Comp. Neurol.,* 84:277–323.

Kuypers, H. G. J. M., Kievit, J., and Groen-Klevant, A. C. (1974): Retrograde axonal transport of horseradish peroxidase in rats forebrain. *Brain Res.,* 67:211–218.

LaVail, J. H., Winston, K. R., and Tish, A. A. (1973): A method based on retrograde intraaxonal transport of proteins for identification of cell bodies of origin of axons terminating within the CNS. *Brain Res.,* 58:470–477.

LaVail, J. H., and LaVail, M. W. (1974): The retrograde intraaxonal transport of horse radish peroxidase in the chick visual system. A light and electron microscopic study. *J. Comp. Neurol.,* 157:303–357.

Lorente de Nó, R. (1949): Cerebral cortex: architecture intercortical connections, motor projections. In: *Physiology of the Nervous System,* edited by J. Fulton, pp. 274–301. Oxford University Press, New York.

Lynch, G., Deadwyler, S., and Gall, C. (1974): Labelling of central nervous system neurons with extracellular recording microelectrodes. *Brain Res.,* 66:337–341.

Morest, D. K. (1969): The growth of dendrites in the mammalian brain. *Z. Anat. Entwicklungsgesch.,* 128:290–317.

Nauta, H. J. W., Pritz, M. B., and Lasek, R. J. (1974): Afferents to the rat caudoputamen studied with horseradish peroxidase: An evaluation of a retrograde neuroanatomical research method. *Brain Res.,* 67:219–238.

Purpura, D. P., Shofer, R. J., Housepean, E. M., and Noback, C. R. (1963): Comparative ontogenesis of structure function relation in cerebral and cerebellar cortex. In: *Progress in Brain Research, Vol. 4: Growth and Maturation of the Brain,* edited by D. P. Purpura and J. P. Schadé, pp. 187–222. Elsevier, New York–Amsterdam.

Schadé, J. P., Van Backer, H., and Colon, E. (1963): Quantitative analysis of neuronal parameters in the maturing cerebral cortex. In: *Progress in Brain Research, Vol. 4: Growth and Maturation of the Brain,* edited by D. P. Purpura and J. P. Schadé, pp. 150–175. Elsevier, New York–Amsterdam.

Scheibel, M. E., and Scheibel, A. B. (1970): Elementary processes in selected thalamic and cortical subsystems—The structural substrates. In: *The Neurosciences: Second Study Program,* edited by F. O. Schmitt, pp. 443–457. Rockefeller University Press, New York.

Turner, P. T., and Harris, A. B. (1974): Ultrastructure of exogenous peroxidase in cerebral cortex. *Brain Res.,* 74:305–326.

Advances in Neurology, Vol. 12, edited by
G. W. Kreutzberg, Raven Press, New York
© 1975.

Dendritic Abnormalities of Purkinje Cells in the Cerebellum of Neurologic Mutant Mice (Weaver and Staggerer)

Constantino Sotelo

*Laboratoire de Neuromorphologie U-106 INSERM, Hôpital de Port Royal, 75014 Paris,
France*

One of the generally accepted concepts in neurogenesis is that the final
dendritic arrangement of neurons is caused by the correlation of genetic
and "epigenetic" factors. Several chapters in this volume are devoted to this
topic (see chapters by Rakic, Privat, and Herndon). Since the identification
and mapping of neurologic mutations affecting the cerebellum of the mouse
by Sidman, Green, and Appel (1965) it is known that some mutations seem
to affect primarily the Purkinje cells, whereas in others the apparent cellular
target of the mutation is the microneuronal population. In both instances
there is a severe alteration of the cerebellar anatomy. In this chapter the
comparative morphology of Purkinje cell dendrites (PCD) in the cerebellum
of two of these neurologic mutant mice, weaver and staggerer, are presented.
In the first case most of the granule cells degenerate before their migration,
completely changing the environment in which the PCD might develop.
In the second case, the Purkinje cells themselves seem to be affected by
the mutation. From this study, the action exerted by the genetic and the
"epigenetic" factors on the morphology of PCD's is discussed.

PURKINJE CELL DENDRITES IN WEAVER CEREBELLUM

Since the morphologic study by Sidman (1968) of the weaver cerebellum
it is known to be characterized by a reduced size and an almost complete
depletion of granule cells. The reason for the agranularity in this cerebellum
is the extensive cellular death observed among postmitotic neuroblasts of
the external granular layer during the first 2 weeks after birth (Sidman,
1968). Rezai and Yoon (1972) have demonstrated that the cerebellar abnormality in weaver mice is transmitted by an incompletely dominant gene.
Using the thymidine labeling method, these investigators have found that
the mitotic rate is similar in mice whether they are affected by the mutation
or not. They suggest that the primary weaver alteration is the retardation in
granule cell migration. Under these circumstances, parallel fibers in the
homozygous weaver are practically not developed, and PCD's must grow

in an abnormal milieu because they are deprived of their most important synaptic input.

The fine structure of Purkinje cells in weaver/weaver cerebellum has been the object of several publications (Hirano and Dembitzer, 1973; Rakic and Sidman, 1973; Sotelo, 1973). From these studies, as from those carried out in other agranular cerebella (Herndon, Margolis, and Kilham, 1971; Altman and Anderson, 1972; Hirano, Dembitzer, and Jones, 1972; Llinás, Hillman, and Precht, 1973) several conclusions can be drawn:

1. Purkinje cell dendrites do not develop spiny branchlets.
2. Their primary and secondary branches are randomly oriented and often their whole dendritic tree is completely inversed.
3. Their primary and secondary branches have an irregular rough surface owing to the presence of numerous spines.

In agreement with these general features, large dendritic trunks belonging to Purkinje cells are widespread within the whole cortical area, from the subpial region to the white matter. These dendritic profiles exhibit all the internal features of PCD's (Palay and Chan-Palay, 1974), but they contain much larger amounts of mitochondria than in normal mice. The electron-microscopic feature that characterizes the weaver cerebellum is the presence of innumerable dendritic spines, which are similar to the normal Purkinje cell tertiary spines, but which are devoid of their presynaptic elements, that is, the parallel fibers (Fig. 1). As described by Hirano and Dembitzer (1973) high magnification of these naked spines discloses the presence of a segment of the spinous membrane that is located in one of the lateral convex sides, undercoated by a fuzzy cytoplasmic material, identical to the normal postsynaptic differentiation, and with an external coating resembling a synaptic cleft material. In the great majority of the cases, these pseudo-postsynaptic and cleft differentiations are facing an apparently normal glial unit membrane. These observations suggest the dependence of the cleft material from the postsynaptic membrane.

Spines exhibiting a shorter stalk and a more rounded head characteristic of normal Purkinje cells of primary and secondary branches also exist in the weaver PCD's. In the latter case as in normal animals, this different category of spines is synaptically contacted by climbing fibers (Larramendi and Victor, 1967). In wv, and probably owing to the large reduction in cerebellar volume, the density of climbing fibers synapsing on PCD's seems higher than in normal animals. Figure 2 illustrates a PCD with naked, apparently tertiary spines and primary spines contacted by a climbing fiber. In addition to these typical PCD spines, atypical forms are also present, although in much-reduced number. These atypical forms can be classified into two well-defined categories according to whether they are (1) branching (Fig. 3) or (2) hypertrophic (Fig. 4). The existence in the weaver cerebellum of all three categories of PCD spines — normal, hypertrophic, and branch-

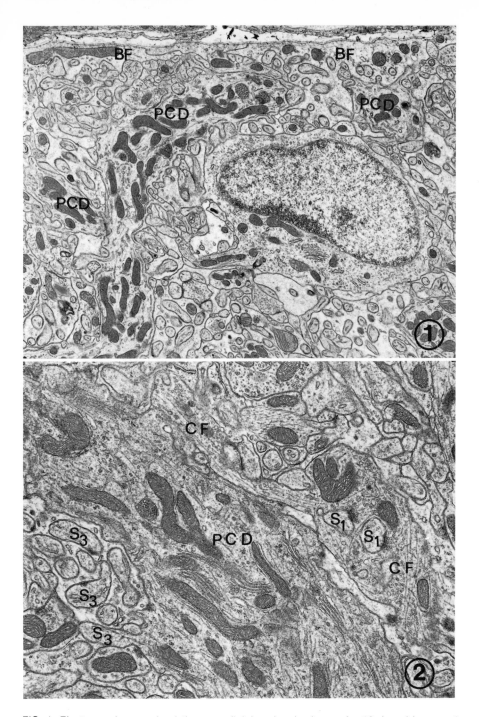

FIG. 1. Electron micrograph of the superficial molecular layer of a 28-day-old weaver/weaver mouse. The surface of the cerebellar cortex is covered by a continuous layer of Bergmann's end feet, BF. Abundant PCD's, cut in longitudinal and cross sections, occupy this superficial region. The dendritic profiles are filled with mitochondria. Note the presence of numerous naked spines encased in the glial cytoplasm. (×8,000.)

FIG. 2. Electron micrograph of a major dendrite of a PCD, in a 22-day-old weaver/weaver mouse. A climbing fiber varicosity, CF, is in synaptic contact with primary-like spines, S_1. In the lower left angle of the micrograph, naked tertiary-like spines, S_3 are in the glial cytoplasm. (×14,000.)

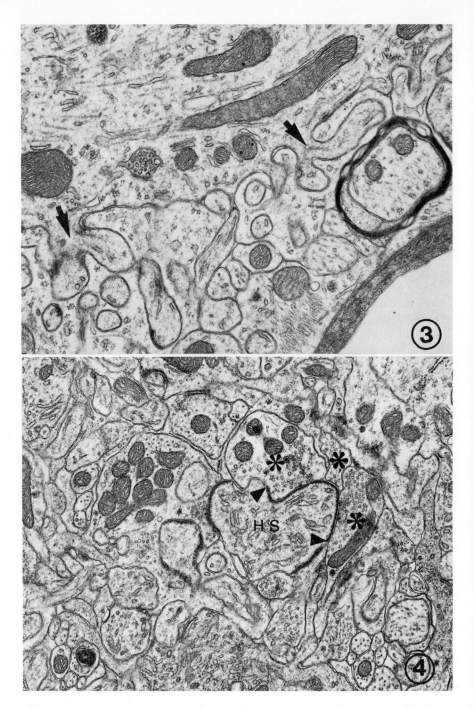

FIG. 3. Electron micrograph of a large dendritic profile belonging to a Purkinje cell in a 22-day-old weaver/weaver mouse. The arrows point to the two branching spines originated from the dendritic trunk. These spines are devoid of presynaptic elements. (×28,000.)

FIG. 4. Electron micrograph of hypertrophic spine, HS, of a PCD in a 28-day-old weaver/weaver mouse. The HS has most of its surface undercoated by a cytoplasmic dense material similar to a postsynaptic specialization. Three different axon terminals (*) innervate the same postsynaptic specialization (*arrow heads*). (×17,000.)

ing—does not fit with the general ideas expressed recently (Eccles, 1973) about use and disuse of spine synapses, as here in an almost complete absence of parallel fibers, the three categories of spines have been encountered free of presynaptic fibers, which, from a morphological viewpoint is the best example of synaptic disuse. Therefore, Purkinje cell dendrites seem to behave in a very different way from, for example, dendrites of pyramidal cells in the visual cortex (for examples, see Valverde, 1967).

Another very important feature of PCD in weaver cerebellum, that has not been reported previously, is the presence of postsynaptic-like dense cytoplasmic material undercoating segments of variable length of the membrane on the smooth surface of the dendrites (Fig. 5). These postsynaptic-like differentiations can face glial elements, naked spines, and more often axon terminals belonging to stellate cells (Figs. 6 and 7). However, in this last instance, the axon terminals do not develop a presynaptic vesicular grid at the level of the postsynaptic differentiation (Fig. 6). The absence of a presynaptic vesicular grid and the great length of the undercoating, which can overpass 4 μm, made these membranous differentiations very distinct from the normal synapses between stellate or basket axon terminals or both, and the smooth surface of PCD's, which occur in the weaver mouse, as Rakic and Sidman (1973) have reported. Occasionally, these hypertrophic postsynaptic thickenings can also undercoat almost the entire membrane of hypertrophic spines (Fig. 4). In all these instances an electron-dense material, similar to the pseudo-synaptic cleft material already described for the naked spines, accompany the external leaflet of the undercoated dendritic membrane (Figs. 5 and 6). The presence of these large postsynaptic differentiations on PCD's is not exclusive in the weaver, but it seems to be a constant feature of agranular cerebella [they have also been illustrated by Altman and Anderson (1972, their Figs. 36 and 37) in irradiated rat cerebellum, and we have observed a similar differentiation in agranular rabbit cerebellum obtained by a combination of antimitotic drugs and X-irradiation, Sotelo and Delhaye-Bouchaud (*unpublished*).]

All the above-mentioned morphologic results can be explained by the following speculation. Purkinje cells seem to have an autonomous development of receptive surfaces. In the normal cerebellum the functional synaptic accomplishment between parallel fibers and PCD spines may serve as a feedback mechanism to regulate the synthesis of receptor protein. In weaver mice, where this synaptic accomplishment does not occur, the Purkinje cells devoid of this regulatory synaptic input pursue the synthesis of receptor protein, which explains the overproduction of postsynaptic differentiations not only at the spine level, but also on the smooth surface of the dendrites. If one imagines this process going on during the life span of the animal, in the adult most of the PCD surface might be undercoated by a postsynaptic-like differentiation; but this is not the case here. This apparent discrepancy may be explained by the fact that in some denervated neurons

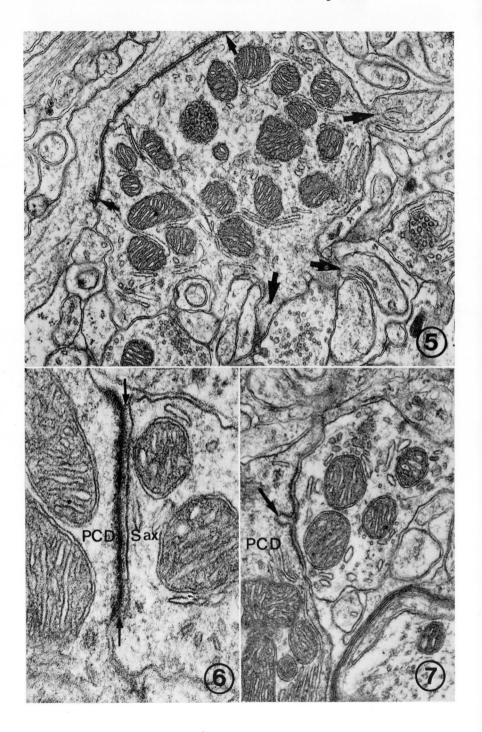

the free postsynaptic differentiation can be removed by a process of membrane sequestration (Gentschev and Sotelo, 1973). The frequent association of free postsynaptic sites with coated vesicles in the weaver (Fig. 7) provides some morphologic evidence in favor of the removal of these membrane segments by a similar process of membrane sequestration.

A different problem concerns the fate of the free spines. Unfortunately, our weaver mice obtained from a stock of mice B6 X CBA/F1 originated from the Jackson Laboratory have an average life span no longer than 1 month. Hence, the information that we have about the fate of the free spines only concerns mice of 20 to 29 days. Generally, the latter are encased by Bergmann glia and survive as free postsynaptic sites until the death of the animal. Rakic and Sidman (1973) in their fine structural study of mice carrying the weaver mutation, but with a genetic background different from ours, have observed that these free spines survive for at least 2 years. These results confirm our previous studies on free postsynaptic differentiations, which were shown by us in some cases to be stable structures capable of having an independent survival (Sotelo, 1968, 1973). By contrast, in the weaver as in other agranular cerebella (Altman and Anderson, 1972), free spines can evolve in a different way. In many instances they tend to converge and form small clusters of 2 to 4 spines where the segments of the spine membrane bearing the postsynaptic densities become closely apposed. Even two spines arising from the same PCD can converge to form a small symmetric junction between them. When the cluster, as it was in the previous case, is formed by only two spines, the undercoated segments of both spine membranes lose their convexity, become straight and parallel, and give rise to an attachment plate, a junction that was never observed between spines in a normal cerebellum (all these features are illustrated in Fig. 4 of the paper by Sotelo, 1973). Nothing is known yet about the mechanism that forces the presumed receptive surfaces of the spines to appose each other. In some instances clusters of spines become very tightly packed inside the glial cytoplasm, a fact that suggests a slow process of spine

---

FIG. 5. Electron micrograph of a cross section of a large dendritic profile belonging to a Purkinje cell in a 19-day-old weaver/weaver mouse. The surface of the dendritic profile at the left of the micrograph is studded with spines (*large arrows*). The smooth surface of the dendrite, in the upper left corner, is undercoated by a very long postsynaptic-like web material (*small arrows*). (×32,000.)

FIG. 6. Higher magnification of another postsynaptic-like specialization on the smooth surface of a PCD (same material as Fig. 5). Note that not only the cytoplasmic dense material undercoating the membrane, but also an extracellular synaptic cleft-like dense material have been differentiated (*arrows*). However, the membrane of a stellate axon terminal, S-ax, has not developed presynaptic specializations. (×83,000.)

FIG. 7. Electron micrograph of a situation similar to that in Fig. 6. The arrow points to the coated vesicle associated with a postsynaptic-like differentiation of the PCD, which is considered to be the morphologic basis for the process of membrane sequestration. (×41,000.)

degeneration. Remnant bodies of dark degenerative debris are occasionally found in the Bergmann fibers.

Occasionally, the free spines can be innervated by axon terminals that never reach such targets in the normal cerebellum. Therefore, mossy fibers establish morphologic synapses with PCD spines (see Fig. 3 in Sotelo, 1973) as they do in the irradiated cerebellum (Altman and Anderson, 1972) and in the ferret cerebellum after infection with panleukopenia virus (Llinás et al., 1973). Hypertrophic spines can be innervated by different types of axon terminals as illustrated in Fig. 4. Finally, in the cerebellar hemispheres, where granule cells are more numerous than in the vermis, PCD spines can be postsynaptic to granule cell somatic synapses. In this respect it can be concluded that the PCD spines in the weaver cerebellum behave as in other agranular cerebella and that furthermore they are able to contribute to the neuronal circuit reorganization.

PCD's IN STAGGERER CEREBELLUM

The cerebellum of staggerer mutant mice (Sidman, Lane, and Dickie, 1962) has been less studied than that of the weaver. For Sidman (1972) the staggerer cerebellum becomes almost agranular by day 33. However, he stressed that the increased cell death between the inner granule cell population does not necessarily mean that these cells are the primary cellular target of the mutation. Indeed, Landis (1971) and Sidman (1972) described another important abnormality in staggerer mice that affects the Purkinje cells, that is, the lack of dendritic spines of the type normally contracted by parallel fibers. In a recent publication we have corroborated the above-mentioned results, and in agreement with Sidman (1972), we have considered the Purkinje cells as the direct site of mutant gene action (Sotelo and Changeux, 1974). The death of the granule cells is probably caused by a retrograde transsynaptic effect.

In young mice (10 days old) the cerebellar cortex of the staggerer consists of a thick external granular layer, a thin molecular layer where some migrating cells can be recognized, a layer of irregularly spaced multipolar neurons arranged in one or two rows, an internal granular layer with apparently normal granule cells and some larger neurons, and the white axis with few myelinated fibers. Because Purkinje cells seem to be directly affected by the sg defect, our first problem was to identify and determine the characteristics of these cells at the ultrastructural level.

Electron-microscopic observations, restricted to the layer of irregularly spaced neurons between the molecular and the internal granular layers where Purkinje cells are normally located, disclose the presence of medium-sized neurons (12 to 16 μm in diameter). These cells do not exhibit the typical features of 10-day-old Purkinje cells, with the exception of the spiny appearance of their perikarya. The basal dendrites are relatively thin and can be in close contact with similar dendritic profiles or perikarya or both. At these contacts, the only observed junctional complex is of the attachment plate type. The most characteristic feature of the cells, which allows us to identify them as Purkinje cells, is the occasional presence of climbing fibers synapsing on the perikaryal and main dendritic spines (Fig. 8) corresponding to the "capuchon" stage described by Ramón y Cajal (1911). The primary and secondary dendrites are much thinner than are those of normal cerebellum, and spiny branchlets are missing. At this age, specialized adhesion zones resembling small attachment plates are numerous between the smooth surface of PCD and the immature nonsynaptic segments of parallel fibers (see Fig. 1 of the paper by Sotelo and Changeux, 1974). Such attachment plates have been considered to be the first morphologic sign of a synaptic contact between parallel fibers and PCD, even in an absence of synaptic vesicles (Altman, 1971). For this reason it can be suggested that the capacity of parallel fibers to "recognize" Purkinje cell surface is preserved. However, in spite of the formation of such attachment plates, these early contacts fail to evolve into the typical synapses. The dendrites have a smooth surface partially covered by thin glial lamellas. In the areas free of glial envelopes nonsynaptic segments of parallel fibers are directly apposed to the dendritic membrane. Golgi staining of 10-day-old staggerer mouse cerebellum has failed to impregnate cells remotely resembling normal Purkinje cells. Only multipolar neurons with smooth thin dendrites spreading mainly into the molecular layer were impregnated (Fig. 9).

In older staggerer mice (20 to 28 days old) the light-microscopic picture of the cerebellar cortex is greatly modified. Only a remnant of the external granular layer persists: the molecular layer is always extremely thin; the Purkinje layer looks very much like the one already described in 10-day-old staggerer; the most important changes occur in the internal granular layer where, according to Sidman's description (1972), many granule cells undergo a degenerative process, followed by cellular death. The ultrastructural features of the granule cell death and its transsynaptic effect have been described in detail (Sotelo and Changeux, 1974).

The electron-microscopic examination of Purkinje cells in these older staggerer mice confirms the multipolar nature of some of these neurons (Fig. 10). Normal mature Purkinje cells (Palay and Chan-Palay, 1974) are characterized not only by the widely dispersed small masses of nissl bodies, with the largest ones lying close to the nucleus, but by the highly developed agranular endoplasmic reticulum, forming at the periphery of the cell the hypolemmal cisterna. This cisterna, which lies subjacent to the cell membrane, is so characteristic that it can be used as a tool to identify not only the Purkinje cell soma, but also its dendritic profiles and even the axon. Unfortunately, in staggerer mature Purkinje cells, the hypolemmal cisterna is very poorly developed, making the ultrastructural identification of Purkinje cell processes very difficult. Moreover, many of the other internal

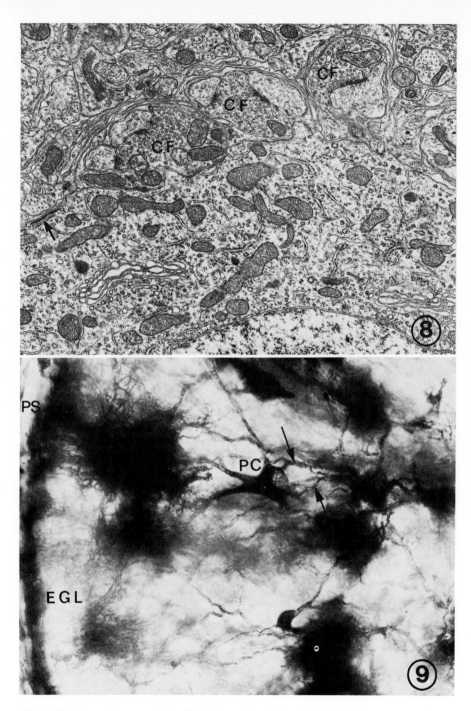

FIG. 8. Electron micrograph of a Purkinje cell body in a 10-day-old staggerer/staggerer mouse. Climbing fiber varicosities, CF, are synapsing on somatic spines. Note the poor development of the hypolemmal cisterna (*arrow*) and the small size of this cell. (×22,000.)

FIG. 9. Light micrograph of a Golgi-impregnated cerebellum from a 10-day-old staggerer/ staggerer mouse. The surface of the cerebellar cortex is at the left of micrograph; PS, pial surface. Cells in the external granular layer, EGL, are not impregnated. The neuron at the center of the micrograph is considered to be an altered Purkinje cell, PC. Note the multipolar appearance of this neuron. The main dendrites are smooth and spread in the molecular layer. However, small dendritic-like processes (*arrows*) spread in the inner granular layer. (×700.)

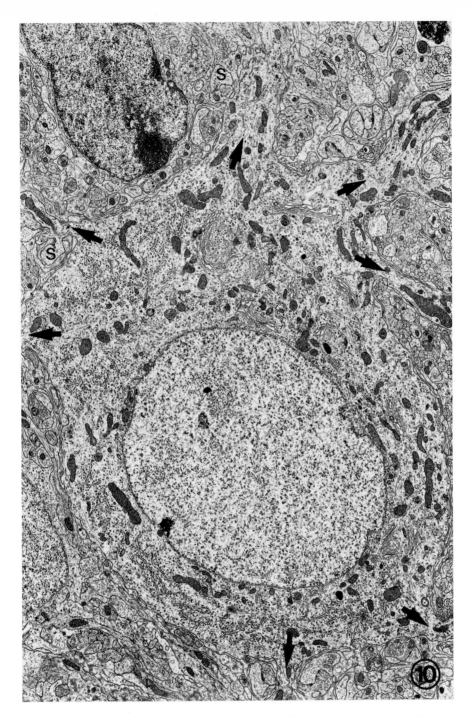

FIG. 10. Electron micrograph of a Purkinje cell in a 20-day-old *sg/sg* mouse. Although the normal cytoplasmic features of Purkinje cells are poorly developed in the staggerer, this cell is identified as an altered Purkinje cell because of its location in the border between the deeper region of the molecular layer and the internal granular layer, and mainly because of the complete glial envelope that surrounds the whole neuron. Seven dendritic profiles of different diameters (*arrows*) originate from the perikaryon. The thicker dendritic trunks are oriented toward the molecular layer. Atypical spines, S, arise from some of the dendrites.

features of normal Purkinje cells are also lacking in the staggerer; therefore, some other criteria must be used. The most important one is the glial investment: in normal cerebellum Purkinje cells are the only cell type that is almost completely ensheathed by astrocytic processes. In staggerer mice this glial sheath is fortunately present at the level of the cell body and main dendritic stem (Fig. 10). A second feature upon which one can rely is the almost constant presence of one or more spines, frequently contacted by axon terminals on the Purkinje cell bodies. The PCD's spread in the molecular layer mainly in a vertical direction, perpendicular to the cerebellar surface. At their origin in the cell body, PCD's can be in synaptic contact with climbing fibers (Fig. 11). These synapses exhibit characteristics similar to those in normal cerebellum. The *boutons en passant* of the climbing fibers establish their synaptic contacts on dendritic spines as illustrated in Fig. 11. The density of climbing fibers is much lower than in the normal cerebellum, making it unlikely that all Purkinje cells are innervated by them. In this respect the electrophysiologic results obtained by Crepel and Mariani (*personal communication*) are relevant. They have found that in staggerer mice after harmaline treatment there are rhythmic burst responses in about only 40% of the tested Purkinje cells.

The primary PCD's, which occupy the deeper third of the molecular layer, are thinner than in the normal cerebellum. They are practically smooth and almost completely ensheathed by glial cytoplasm (Fig. 12). The absence of tertiary-like spines is not absolute, and at this deep region of the molecular layer, occasionally there are small areas in which parallel fibers are in synaptic contact with what appear to be PCD spines. Intriguingly enough, some of these sparse spines can be devoid of their presynaptic elements, appearing as naked spines provided, however, with clear postsynaptic differentiations.

The superficial two-thirds of the molecular layer are mainly occupied by clusters of closely packed parallel fibers. Each cluster is separated from a neighboring one by glial processes with abundant gliofilaments (Fig. 13). In this superficial region, dendritic profiles are infrequent. They generally have a diameter measuring in between 0.5 to 1 μm and they are devoid of spines. As illustrated in Fig. 13 (arrow), spines in synaptic contact with parallel fibers are more infrequently observed than in deeper regions. Most of the dendrites lying in the superficial molecular layer run in a vertical direction perpendicular to the cerebellar surface; the great majority of them are partially covered by thin glial processes, but parallel fibers synapsing on their smooth surface (Fig. 14) are numerous. In Golgi preparations there are two main types of dendrites spreading in the superficial molecular layer: (1) thin dendrites arising from Purkinje cells, and (2) thin dendrites arising from Golgi cells. The dendrites observed in the electron micrographs must belong to these two categories of neurons. In a recent electrophysiologic study, Crepel, Mariani, Korn, and Changeux (1973) described that,

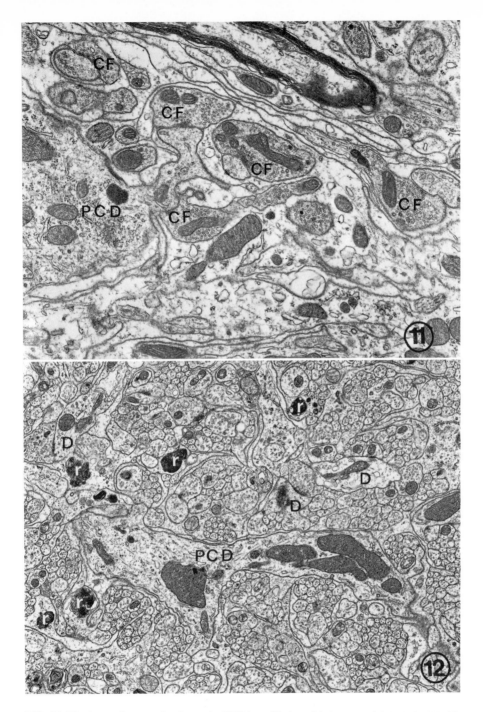

FIG. 11. Electron micrograph of a main PCD in a 22-day-old staggerer/staggerer mouse. Climbing fiber varicosities, CF, establish synaptic contacts with spines originated from this dendrite. Note the large amount of glial processes surrounding the dendritic profile and the synapses. (×14,000.)

FIG. 12. Deep region of the molecular layer in the same mouse as Fig. 11. A thin PCD is almost covered by glial processes. Nonsynaptic segments of parallel fibers are abundant. Smaller dendrites, D, probably belonging to interneurons are contacted by parallel fibers. Numerous dense bodies, r, remnants, of degenerated parallel fibers, are present in the glial cytoplasm. (×10,000.)

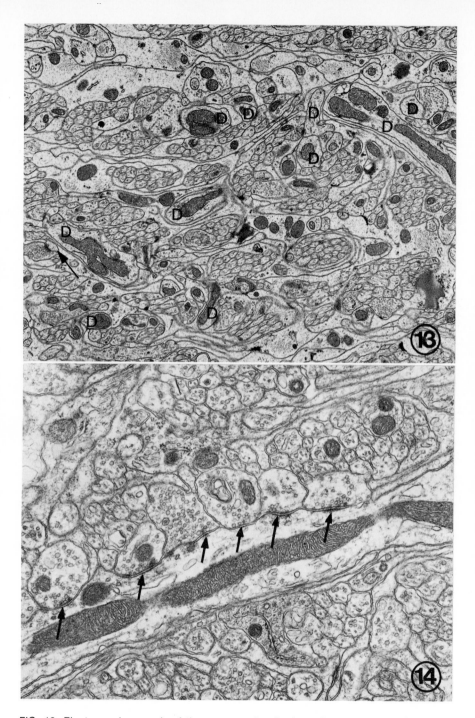

FIG. 13. Electron micrograph of the upper molecular layer in a 26-day-old staggerer/
staggerer mouse. This region is composed of some small dendritic profiles, D, and by
numerous parallel fibers clustered in small groups by astrocytic processes. Some parallel
fiber axon terminals are in synaptic contacts with the smooth surface of the dendrites.
Occasionally, the parallel fibers synapse on dendritic spines (*arrow*). (×8,000.)
FIG. 14. Higher magnification of the upper molecular layer of a 20-day-old staggerer/
staggerer mouse. A dendritic profile, running perpendicular to the cerebellar surface, is
completely ensheathed by glial processes, with the exception of the regions in which
parallel fibers (*arrows*) synapse on the smooth surface of the dendrite. (×20,000.)

after local stimulation and on beam recording in the staggerer cerebellum, there are simple orthodromic responses of Purkinje cells with latencies very similar to those occurring in the normal cerebellum after parallel fiber stimulation. Because the number of residual synapses between parallel fibers and PCD spines (their quantitative analysis is now under study) is too low to explain the physiologic results, and because most of the dendritic profiles in the superficial molecular layer are contacted on their smooth surface by parallel fibers, it can be argued that these fibers may succeed in establishing a small number of atypically located synapses with the smooth surface of PCD's. The glial envelope that ensheaths the nonsynaptic surface of some dendritic profiles (Fig. 14) lends further support to the identification of these profiles as those of Purkinje cells.

GENERAL CONSIDERATIONS AND CONCLUSIONS

The cerebella of the two neurologic 1-month-old mutant mice described in this chapter are agranular. However, the presumptive mechanism for this agranularity is different in each mutant. In weaver, granule cell axons do not develop. In staggerer mice, the receptive surface of Purkinje cells appears to be altered.

The dendritic tree of Purkinje cells in weaver mice is very similar to that described in other agranular cerebella (Shofer, Pappas, Purpura, 1964; Herndon et al., 1971; Altman and Anderson, 1972; Hirano et al., 1972; Llinás et al., 1973). The similarity of Purkinje cell dendritic arborization in all agranular cerebella provides morphologic proof that the size, shape, and orientation of PCD's depend on the microenvironment of these cells, i.e., the dendritic pattern of normal Purkinje cells is directly dependent upon its interaction with parallel fibers. But another important conclusion that can be drawn from these studies is that the Purkinje cell is nevertheless capable of developing autonomously its dendritic spines. However, a different interpretation has been reported by Hámori (1973), who postulates for an indirect or heterotopic induction of PCD spines by "afferent elements [climbing fibers] contacting other postsynaptic sites of the same neuron." A final proof in confirmation of this hypothesis is yet to be found. In fact, there are some indications, chiefly arising from tissue culture experiments (see the chapter by Privat, this volume), against the validity of this hetero-topic induction. This is because Purkinje cells explanted from 16-day-old embryos to newborn rats develop dendritic spines in the absence of climbing fibers. The concluding *in vivo* experiment will be the study of PCD's in an animal in which the inferior olives were destroyed at birth. Work is presently in progress in our laboratory to study the adult cerebellum of such animals.

The Purkinje cells in staggerer mice display a wide spectrum of shapes from cells that give off only one main dendritic trunk, to real multipolar neurons giving rise to as many as eight dendritic trunks. In the latter instance, most of the dendritic branches curve in such a way that they spread in the molecular layer. However, occasionally tiny dendritic processes can spread within the granular layer. The multipolar appearance of some Purkinje cells may indicate a remnant of their immature shape, in which the filopodia-like somatic processes were not reabsorbed, but evolved into real dendrites. Even in cells in which the dendritic tree arborizes from one to three main dendrites, the cell body retains its spiny appearance. Some of the main dendritic trunks are also provided with spines, which are synaptically contacted by climbing fibers. Thinner dendritic branches are almost smooth, and tertiary-like spines are a rare observation. From these facts it can be concluded that the development of the two categories of dendritic spines present in Purkinje cells is controlled by different genes; for example, the gene controlling tertiary spines seems to be the one that is altered in staggerer mice.

The comparative study of the PCD abnormalities in these mutant mice provides some new evidence that the final dendritic arrangement of Purkinje cells is caused by genetic and "epigenetic" factors. The development of postsynaptic structures, such as spines and postsynaptic densities, which probably represent the receptive surface, might depend on autonomous factors. Conversely, the dendritic pattern is modulated by the synaptic interactions of granule cells—through parallel fibers—with Purkinje cells.

ACKNOWLEDGMENTS

The author wishes to express his sincere thanks to Drs. J.-P. Changeux, F. Crepel, and J. Mariani for useful discussions and suggestions. This research was supported in part by A.T.P. 6–74–27 (grant number 20) from the I.N.S.E.R.M. (Institut National de la Santé et de la Recherche Médicale).

REFERENCES

Altman, J. (1971): Coated vesicles and synaptogenesis. A developmental study in the cerebellar cortex of the rat. *Brain Res.*, 30:311–322.
Altman, J., and Anderson, W. J. (1972): Experimental reorganization of the cerebellar cortex. I.
Morphological effects of elimination of all microneurons with prolonged X-irradiation started at birth. *J. Comp. Neurol.*, 146:355–406.
Crepel, F., Mariani, J., Korn, H., and Changeux, J. P. (1973): Electrophysiologie du cortex cérébelleux chez la souris mutante "staggerer." *C. R. Acad. Sci.* [D] (*Paris*), 277:2761–2763.
Eccles, J. C. (1973): *The Understanding of the Brain*. McGraw-Hill, New York.
Gentschev, T., and Sotelo, C. (1973): Degenerative patterns in the ventral cochlear nucleus of the rat after primary deafferentation. An ultrastructural study. *Brain Res.*, 62:37–60.
Hámori, J. (1973): Developmental morphology of dendritic postsynaptic specializations. In: *Recent Developments of Neurobiology in Hungary, Vol. IV: Results in Neuroanatomy, Neuroendocrinology, Neurophysiology and Behavior, Neuropathology*, edited by K. Lissak, pp. 9–32. Akadémiai Kiado, Budapest.

Herndon, R. M., Margolis, G., and Kilham, L. (1971): The synaptic organization of the malformed cerebellum induced by perinatal infection with the feline panleukopenia virus (PLV). II. The Purkinje cell and its afferents. *J. Neuropathol. Exp. Neurol.,* 30:557–570.

Hirano, A., and Dembitzer, H. M. (1973): Cerebellar alterations in the weaver mouse. *J. Cell Biol.,* 56:478–486.

Hirano, A., Dembitzer, H. M., and Jones, M. (1972): An electron microscopic study of cycasin-induced cerebellar alterations. *J. Neuropathol. Exp. Neurol.,* 31:113–125.

Landis, D. (1971): Cerebellar cortical development in the staggerer mutant mouse. *J. Cell Biol.,* 51:159a.

Larramendi, L. M. H., and Victor, T. (1967): Synapses on Purkinje cell spines in the mouse. An electron microscopic study. *Brain Res.,* 5:15–30.

Llinás, R., Hillman, D. E., and Precht, W. (1973): Neuronal circuit reorganization in mammalian agranular cerebellar cortex. *J. Neurobiology,* 4:69–94.

Palay, S. L., and Chan-Palay, V. (1974): *Cerebellar Cortex. Cytology and Organization.* Springer-Verlag. Berlin, Heidelberg, New York.

Rakic, P., and Sidman, R. L. (1973): Organization of cerebellar cortex secondary to deficit of granule cells in weaver mutant mice. *J. Comp. Neurol.,* 152:133–162.

Ramón y Cajal, S. (1911): *Histologie du système nerveux de l'homme et des vertébrés,* Vol. II. Maloine, Paris.

Rezai, Z., and Yoon, C. H. (1972): Abnormal rate of granule cell migration in the cerebellum of "weaver" mutant mice. *Dev. Biol.,* 29:17–26.

Shofer, R. J., Pappas, G. D., and Purpura, D. P. (1964): Radiation-induced changes in morphological and physiological properties of immature cerebellar cortex. In: *Response of the Nervous System to Ionizing Radiation, Second International Symposium,* edited by T. J. Haley and R. S. Snider, pp. 476–508. Little, Brown, Boston, Massachusetts.

Sidman, R. L. (1968): Development of interneuronal connections in brains of mutant mice. In: *Physiological and Biochemical Aspects of Nervous Integration,* edited by F. D. Carlsson, pp. 163–193. Prentice-Hall, Englewood Cliffs, New Jersey.

Sidman, R. L. (1972): Cell interactions in developing mammalian central nervous system. In: *Cell Interactions, Proceedings of the Third Lepetit Colloquium,* edited by L. G. Silvestri, pp. 1–13. North-Holland, Amsterdam and London.

Sidman, R. L., Green, M. C., and Appel, S. H. (1965): *Catalog of Neurological Mutants of the Mouse.* Harvard University Press, Cambridge, Massachusetts.

Sidman, R. L., Lane, P., and Dickie, M. (1962): Staggerer, a new mutation in the mouse affecting the cerebellum. *Science,* 137:610–612.

Sotelo, C. (1968): Permanence of postsynaptic specializations in the frog sympathetic ganglion cells after denervation. *Exp. Brain Res.,* 6:294–305.

Sotelo, C. (1973): Permanence and fate of paramembranous synaptic specializations in "mutants" and experimental animals. *Brain Res.,* 62:345–351.

Sotelo, C., and Changeux, J. P. (1974): Trans-synaptic degeneration "en cascade" in the cerebellar cortex of staggerer mutant mice. *Brain Res.,* 67:519–526.

Valverde, F. (1967): Apical dendritic spines of the visual cortex and light deprivation in the mouse. *Exp. Brain Res.,* 3:337–352.

Advances in Neurology, Vol. 12, edited by
G. W. Kreutzberg, Raven Press, New York
© 1975.

Aberrant Development of the Purkinje Cell Dendritic Spine

Asao Hirano and Herbert M. Dembitzer

Montefiore Hospital and Medical Center, Bronx, New York 10467

One of the principal contributions of the electron microscope has been the elucidation of the structure of the synapse. These observations have finally laid to rest the classic controversy between the reticular and neuronal theories of the nervous system.

When applied to the development of the synapse, however, the results of electron-microscopic observation have been, to some extent at least, disappointing. To date, the precise sequence of events leading to the formation of the mature synapse is still obscure (Hirano and Zimmerman, 1973). It cannot with certainty be stated at this time whether the presumptive presynaptic process seeks out its postsynaptic mate and induces the latter to specialize, or vice versa.

In virtually all attempts to investigate this problem, one fact has been tacitly assumed. Almost all the authors working in the field seem to agree that the full maturation of either component of the synapse requires communication between two neuronal elements on a one-to-one basis. That is, for any single postsynaptic structure to differentiate into its mature form, a presynaptic element must be in some kind of contact, and likewise the full development of a presynaptic structure requires the presence and active participation of a developing (or developed) postsynaptic element.

We have investigated a number of animal models that suggest to us that this assumption may not be valid. Our studies began with the cycasin-treated mouse. Hirono, Shibuya, and Hayashi (1969), using the optical microscope, demonstrated that when cycasin was administered to perinatal mice, the cerebellar granule cells were destroyed before they formed an internal layer. When we examined similarly treated mice with the electron microscope, we confirmed Hirono's observations; we also noticed that unattached dendritic spines of the Purkinje cells remained apparently intact (Hirano, Dembitzer, and Jones, 1972). These spines showed all the features of those seen in the normal animal except that they were embedded within a matrix of astrocytic cytoplasm rather than being in synaptic contact with a parallel fiber (Fig. 1). They had a postmembranous thickening, and the apposing extracellular space was somewhat widened and contained a relatively dense cleft material. Soon thereafter, we detected similar changes (Fig. 2) in what

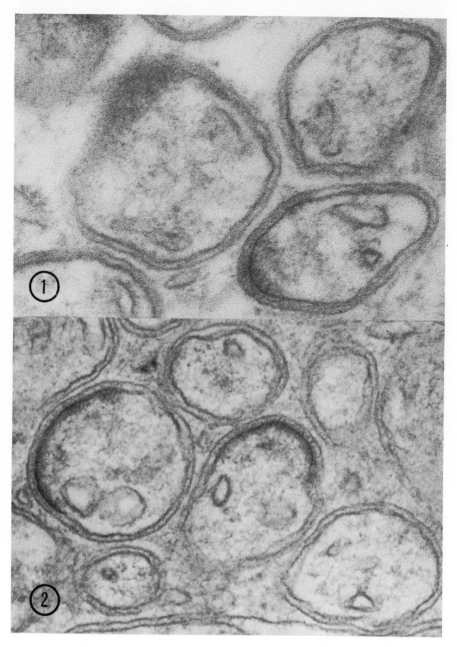

FIG. 1. Unattached dendritic spines in the cerebellum of a cycasin-treated mouse. (×96,000.)
FIG. 2. Unattached dendritic spines in the cerebellum of a weaver mouse. (×80,000.)

seems to be a genetic model of cycasin intoxication, the weaver mouse (Hirano and Dembitzer, 1973). Again, in this animal granule cells are virtually absent but the dendritic spines of the Purkinje cells remain behind (Llinás, Hillman, and Precht, 1973; Rakic and Sidman, 1973a,b,c; Sotelo, 1973). Similar results had previously been described in animals that had been inoculated with feline panleukopenia virus (Herndon, Margolis, and Kilham, 1971). We assumed at that point that in all three cases, the unattached dendritic spines represented the remains of an intact synapse that had lost its presynaptic element when the granule cells degenerated. Herndon had treated adult animals with thiophene and, indeed, was able to demonstrate precisely this effect. That is, after thiophene administration, the parallel fibers degenerated leaving the intact dendritic spine behind (Herndon, 1968).

We thought it would be a relatively simple task to demonstrate the same effect in the weaver mouse. We were somewhat troubled, however, by the fact that in normal animals, according to Larramendi, the bulk of the dendritic spine-parallel fiber synapses formed during the second or third postnatal week (Larramendi, 1969), whereas the weaver trait was detectable before the tenth day (Sidman, 1968). When we examined the youngest weavers we could find, we were unable to demonstrate any degenerating parallel fibers attached to dendritic spines (Hirano and Dembitzer, 1974). Things apparently were not as simple as we had first suspected.

How, then, did the spines develop? We thought that it might be best to first determine just how similar the unattached spines of the weaver mice were to the attached spines of the normal mouse. To this end, we applied several simple cytochemical techniques using uranyl acetate, phosphotungstic acid (Figs. 3 and 4), and bismuth iodide. In all cases we were unable to detect any difference in staining reaction between the dendritic spines within the intact synapses of the normal mouse and those of the weaver mouse (Hirano and Dembitzer, 1973).

If the Purkinje cell dendritic spines did not arise under the influence of a presynaptic element, how did they come to be? Hámori had been working with virus-infected animals and he suggested that it was the climbing fiber input that acted as a signal for the production of spines over the entire dendritic tree (Hámori, 1973a,b). Climbing fibers were, in fact, present in weaver, so that this theory seemed very attractive at first.

However, there appeared to be some serious reservations concerning Hámori's ingenious idea. In order to test his theory, Hámori had undercut the cerebellar cortex of untreated animals, thereby presumably severing climbing fiber input. As he predicted, dendritic spines were absent, although parallel fibers were abundant (Hámori, 1973a). Unfortunately, however, when the cortex is undercut, the Purkinje cell axon is inevitably destroyed. How can one be sure that it is not this loss that results in the failure to

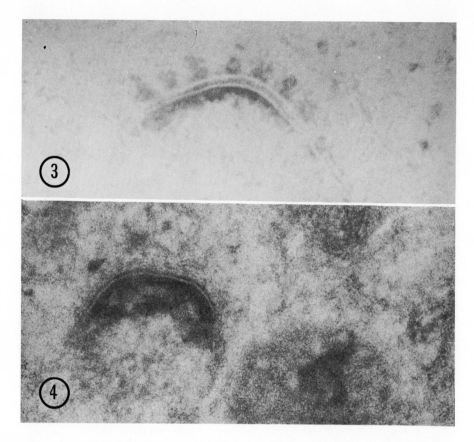

FIG. 3. An intact synapse in the cerebellum of a mouse. Phosphotungstic acid stain. (×112,000.)

FIG. 4. An unattached dendritic spine in the cerebellum of a weaver mouse. Phosphotungstic acid stain. (×112,000.)

produce dendritic spines? More recently, Hámori addressed himself to this problem (Hámori, 1973*b*), and, using the adult animal, he severed the climbing fiber input at the level of the restiform body, which is believed to be the source of the climbing fibers from the inferior olive (Eccles, 1974). As his theory predicted, this resulted in severely reducing the number of dendritic spines. (Some authors maintain that at least some climbing fibers are from sources other than the inferior olives (Riviera-Dominguez, Mettler, and Noback, 1974). Presumably, these may be responsible for the remaining spines.) In any event, Hámori concluded that the climbing fiber is required not only for the induction of the spines but also for their maintenance. Nevertheless, one must consider the results of the tissue culture experiments of Seil and Herndon (1970) and of S. U. Kim (1974, *personal com-*

munication). These authors were able to culture Purkinje cells and to demonstrate unattached dendritic spines as well as some in synaptic contact with parallel fibers in preparations clearly free of influence from the inferior olives. Could it be that some nucleus intrinsic to the cerebellum gives rise to climbing fibers?

It occurred to us that the question of the influence of climbing fibers might be approached by examination of another murine mutant, the staggerer mouse (Sidman, Lane, and Dickie, 1962). This animal also loses its granule cells during development (although somewhat later than the weaver), but was reported to be free of dendritic spines, attached or unattached (Landis, 1971; Landis and Sidman, 1974; Sotelo and Changeux, 1974). We examined these animals and found climbing fibers, as had been previously reported by Sidman (1972). Unfortunately, we also found occasional dendritic spines. Although it is true that they are absent in the younger animal (under 2 weeks) and in the adult, somatic spines may be found at 3 to 4 weeks, and occasional dendritic spines arise slightly later, a few of which were unattached. Therefore, the staggerer is not a suitable test object for Hámori's theory.

It occurred to us that a simple variation on Hámori's idea might serve to explain some of these results. In our observations of the young weaver, we occasionally came across an intact synapse between parallel fibers and dendritic spines. Could it be that these rare, ephemeral contacts serve as the trigger mechanism (Hirano and Dembitzer, 1974). This would explain the presence of spines not only in weaver, but also in the cycasin-treated animals in which a few such synapses were also found, and perhaps in the virus-treated animals as well. It would also allow us to explain the presence of spines in the cultures of cerebellum. However, we have no test for this hypothesis and it seems to be in conflict with Hámori's more recent experiment in which he was able to reduce the number of dendritic spines in the presence of parallel fibers, by cutting the inferior olive input.

Apparently all that we can safely conclude at this point is that the dendritic spines do not seem to require a one-to-one induction of a presynaptic element. This is not to say that the parallel fiber is totally without influence on the development of the dendritic spines. When we examine the unattached spines in the weaver or in the cycasin-treated mouse in detail, several minor but interesting differences appear. First, they are more common on the larger dendritic branches than in the normal (Fig. 5 in Hirano et al., 1972). In addition, some are quite elongated with narrow necks and bulbous endings. Others show branching at their origin and some show more than one postsynaptic membranous thickening (Fig. 5). It seems as though the formation of the spine might be induced by some generalized stimulus but that the resulting structures, in the absence of their normal presynaptic mates, remain unfulfilled and aberrant.

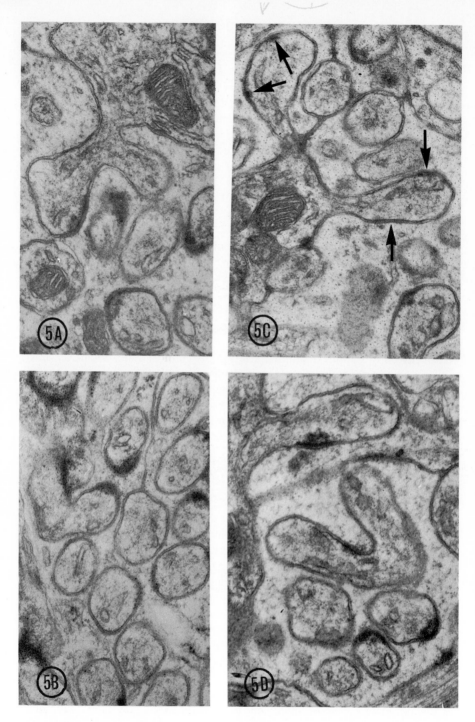

FIG. 5. Aberrant dendritic spines in the cerebellum of the cycasin-treated mouse. (×34,000.) (A) A branching spine; (B) a branching spine with two postmembranous thickenings. One is apparently in synaptic contact; (C) spines with two postmembranous thickenings (arrows); (D) a branching spine with a postmembranous thickening near the origin of the spine.

ACKNOWLEDGMENT

This work was supported by grant 1 RO 1 NS 10427–01 NEUA.

REFERENCES

Eccles, J. C. (1974): Trophic interactions in the mammalian central nervous system. *Ann. NY Acad. Sci.,* 228:406–423.

Hámori, J. (1973*a*): Developmental morphology of dendritic postsynaptic specializations. In: *Recent Developments of Neurobiology in Hungary, Vol. IV: Results in Neuroanatomy, Neuroendocrinology, Neurophysiology and Behavior, Neuropathology,* edited by K. Lissak. Akadémiai Kiadó, Budapest.

Hámori, J. (1973*b*): The inductive role of presynaptic axons in the development of post-synaptic spines. *Brain Res.,* 62:337–344.

Herndon, R. M. (1968): Thiophen induced granule cell necrosis in the rat cerebellum. An electron microscopic study. *Exp. Brain Res.,* 6:49–68.

Herndon, R. M., Margolis, G., and Kilham, L. (1971): The synaptic organization of malformed cerebellum induced by perinatal infection with the feline panleukopenia virus (PLV). *J. Neuropathol. Exp. Neurol.,* 30:557–580.

Hirano, A., and Dembitzer, H. M. (1973): Cerebellar alterations in the weaver mouse. *J. Cell Biol.,* 56:478–486.

Hirano, A., and Dembitzer, H. M. (1974): Observations on the development of the weaver mouse cerebellum. *J. Neuropathol. Exp. Neurol.* 33:354–364.

Hirano, A., Dembitzer, H. M., and Jones, M. (1972): An electron microscopic study of cycasin-induced cerebellar alterations. *J. Neuropathol. Exp. Neurol.,* 31:113–125.

Hirano, A., and Zimmerman, H. M. (1973): Aberrant synaptic development: A review. *Arch. Neurol.,* 28:359–366.

Hirono, I., Shibuya, C., and Hayashi, K. (1969): Induction of a cerebellar disorder with cycasin in newborn mice and hamsters. *Proc. Soc. Exp. Biol. Med.,* 131:593–599.

Landis, D. (1971): Cerebellar cortical development in the staggerer mutant mouse. Eleventh Annual Meeting. The American Society for Cell Biology. Abstr. 159.

Landis, D., and Sidman, R. L. (1974): Cerebellar cortical development in the staggerer mouse. *J. Neuropathol. Exp. Neurol.,* 33:180 (Abstr.).

Larramendi, L. M. H. (1969): Analysis of synaptogenesis in cerebellum of the mouse. In: *Neurobiology of Cerebellar Evolution and Development,* edited by R. R. Llinás. American Medical Association/Education and Research Foundation, Chicago, Illinois.

Llinás, R., Hillman, D. E., and Precht, W. (1973): Neuronal circuit reorganization in mammalian agranular cerebellar cortex. *J. Neurobiol.,* 4:69–94.

Rakic, P., and Sidman, R. L. (1973*a*): Weaver mutant mouse cerebellum: Defective neuronal migration secondary to abnormality of Bergmann glia. *Proc. Natl. Acad. Sci. USA,* 70:240–244.

Rakic, P., and Sidman, R. L. (1973*b*): Sequence of development abnormalities leading to granule cell deficit in cerebellar cortex of weaver mutant mice. *J. Comp. Neurol.,* 152:103–132.

Rakic, P., and Sidman, R. L. (1973*c*): Organization of cerebellar cortex secondary to deficit of granule cells in weaver mutant mice. *J. Comp. Neurol.,* 152:133–162.

Riviera-Dominguez, M., Mettler, F. A., and Noback, C. R. (1974): Origin of cerebellar climbing fibers in the Rhesus monkey. *J. Comp. Neurol.,* 155:331–336.

Seil, F. J., and Herndon, R. M. (1970): Cerebellar granule cells *in vitro.* A light and electron microscope study. *J. Cell Biol.,* 45:212–220.

Sidman, R. L. (1968): Development of interneuronal connection in brains of mutant mice. In: *Physiological and Biochemical Aspects of Nervous Integration,* edited by F. D. Carlsson. Prentice-Hall, Englewood Cliffs, New Jersey.

Sidman, R. L. (1972): Cell interactions in developing mammalian central nervous system. In: *Cell Interactions. Proceedings of the Third Lepetit Colloquium,* edited by L. G. Silvestri. North-Holland, Amsterdam.

Sidman, R. L., Lane, P. W., and Dickie, M. M. (1962): Staggerer, a new mutation in the mouse affecting the cerebellum. *Science,* 137:610–612.

Sotelo, C. (1973): Permanence and fate of paramembranous synaptic specializations in "mutants" and experimental animals. *Brain Res.,* 62:345–351.

Sotelo, C., and Changeux, J. P. (1974): Trans-synaptic degeneration "en cascade" in the cerebellar cortex of staggerer mutant mice. *Brain Res.,* 67:519–526.

Advances in Neurology, Vol. 12, edited by
G. W. Kreutzberg, Raven Press, New York
© 1975.

Effect of Granule Cell Destruction on Development and Maintenance of the Purkinje Cell Dendrite

Robert M. Herndon and Mary Lou Oster-Granite

Department of Neurology, Johns Hopkins University School of Medicine, Baltimore, Maryland 21205

Morphologic descriptions of mature neuronal systems or of the sequence of morphogenetic events that occur in a developing system give us some idea of the complexity of the interactions in the system. Unfortunately, they provide us with little information regarding the types of forces involved in the development of the system or of the interdependence of the various elements involved. In order to understand the extent of such interdependence, we must remove one or another element from the system and observe the behavior of the remaining elements. The purpose of this chapter is to discuss the effect of cerebellar granule cell destruction on the developing and on the mature Purkinje cell and on basket-stellate cell dendrites and then to discuss some theoretical considerations and hypotheses relating to dendritic development and maintenance in the cerebellar molecular layer.

More or less selective destruction of mature cerebellar granule cells has been described as occurring (1) following roentgen irradiation (Vogel, 1960; Pitcock, 1962), (2) in the homozygous leaner mutant mouse (Sidman, 1968), (3) following exposure to organomercurial halides and sulfides (Hunter, Bomford, and Russell, 1940; Tokoumi and Okajimo, 1961), and (4) following exposure to thiophene (Herndon, 1968).

Of these, roentgen irradiation and the organomercurials have the disadvantage of producing directly observable effects on other cellular elements, including the Purkinje cells. In addition, radiation in doses that cause adequate destruction of mature granule cells produces delayed changes in the vascular bed. The leaner mutant produces a selective but very incomplete destruction of the granule cells and is therefore unsatisfactory, although it remains interesting from a number of points of view, particularly as regards the possible study of regenerative sprouting by surviving parallel fibers.

Thiophene (thiofuran) is a noxious industrial solvent which, when injected intramuscularly into experimental animals, causes extensive necrosis of cerebellar granule cells while having little apparent effect on other elements in the nervous system (Christomanos and Scholtz, 1933; Upners,

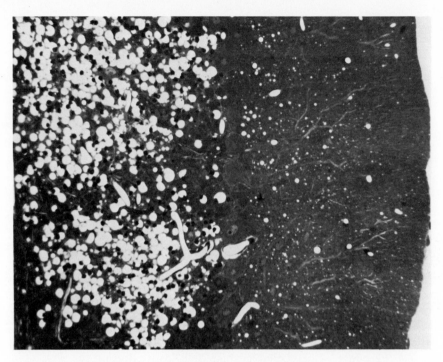

FIG. 1. Cerebellar cortex of a rat 13 days after the beginning of a 7-day course of thiophene injections. There is severe granule cell destruction. The small vacuoles in the molecular layer are caused by parallel fiber destruction. (×225.)

1939; Ule and Rossner, 1960; Herndon, 1968). In some folia, this re-sults in virtually complete selective destruction of the granule cell popu-lation (Figs. 1 and 2). Whereas some late loss of Golgi type II cells may occur, this is not extensive and other cerebellar elements appear to be little affected. This extensive destruction of the granule cells and their axons—the parallel fibers—has surprisingly little effect on the Purkinje cell den-drites. Although they become a little shorter and thicker than normal, they retain their dendritic spines. These spines are slightly elongated, but appear otherwise normal. A postsynaptic web persists, even though the parallel fiber contacts have been replaced by hypertrophic glial processes. The dendrites retain a relatively normal espaliered shape and the spines persist for periods of at least 5 months following the granule cell destruction. Therefore, it appears that once the Purkinje cell dendrite is fully developed, elimination of its parallel fiber input has relatively little effect on its mor-phology.

The destruction of the granule cell precursors—the external germinal cells—in the developing cerebellum can be accomplished in a variety of ways. These include (1) the use of genetic mouse mutants weaver (Sidman,

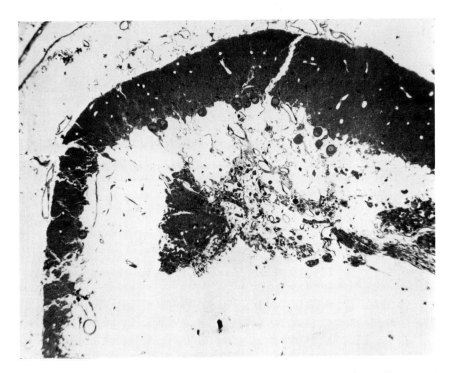

FIG. 2. Cerebellar cortex 5 months after a series of thiophene injections. The granular layer has been replaced by a cystic cavity. Intact Purkinje cells can be seen hanging from the molecular layer. (×100.)

1968; Rezai and Yoon, 1972; Hirano and Dembitzer, 1973; Rakic and Sidman, 1973a,b,c) and staggerer (Sidman, 1968; Sotelo and Changeaux, 1974); (2) the use of toxins such as cycasin (Hirano, Dembitzer, and Jones, 1972), cyclophosphamide (Nathanson, Cole, and VanderLoos, 1969), and floxuridine (Langman, Shimada, and Rodier, 1972); (3) roentgen irradiation (Shofer, Pappas, and Purpura, 1964; Altman, Anderson, and Wright, 1967, 1968, 1969); (4) surgical extirpation of the rhombic lip (Forstronen, 1963); and (5) parvovirus infection (Herndon, Margolis, and Kilham, 1971a,b; Llinás, Hillman, and Precht, 1973; Oster-Granite, 1974).

Each of these systems has certain inherent advantages and disadvantages for studying the effect of granule cell destruction on the developing cerebellum. The genetic mutants—weaver and staggerer—result from single gene mutations that cause a relatively clean destruction of the cerebellar granule cells. However, the mechanism of the gene action is not known in either case. The main locus of the effect in the homozygous staggerer mouse may be the Purkinje cell. These fail to develop dendritic spines and retrograde transsynaptic degeneration of the granule cells results (Sotelo and Changeaux, 1974). This makes the model unsuitable for the study of the influence of granule cell destruction on Purkinje cell development. In the homozygous weaver mouse, the abnormality may lie in the Bergmann astrocytes, resulting in a failure of migration of the granule cells and their subsequent death in the external germinal layer. Thus, the main locus of effect is the glial cell, which is intimately related to the developing Purkinje cells. It is difficult to be sure which, if any, of the changes in dendritic development may be related to the glial abnormality rather than the absence of granule cells. Nevertheless, these are very useful experimental systems that have yielded a considerable amount of information on cerebellar development.

Of the toxins, only one, cycasin (Hirano et al., 1972), appears to produce extensive granule cell destruction. Floxuridine (Langman et al., 1972) and cyclophosphamide (Nathanson et al., 1969) act only during a specific part of the cell cycle and produce inadequate destruction of the granule cells unless repeated dosage is used. The surviving germinal cells remain mitotic and partially reconstitute the external germinal layer, although the directional specificity of their axons—the parallel fibers—may be disrupted. The result is a partial granule cell destruction with regeneration, granule cell heterotopia, and parallel fiber misdirection. Cycasin appears to act over a longer period of time than the other toxins, producing a more complete destruction without regeneration. Because it induces profound changes in the nucleolar RNA synthesis in liver cells (Zedeck, Sternberg, McGowan, and Poynter, 1972), it may produce significant direct effects on cerebellar elements other than granule cells.

Roentgen irradiation (Shofer et al., 1964; Altman et al., 1967, 1968, 1969) can, by varying timing and dosage, be used to produce partial or complete destruction of the external germinal layer of the cerebellum. Such flexibility of protocol has proven very useful for the study of the development of the granuloprival cerebellum, despite the known delayed effects of radiation. Such effects raise the possibility that some of the changes seen, especially the delayed Purkinje cell alterations and loss, may be a direct, rather than indirect, result of the radiation.

Surgical extirpation of the rhombic lip (Forstronen, 1963) is perhaps the cleanest and most interesting method of removing the granule cell precursors and deserves further detailed study. Unfortunately, it has not, thus far, been studied except by routine histologic methods, and the details of the Purkinje cell changes have not been described.

Parvoviruses (Herndon et al., 1971a,b; Llinás et al., 1973; Oster-Granite, 1974) are a group of very small DNA viruses that have an affinity for certain dividing cell populations that they infect and destroy. In the newborn animal, the external germinal cells of the cerebellum are selectively infected and destroyed. There is very little, if any, inflammatory response to the viral infection, and it is possible to verify the locus of infection by both immunofluorescent staining and electron microscopy. We have studied infection of the neonatal hamster with Kilham rat virus strain PRE 308 (Oster-Granite, 1974) and have shown that, in the cerebellum, the infection is limited to the external germinal cells and a few infected granule cells that have succeeded in migrating after becoming infected. Viruses have not been seen in the Purkinje cells, and in the Bergmann glia they appear to be limited to vacuoles containing phagocytized debris. In hamsters infected within 6 hr after birth, there is virtually complete destruction of the external germinal layer by the eighth postinoculation day.

The Purkinje cell dendrites undergo normal development up to the eighth day; thereafter, however, dendritic growth is retarded and tertiary branches are either absent or poorly developed. Nevertheless, dendritic spines form, develop a normal postsynaptic web and apparently normal cleft material, and persist even though the presynaptic terminals never develop (Fig. 3). These "naked" spines become encased by glial processes and are morphologically identical to the "naked" spines originally described following destruction of the granule cells in the mature cerebellum (Herndon, 1968).

Beginning about the thirteenth postnatal day, further changes appear in

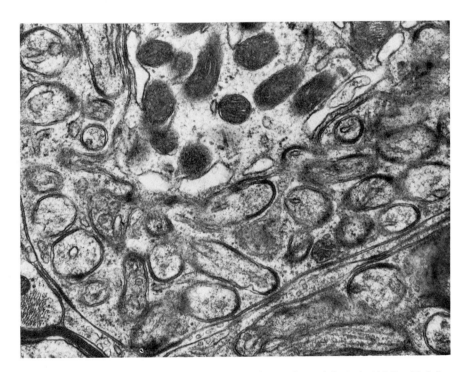

FIG. 3. Electron micrograph of cerebellar cortex from a ferret infected at birth with feline panleukopenia virus. Numerous elongate dendritic spines can be seen enveloped by the hypertrophic glial process that surrounds the Purkinje cell dendrite. A normal-appearing postsynaptic web can be seen on many of these unattached spines. (×32,000.)

the developing dendrites. They fail to assume their normal espaliered shape and spread out in all directions. The tips of the dendrites begin to droop progressively about the soma in a weeping willow fashion until some of the Purkinje cells become completely inverted. Others have stunted, drooping dendritic trees. Thus, in the absence of the parallel fibers, which normally play an important role in maintaining the orientation and shape of the Purkinje cell dendrite, the dendrites appear to reorient themselves to a greater or lesser extent toward the incoming climbing fibers.

Synapse formation is normal within this altered system as long as both the pre- and postsynaptic elements are present in relatively normal numbers; however, occasional abherent synapses are seen between true mossy fiber terminals and Purkinje cells (Llinás et al., 1973; Oster-Granite, 1974).

What conclusions can be drawn from these studies regarding (1) synaptic specificity and (2) the forces responsible for shaping the Purkinje and basket-stellate cell dendrites?

In these systems, despite gross disorganization and displacement of the various elements, synaptic specificity is maintained as long as the pre- and postsynaptic elements are present in reasonably normal numbers. The circuitry of the residual elements in the granuloprival cerebellum is thus relatively normal. Irrespective of the method used to eliminate the granule cells and their processes, abherent synapse formation appears only when there is a marked disproportion between the residual developing presynaptic elements and available postsynaptic surface to be contacted. In the absence of granule cells, mossy fibers occasionally contact Purkinje cells directly. Even displaced granule cells at the pial surface are regularly contacted by mossy fiber endings extending through the upper molecular layer to form glomeruli (Palay and Chan-Palay, 1974). Therefore, synaptic specificity appears to involve some type of contact recognition occurring between pre- and postsynaptic elements rather than mechanical factors related to histologic organization.

Recently, various investigators have described several new ways to destroy the external germinal layer of the cerebellum, all of them leading to essentially similar malformations. Thus, the effect of perinatal granule cell destruction on the shape of the basket-stellate cell and Purkinje cell dendrites is essentially independent of the method used and depends only on the timing and the extent of the destruction. It is thus clear that most of the effects seen are secondary to the granule cell destruction and not direct toxic effects on the Purkinje and basket-stellate cells.

It is now time to move beyond this descriptive stage and to develop testable hypotheses regarding the interactions of the various cellular elements which result in the growth of Purkinje cell and basket-stellate cell dendrites so that they follow the "rule" of spreading in such a way as to maximize the number of parallel fibers they can contact (Rakic, 1972, 1974). Considering their relatively straight course, neurotubule content, and mutual reinforcement, we can conclude that the parallel fibers are moderately "rigid" structures. Altman (1973) has shown that after partial granule cell destruction, regenerating parallel fiber bundles are often misoriented and that Purkinje cell and basket-stellate cell dendrites align themselves orthogonal to these abherent parallel fiber bundles. Thus, we can conclude, as did Ramon y Cajal (1929), that the parallel fibers are an important, perhaps principal, organizing element in the developing molecular layer.

What type of cellular interactions could induce this orthogonal dendritic alignment? The three mechanisms classically proposed for directed cell growth are (1) Contact guidance, such as that which appears to control granule cell migration in the cerebellum (Rakic, 1974), (2) electrical gradients, and (3) chemical gradients. To these we should add (4) random growth with contact recognition and withdrawal of noncontacting processes.

A number of approaches have been used to attempt to establish which of these mechanisms may be important in neurogenesis. In his classic *in vitro* studies, Weiss (1934) found no evidence that electrical or chemical gradients played a role in directing the growth of axonal processes and concluded that mechanical factors were responsible for directed growth. Since that time numerous studies have been carried out and there is, as yet, no convincing evidence for directed neural growth under the control of chemical gradients, although the recent work of Levi-Montalcini and Chen (1971) is perhaps suggestive.

It is unlikely that a chemical gradient set up by the parallel fibers could cause orthogonal dendritic growth. Such a gradient would have to have a very short effective range not exceeding a few times the diameter of the parallel fibers or the gradients would overlap extensively and cancel each other out. In addition, it would be necessary to postulate that contact between the dendrite and parallel fiber "shuts the gradient off" for a finite segment. Otherwise, the growing fiber would follow the parallel fiber where the concentration of the growth directing substance should be highest. If the parallel fibers were shut off one would expect parallel fiber terminals to be regularly separated by a certain minimal distance as suggested by Palkovits and Szentagothai (Palkovits, Magyar, and Szentagothai, 1971*a,b*) who calculated that a given parallel fiber contacts only every fifth Purkinje cell. However, recent studies of parallel fibers in the rat indicate that terminal separation is irregular and most of the terminals are separated by distances of less than 1 μm (Palay and Chan-Palay, 1974). Because the majority of these terminals are parallel fiber-Purkinje cell dendrite synapses the hypothesis would require considerable modification to be tenable.

We would like to propose a new hypothesis here which we shall refer to as the "slippery fiber hypothesis." Let us assume that the portion of the developing dendrite proximal to the growth cone has a tendency to retract. Further assume that the growth cones use the parallel fibers as relatively fixed but slippery rods, which they climb by first insinuating processes between the fibers, and then by expanding them distally, thus pulling the processes out from the soma. Fibers growing out parallel to the parallel fibers could not anchor themselves and would slide back much like someone trying to climb a greased pole. Fibers growing out at an angle would tend to retract and slide along the parallel fiber until the angle between the dendrite and the parallel fiber approached 90°. Thus, an orthogonal orientation would develop which would maximize synaptic contacts between parallel fibers and Purkinje cell dendrites. Only after the dendrites are anchored on the parallel fibers, does the soma migrate downward toward the granular layer (Hendleman and Rouf, 1974) and assume its kohlrabi shape (Palay and Chan-Palay, 1974).

This hypothesis allows us to make several predictions as follows:

1. In the absence of parallel fibers on which to anchor themselves, the dendrites would retract and become shortened and thickened unless they found alternative structures on which to anchor themselves. This may explain why inverted Purkinje cell dendrites expand more than their upright counterparts in the granuloprival cerebellum, i.e., the incoming axons, Golgi cell processes, and Purkinje axons could serve as "anchors" on which the dendrite can expand.

2. The growth cones will invariably have bulbous enlargements near their tips. Constrictions within these bulbs (Fig. 4) will be fairly common and represent necessary transition forms as the growing fiber "climbs" between the parallel fibers. They will also contain some apparatus of locomotion to control the shape and motion of the growing tip—most likely actin filaments (Luduena and Wessells, 1973) in the growth cone pseudopod—with micro- or neutrotubules developing later in the more proximal, stable regions.

3. The growing dendritic tips will be free of junctional complexes and synapses. Synapses should develop on the dendritic stems behind the growing tip.

4. The parallel fibers behind the shoulder of the growth cone will be bent back toward the origin of the fiber as a result of tension on the growth cone. Fibers in front of the growing tip should not be bent. Where not surrounded by abundant extracellular space, those on either side of the growth cone will, of course, be bent outward slightly by expansion of the tip.

5. Purkinje cell and basket-stellate cell dendrites will reorient even a small portion of their dendritic tree orthogonally to any nearby abherent bundle of parallel fibers.

This hypothesis puts no constraints on the number or distribution of the synaptic enlargements which form on the parallel fibers. It does predict that they would not yet be present in regions being invaded by dendritic growth cones and would form only after coming into contact with receptive areas on the dendrites behind the growth cones.

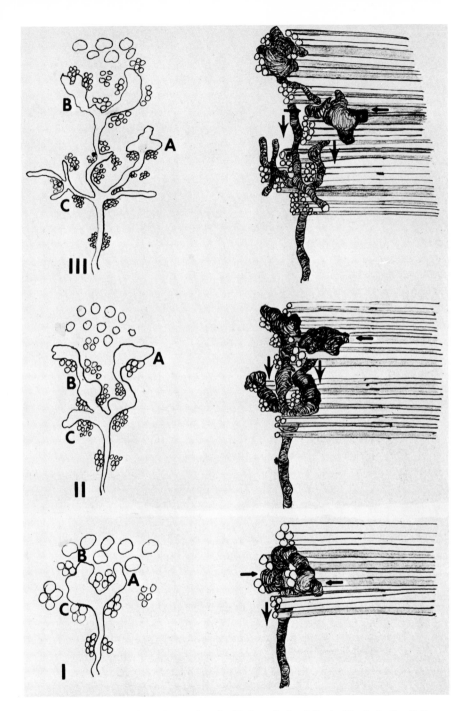

FIG. 4. Schematic drawing of growing Purkinje cell dendrite to illustrate the "slippery fiber" hypothesis. The large arrows indicate the direction of tension on the growing fiber. The small arrows indicate the direction in which the bulbous tips would slide because of the horizontal component of the force, thereby producing orthogonal alignment. The bulbous enlargements overhang the parallel fibers, thus preventing further retraction.

This rather simple "slippery fiber" hypothesis thus appears to be compatible with what is known about the shape, orientation, and development of both normal and abnormal dendritic trees in the cerebellar molecular layer and it predicts the occurrence of certain features during development that are testable by direct observation. These considerations should, however, be regarded only as a starting point. To develop an understanding of the forces that shape dendrites in the cerebellum further experimentation will be necessary to validate or invalidate this hypothesis or to develop new ones to explain the development of these relationships.

ACKNOWLEDGMENTS

This research was supported by U.S. Public Health Service Grant NS-08997 and by National Institutes of Health Program Project Grant 5P01 NS10920–02.

REFERENCES

Altman, J. (1973): Experimental reorganization of the cerebellar cortex. IV. Parallel fiber reorientation following regeneration of the external germinal layer. *J. Comp. Neurol.*, 149: 181–192.

Altman, J., Anderson, W. J., and Wright, K. A. (1967): Selective destruction of precursors of microneurons of the cerebellar cortex with fractionated low dose x-ray. *Exp. Neurol.*, 17: 481–497.

Altman, J., Anderson, W. J., and Wright, K. A. (1968): Gross morphological consequences of irradiation of the cerebellar in infant rats with repeated doses of low dose x-ray. *Exp. Neurol.*, 21:69–91.

Altman, J., Anderson, W. J., and Wright, K. A. (1969): Reconstitution of the external granular layer of the cerebellar cortex in infant rats after low level x-irradiation. *Anat. Rec.*, 163: 453–472.

Christomanos, A., and Scholtz, W. (1933): Klinische Beobachtungen und Pathologische-anatomische Befundm Zentralnervensystem bei mit Thiophen vergifteten Hunden. *Z. Neurol.*, 144:1–20.

Forstronen, R. F. (1963): The origin and morphogenetic significance of the external granular layer of the cerebellum, as determined experimentally in chick embryo. *Acta. Neurol. Scand. (Suppl.)* 39, 4:314–316.

Hendleman, W., and Rouf, R. (1974): The development of the Purkinje cell in the mouse: A Golgi study. *Anat. Rec.*, 178:372.

Herndon, R. M. (1968): Thiophen-induced granule cell necrosis in the rat cerebellum: An electron microscopic study. *Exp. Brain Res.*, 6:49–68.

Herndon, R. M., Margolis, G., and Kilham, L. (1971a): The synaptic organization of the malformed cerebellum induced by perinatal infection with the feline panleukopenia virus (PLV). I. The Purkinje cell and its afferents. *J. Neuropathol. Exp. Neurol.*, 30:196–205.

Herndon, R. M., Margolis, G., and Kilham, L. (1971b): The synaptic organization of the malformed cerebellum induced by perinatal infection with the feline panleukopenia virus (PLV). II. The Purkinje cell and its afferents. *J. Neuropathol. Exp. Neurol.*, 30:557–569.

Hirano, A., and Dembitzer, H. M. (1973): Cerebellar alterations in the weaver mouse. *J. Cell Biol.*, 56:478–486.

Hirano, A., Dembitzer, H., and Jones, M. (1972): An electron microscopic study of cycasin-induced cerebellar alterations. *J. Neuropathol. Exp. Neurol.*, 31:113–125.

Hunter, D., Bomford, R. R., and Russell, D. S. (1940): Poisoning by methyl mercury compounds. *Quart. J. Med.*, 9:193–213.

Langman, J., Shimada, M., and Rodier, P. (1972): Floxuridine and its influence on postnatal cerebellar development. *Pediatr. Res.*, 6:758–764.

Levi-Montalcini, R., and Chen, R. S. (1971): Selective outgrowth of nerve fibers *in vitro* from embryonic ganglia of *Periplaneta americana*. *Arch. Ital. Biol.,* 109:307–337.

Llinás, R., Hillman, D. E., and Precht, W. (1973): Neuronal circuit reorganization in mammalian agranular cerebellar cortex. *J. Neurobiol.,* 4:69–94.

Luduena, M. A., and Wessells, N. K. (1973): Cell locomotion nerve elongation and microfilaments. *Dev. Biol.,* 30:427–440.

Nathanson, N., Cole, G. H., and Van der Loos, H. (1969): Heterotopic cerebellar granule cells following administration of cyclophosphamide to suckling rats. *Brain Res.,* 15:532–536.

Oster-Granite, M. L. (1974): *The pathogenesis of rat virus induced cerebellar hypoplasia in the Syrian hamster, Mesocricetus auratus. A light Golgi, and electron microscopic study.* Ph.D. thesis, Johns Hopkins University, Baltimore, Maryland.

Palay, S. L., and Chan-Palay, V. (1974): *Cerebellar Cortex: Cytology and Organization.* Springer-Verlag, New York.

Palkovits, M., Magyar, P., and Szentagothai, J. (1971*a*): Quantitative histological analysis of the cerebellar cortex in the cat. I. Number and arrangement in space of the Purkinje cells. *Brain Res.,* 32:1–13.

Palkovits, M., Magyar, P., and Szentagothai, J. (1971*b*): Quantitative histological analysis of the cerebellar cortex in the cat. II. Structural organization of the molecular layer. *Brain Res.,* 34:1–18.

Pitcock, J. A. (1962): An electron microscopic study of acute radiation injury of the rat brain. *Lab. Invest.,* 2:32–44.

Rakic, P. (1972): Extrinsic cytological determinants of basket and stellate cell dendritic patterns in the cerebellar molecular layer. *J. Comp. Neurol.,* 146:335–354.

Rakic, P. (1974): Intrinsic and extrinsic factors influencing the shape of neurons and their assembly into neuronal circuits. In: *Frontiers in Neurology and Neuroscience,* edited by P. Seeman and G. M. Brown, pp. 112–132. Univ. of Toronto Press, Toronto.

Rakic, P., and Sidman, R. L. (1973*a*): Sequence of abnormalities leading to granule cell deficit in cerebellar cortex of weaver mutant mice. *J. Comp. Neurol.,* 152:103–132.

Rakic, P., and Sidman, R. L. (1973*b*): Organization of cerebellar cortex secondary to deficit of granule cells in weaver mutant mice. *J. Comp. Neurol.,* 152:133–162.

Rakic, P., and Sidman, R. L. (1973*c*): Weaver mutant mouse cerebellum: Defective neuronal migration secondary to abnormality of Bergmann glia. *Proc. Natl. Acad. Sci. USA,* 70:240–244.

Ramon y Cajal, S. (1929): *Studies on Vertebrate Neurogenesis.* Thomas, Springfield, Illinois. (Translated by L. Guth, 1960.)

Rezai, T., and Yoon, C. H. (1972): Abnormal rate of granule cell migration in the cerebellum of the weaver mouse. *Dev. Biol.,* 29:17–26.

Shofer, R. J., Pappas, G. D., and Purpura, D. P. (1964): Radiation-induced changes in morphological and physiological properties of immature cerebellar cortex. In: *Response of the Nervous System to Ionizing Radiation,* edited by T. J. Haley and R. S. Snider, pp. 476–508. Little, Brown, Boston, Massachusetts.

Sidman, R. L. (1968): Development of interneuronal connections in the brains of mutant mice. In: *Physiological and Biochemical Aspects of Nervous Integration,* edited by F. D. Carlsson, pp. 163–193. Prentice-Hall, Englewood Cliffs, New Jersey.

Sotelo, C., and Changeux, J. P. (1974): Transsynaptic degeneration "en cascade" in the cerebellar cortex of staggerer mutant mouse. *Brain Res.,* 67:519–526.

Tokoumi, H., and Okajimo, T. (1961): Minamata disease. *World Neurol.,* 2:536–545.

Ule, G., and Rossner, J. A. (1960): Elektronenmikroskopische Studien zum akuten Kornerzellnekrose in Kleinhirn. *Verh. Dtsch. Ges. Pathol.,* 44:210–214.

Upners, T. (1939): Experimentelle Untersuchungen uber die lokale Einwirkung des Thiophen im Zentralnervensysten. *Z. Neurol.,* 166:623–645.

Vogel, F. S. (1960): Effects of high-dose gamma radiation on the brain and on individual neurons. In: *Response of the Nervous System to Ionizing Radiation,* edited by T. J. Haley and R. S. Snider, p. 249. Little, Brown, Boston, Massachusetts.

Weiss, P. (1934): *In vitro* experiments on the factors determining the course of the outgrowing nerve fiber. *J. Exp. Zool.,* 68:393–448.

Zedeck, M. S., Sternberg, S. S., McGowan, J., and Poynter, R. W. (1972): Methylazoxymethanol acetate: Induction of tumors and early effects on RNA synthesis. *Fed. Proc.,* 31:1485–1492.

Advances in Neurology, Vol. 12, edited by
G. W. Kreutzberg, Raven Press, New York
© 1975.

Retrograde Dendritic Degeneration[1]

Gunnar Grant

Department of Anatomy, Karolinska Institute, Stockholm 60, Sweden

In the adult central nervous system of vertebrates the initial retrograde neuronal reaction to peripheral nerve lesions is usually followed by restitution of the neuron. The primary reaction may, however, be followed by degeneration and rapid dissolution of the neuron. Such degeneration may also occur in intrinsic neurons of the central nervous system, i.e., in neurons whose axons do not project outside the central nervous system.

Although this type of neuronal degeneration may occur in the adult, it seems to be much more easily provoked in immature animals (Grant, 1970). This most probably results from the fact that the retrograde reaction after axonal lesion seems to be much more intense in immature than in adult neurons (Brodal, 1940; La Velle and La Velle, 1958). This circumstance has been exploited in a series of studies on retrograde neuronal degeneration in our laboratory (Grant, 1965, 1968; Grant and Aldskogius, 1967; Grant and Westman, 1968, 1969; Aldskogius, 1974*a,b;* see also Grant, 1970, 1974; Grant and Wallberg, 1974). Kittens of various ages were subjected to peripheral nerve transections or to lesions in the central nervous system. The ensuing degeneration was studied primarily at the light-microscopic level, but electron microscopy was also carried out. For the light-microscopic studies "suppressive" silver techniques, such as those of Nauta (1957) and Fink and Heimer (1967) were used. In central nerve nuclei deprived of their efferent projections in this way, we found degeneration not only of cell bodies but also of dendrites and axons.

The finding of degenerating dendrites (Grant, 1965; Grant and Westman, 1968), which is of special interest in this context, was rather unexpected. Such structures did not seem to have been shown before.

It was known that structural changes could occur in dendrites in connection with the retrograde cellular response to axonal lesion. Early studies

---

[1] The Chapter by Dr. Lynch and his colleagues in this volume, as well as discussions at the symposium, raises the question of whether the term retrograde dendritic degeneration, which has been used for describing dendritic degeneration in connection with retrograde neuronal degeneration after axonal lesions (Grant, 1970, p. 185), can be regarded as precise enough any longer. It appears that this term could possibly be misinterpreted as characterizing degeneration beginning peripherally in dendrites and proceeding in a cellipetal direction. It might therefore be better to use a more descriptive terminology, e.g., degeneration of dendrites, in connection with retrograde neuronal degeneration.

(Nissl, 1892; Nicholson, 1924) had shown that the nissl substance occurring in the proximal part of dendrites could be involved in the chromatolytic process. Likewise, the neurofibrils in the basal part of the cell processes had been reported to show changes in connection with the retrograde cellular response (Bethe, 1903; Marinesco, 1904). Cerf and Chacko (1958) seem to have been the first to devote their interest more specifically to the retrograde reaction of dendrites. They studied spinal motor neuron dendrites of frogs 8 to 11 days after ventral root transections. In association with chromatolytic changes in the parent cell bodies, they found, in the dendrites, a decrease in the affinity for silver in Protargol-stained sections and an increase in acid phosphatase activity.

Our demonstration of degenerating dendrites at the light-microscopic level was undoubtedly rendered possible by virtue of the superiority of the suppressive silver techniques over previously used methods for demonstrating neuronal degeneration. It was interesting to find that these methods, widely used for staining degenerating axons, were also capable of impregnating degenerating dendrites and cell bodies.

Typical examples of silver-impregnated degenerating neurons are seen in Figs. 1–3. Degenerating dendrites are especially well seen in Figs. 2 and 3. The degenerating dendrites generally have a rather characteristic appearance. They may look like beaded or fragmented strands radiating from impregnated cell bodies. Sometimes the fragmentation is not especially well pronounced, and the neuron may then look very much like a Golgi-impregnated neuron (cf. Fig. 3). In cases in which dendrites can be followed for longer distances, branching can be seen to take place. In some instances we have followed dendrites far enough to include branches of the third order. The diameter of the dendritic branches have then been found to be smaller distal to the branching points.

The fact that, for technical reasons, the thickness of the Nauta and Fink-Heimer sections has to be kept below 20 to 30 μm restricts the possibility of tracing individual dendrites over longer distances in single sections. If the topographic distribution of degenerating dendrites is to be studied, one would therefore have to rely upon reconstructions from serial sections.

The silver impregnation during retrograde degeneration of hypoglossal neurons was found to appear earlier in the cell bodies and their closest fiber ramifications than in the intramedullary root fiber axons at some distance from the nerve cells (Grant and Aldskogius, 1967). Therefore, it would not be surprising if there is a temporal development of the impregnation of dendrites in a cellulifugal direction. The observations made so far, however, do not permit any conclusions regarding this question.

In electron-microscopic studies on retrograde neuronal degeneration in the lateral cervical nucleus of kittens (Grant and Westman, 1968, 1969) degenerating dendrites were found (Figs. 4 and 5). They were characterized by an increased interior electron density very similar to that found during

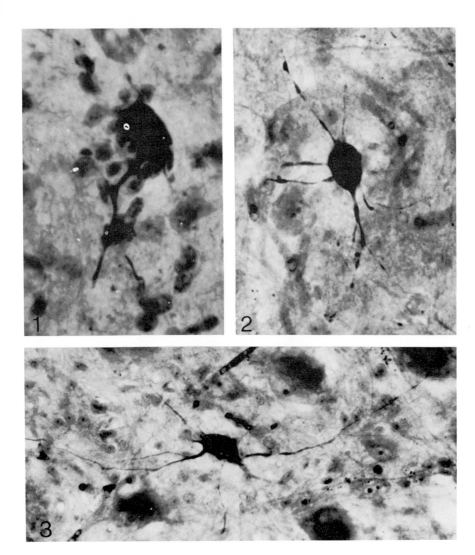

FIG. 1. Photomicrograph showing impregnated spinal motor neuron. Note the glial cells aggregated around the cell body. Sciatic nerve transection. Kitten operated at 1 day of age. Seven days postoperative survival. Nauta preparation. ×700. [From *Exp. Brain Res.,* 6 (1968), with permission.]

FIG. 2. Photomicrograph showing impregnated spinal motor neuron. Note the branching of the dendrite below. Ventral root transection. Kitten operated at 1 day. Seven days postoperative survival. Nauta preparation. ×350. [From *Exp. Brain Res.,* 6 (1968), with permission.]

FIG. 3. Photomicrograph showing impregnated spinal motor neuron. Note the branching of the dendrite at left. Ventral root transection. From the same case as Fig. 2. Nauta preparation. ×350. [From *Exp. Brain Res.,* 6 (1968), with permission.]

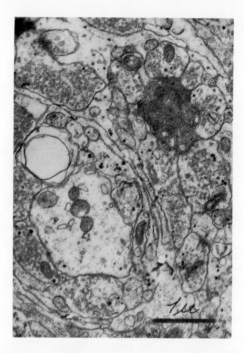

FIG. 4. Electron micrograph showing degenerating dendrite at upper right and normal dendrite at lower left from the lateral cervical nucleus. Note the enlarged fragmented mitochondria filling most of the degenerating dendrite and the apparently normal boutons surrounding it. Cervicothalamic tract lesion. Kitten operated at 3 days. Ten days postoperative survival. [From *Exp. Brain Res.,* 7 (1969), with permission.]

the orthograde type of fiber degeneration. These dendrites contained large mitochondria, which were sometimes fragmented. Occasionally they showed bundles of filaments and small dense granules. After short postoperative survival periods they were found to be contacted by apparently normal synaptic boutons. At later postoperative stages a larger part of the dendritic surface seemed to be covered with astroglial cell processes. Even in these instances, however, the boutons appeared to be normal. Degenerating dendrites of a similar type have also been found in the hypoglossal nucleus of kittens subjected to hypoglossal nerve transections (H. Aldskogius, *unpublished observations*).

The fact that degenerating dendrites may be demonstrated in association with retrograde neuronal degeneration in young animals is of interest, primarily perhaps for experimental neuroanatomy. At the light-microscopic level the retrograde neuronal reaction has long been used for "marking" cells of origin of various neuronal systems. This has been especially successful in young animals. It now seems that dendrites can also be marked. The possibility that this could be done also at the ultrastructural level is of special interest, the more so because it seems that normal-appearing boutons can under certain conditions retain their synaptic contacts with the de-

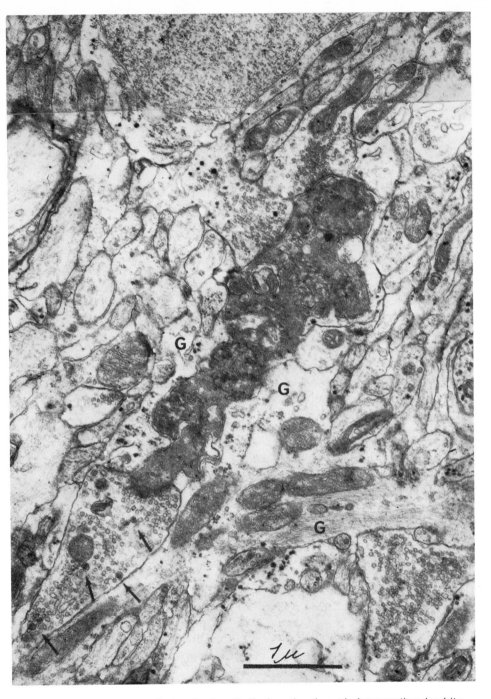

FIG. 5. Electron micrograph showing longitudinal section through degenerating dendrite from the lateral cervical nucleus. Note the fragmented mitochondria in the dendrite. Note also the three apparently normal boutons contacting it and the astroglial cell processes, G, surrounding it. Cervicothalamic tract lesion. Kitten operated at 3 days. Ten days postoperative survival. [From *Exp. Brain Res.,* 7 (1969), with permission.]

generating dendrites (see above). Therefore it might be possible to study synaptic connections of neurons marked by retrograde neuronal degeneration. For studies of synaptic connections in the central nervous system it would, however, be more fruitful if the retrograde degeneration could be combined with selective marking of various afferent systems in contact with the dendrites. This should be made possible by transection of afferents at a second operation.

The possible usefulness of retrograde dendritic degeneration as a tool in studies on neuronal connections would naturally be extended considerably if it could also be applied to adult animals. Several recent papers including observations on retrograde degenerative changes morphologically very similar to those found in immature animals and affecting both perikarya (Campos-Ortega, Hayhow, and Clüver, 1970; Torvik and Skjörten, 1971; Wong-Riley, 1972; Barron, Means, and Larsen, 1973) and dendrites (Campos-Ortega et al., 1970; Barron et al., 1973) indicate that this might well be the case. Campos-Ortega et al. (1970) investigated thalamocortical connections to the visual cortex in young adult monkeys. They found strongly argyrophilic cells with fragmented dendrites in Nauta- and Fink-Heimer-stained sections from the inferior and lateral pulvinar nuclei and from the lateral geniculate nucleus after cortical lesions. After the same type of lesions they also found, in electron micrographs from the lateral geniculate nucleus, electron-dense profiles with a characteristic postsynaptic location, which they considered as degenerating dendrites. Barron et al. (1973) made an ultrastructural study of the lateral thalamic nucleus of the rat after localized unilateral decorticotomy. They found "dark" degenerating neurons, including dark degenerating processes presumed to be dendrites. In addition, they described a type of "pale" neuron, which they also believed to represent lethally injured neurons.

One possible explanation for the fact that in these two studies in adult animals the lesions resulted in neuronal degeneration could be the reciprocal connections that exist between the thalamus and the cerebral cortex. The degeneration of the neurons may have been caused by a combination of retrograde and transneuronal effects (cf. Glees, Soler, and Bailey, 1951; see also Grant, 1970, 1975; Matthews, 1973).

It is possible that retrograde neuronal degeneration, including degeneration of dendrites, may be brought about more widely in adult animals if the factors influencing the retrograde cellular response to axonal lesion could be exploited to provoke a retrograde cellular response severe enough to result in a metabolic collapse in the neuron.

REFERENCES

Aldskogius, H. (1974a): Indirect and direct Wallerian degeneration in the intramedullary root fibres of the hypoglossal nerve. An electron microscopical study in the kitten. *Adv. Anat. Embryol. Cell Biol.,* 50:7–78.

Aldskogius, H. (1974b): Indirect Wallerian degeneration in intramedullary root fibres of the kitten hypoglossal nerve. Light and electron microscopical observations on silver impregnated sections. *Neurobiology,* 4:132–150.

Barron, K. D., Means, E. D., and Larsen, E. (1973): Ultrastructure of retrograde degeneration in thalamus of rat. I. Neuronal somata and dendrites. *J. Neuropathol. Exp. Neurol.,* 32: 218–244.

Bethe, A. T. J. (1903): *Allgemeine Anatomie und Physiologie des Nervensystems.* Thieme, Leipzig.

Brodal, A. (1940): Modification of Gudden method for study of cerebral localization. *Arch. Neurol.,* 43:46–58.

Campos-Ortega, J. A., Hayhow, W. R., and Clüver, P. F. De V. (1970): The descending projections from the cortical visual fields of Macaca mulatta with particular reference to the question of a cortico-lateral geniculate-pathway. *Brain Behav. Evol.,* 3:368–414.

Cerf, J. A., and Chacko, L. W. (1958): Retrograde reaction in motoneuron dendrites following ventral root section in the frog. *J. Comp. Neurol.,* 109:205–220.

Fink, R. P., and Heimer, L. (1967): Two methods for selective silver impregnation of degenerating axons and their synaptic endings in the central nervous system. *Brain Res.,* 4:369–374.

Glees, P., Soler, J., and Bailey, R. A. (1951): Retrograde axonal changes of the de-afferentated nucleus gracilis following mid-brain tractotomy. *J. Neurol. Neurosurg. Psychiat.* 14:281–286.

Grant, G. (1965): Degenerative changes in dendrites following axonal transection. *Experientia,* 21:722.

Grant, G. (1968): Silver impregnation of degenerating dendrites, cells and axons central to axonal transection II. A Nauta study on spinal motor neurones in kittens. *Exp. Brain Res.,* 6:284–293.

Grant, G. (1970): Neuronal changes central to the site of axon transection. A method for the identification of retrograde changes in perikarya, dendrites and axons by silver impregnation. In: *Contemporary Research Methods in Neuroanatomy,* edited by W. J. H. Nauta and S. O. E. Ebbesson, pp. 173–185. Springer-Verlag, Berlin.

Grant, G. (1975): Retrograde neuronal degeneration. In: *Golgi Centennial Symposium. Perspectives in Neurobiology,* edited by M. Santini, pp. 195–200. Raven Press, New York.

Grant, G., and Aldskogius, H. (1967): Silver impregnation of degenerating dendrites, cells and axons central to axonal transection. I. A. Nauta study on the hypoglossal nerve in kittens. *Exp. Brain Res.,* 3:150–162.

Grant, G., and Walberg, F. (1974): The light and electron microscopical appearance of anterograde and retrograde neuronal degeneration. In: *Dynamics of Degeneration and Growth in Neurons,* edited by K. Fuxe, L. Olson, and Y. Zotterman, pp. 5–18. Pergamon, Oxford.

Grant, G., and Westman, J. (1968): Degenerative changes in dendrites central to axonal transection. Electron microscopical observations. *Experientia,* 24:169–170.

Grant, G., and Westman, J. (1969): The lateral cervical nucleus in the cat IV. A light and electron microscopical study after midbrain lesions with demonstration of indirect Wallerian degeneration at the ultrastructural level. *Exp. Brain Res.,* 7:51–67.

La Velle, A., and La Velle, F. W. (1958): Neuronal swelling and chromatolysis influenced by the state of cell development. *Am. J. Anat.,* 102:219–241.

Marinesco, G. (1904): Recherches sur la structure de la partie fibrillaire des cellules nerveuses à l'état normal et pathologique. *Rev. Neurol.,* 12:405–428.

Matthews, M. A. (1973): Death of the central neuron: An electron microscopic study of thalamic retrograde degeneration following cortical ablation. *J. Neurocytol.,* 2:265–288.

Nauta, W. J. H. (1957): Silver impregnation of degenerating axons. In: *New Research Techniques of Neuroanatomy,* edited by W. F. Windle, pp. 17–26. Charles C Thomas, Springfield, Illinois.

Nicholson, F. M. (1924): Morphologic changes in nerve cells following injury to their axons. *Arch. Neurol. Psychiatry,* 11:680–697.

Nissl, F. (1892): Ueber die Veränderungen der Ganglienzellen am Facialiskern des Kaninchens nach Ausreissung der Nerven. *Allg. Z. Psychiatrie,* 48:197–198.

Torvik, A., and Skjörten, F. (1971): Electron microscopic observations on nerve cell regeneration and degeneration after axon lesions. I. Changes in the nerve cell cytoplasm. *Acta Neuropathol.,* 17:248–264.

Wong-Riley, M. T. T. (1972): Changes in the dorsal lateral geniculate nucleus of the squirrel monkey after unilateral ablation of the visual cortex. *J. Comp. Neurol.,* 146:519–548.

Advances in Neurology, Vol. 12, edited by
G. W. Kreutzberg, Raven Press, New York
© 1975.

Ultrastructural Changes in Dendrites of Central Neurons during Axon Reaction

Kevin D. Barron

*Veterans Administration Hospital, Research Service (Neuropathology), Albany, New York
and the Department of Neurology, Albany Medical College, Albany, New York 12208*

Previous reports from this laboratory on the ultrastructure of retrograde axonal reaction of rat thalamic neurons (Barron, Means, and Larsen, 1973; Barron, Means, Feng, and Harris, 1974) and feline lateral geniculate and red nucleus nerve cells (Barron and Doolin, 1968, 1969; Barron, Dentinger, Nelson, and Mincy, 1975), have emphasized description of the alterations that occur in neuronal perikarya and adjacent blood vessels (Barron et al., 1974). This chapter details the pathologic changes that take place in the dendrites of reacting nerve cells in the lateral nuclear complex of rat thalamus after corticectomy, and in red nucleus of cat after high cervical lateral funiculotomy.

MATERIALS AND METHODS

The surgical procedure, mode of fixation, and other technical details in rat studies are provided in earlier communications (Barron et al., 1973, 1974). Two control (unoperated) and 15 operated rats were used. Two or three animals were killed at each survival period (1, 2, 3, 4, 5, and 10 days). Adult cats underwent lateral funiculotomy at C-2 segmental level, and were killed 2 to 65 days postoperatively (Barron et al., 1975). Unoperated cats were sacrificed also. In both sets of animals "thick" sections were stained with toluidine blue prior to "thin" sectioning of blocks and "electron staining" in lead and uranyl salts and examination in a Joelco JEM-100B electron microscope. All operations were unilateral. The side unaffected by operation served as an additional control as alterations did not occur in the thalamus contralateral and in the red nucleus ipsilateral to operation.

RESULTS

Rat Thalamus

Normal Thalamus

The ultrastructure of rat thalamic neuropil was described recently by Spacek and Lieberman (1974) in their report on ventrobasal nuclei. The normal fine structure of the neuropil of the thalamic area reported on in this chapter did not differ significantly except that no bouton–bouton synapses were identified in our control material. Rare dendritic profiles contained round or flattened or dense-cored vesicles identical to those of axonic termini, but these processes made no identifiable synaptic connections. Tissue from unoperated animals and from the side contralateral to corticectomy was identical.

Normal dendrites have a relatively lucent hyaloplasm, occasional vacuoles (generally not more than 400 nm and rarely 600 nm in diameter), mitochondria with a width usually approximating 0.4 μm (but not more than 0.8 μm), more-or-less abundant microtubules (greater in number the closer to the cell body), scattered profiles of endoplasmic reticulum (ER) (predominantly smooth), occasional clusters of ribosomes, and some multivesicular bodies. The last may have an electron-dense matrix. Significantly, glycogen granules are absent. Synaptic formations have the expected postsynaptic membranous thickenings or specializations. Direct appositions of dendrites to plasma membranes of neuronal perikarya occur, but most often a thin astrocytic slip intervenes. The cytoplasm of the largest dendrites most closely resembles that of cell bodies. These electron-microscopic features of normal thalamic dendrites do not need illustration.

Atrophying Thalamus

Dispersion of dendritic ribosomal clusters into single units was observed in some dendrites 2 days after surgery (Barron et al., 1973). Its relation to development of the dark and lucent dendrites described below is uncertain but may precede each type of dendritic abnormality.

Electron-dense (dark) dendrites: Degenerating electron-dense neurons first were encountered in 3-day survivals (Barron et al., 1973) when they were relatively numerous and gave rise to primary dendrites of similar appearance (Fig. 1). Some degenerating neurons (Barron et al., 1973) and dendrites (e.g., Fig. 2) had a density of intermediate degree and contained recognizable multivesicular bodies (Fig. 1, inset), dispersed ribosomes (Fig. 1, inset; Figs. 2 and 3), profiles of smooth ER (Figs. 2 and 3) and abundant microtubules (Fig. 2). Although electron-dense dendritic profiles were most numerous 3 and 4 days postoperatively (as were dark neuronal perikarya), they persisted with increasing rarity to 10 days after surgery. Profiles of *intermediate* density may or may not have pre- and postsynaptic membranous thickenings (Figs. 2 and 3). Cytoplasmic organelles were unrecognizable, or virtually so, against the dense hyaloplasmic background (Fig. 4) or large dark mitochondria (up to 1 μm in diameter) with bizarre cristal arrangements were encountered (Fig. 5). On the average, the diameter of mitochondria associated with dense dendrites appeared greater than the normal. Attenuated processes associated with some dark dendrites sug-

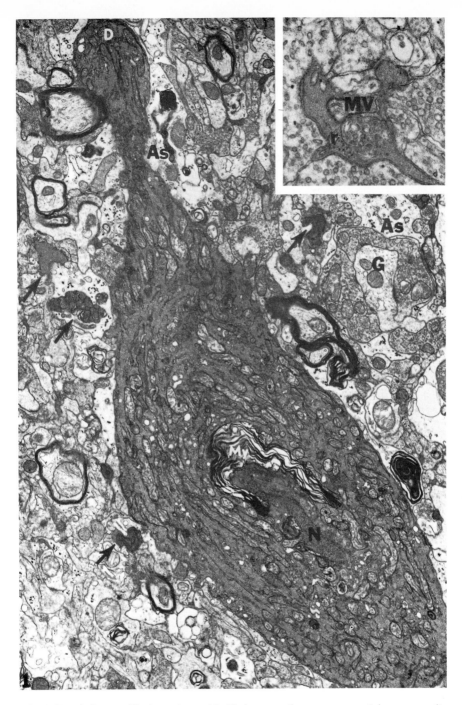

FIG. 1. Rat thalamus. Electron-dense (dark) degenerating neuron contains many mito-chondria, discernible against electron-opaque cytoplasmic matrix. Note granular remnant of nucleus, N, and myeloid body, My, closely apposed to nucleus. Arrows point to dark dendritic profiles in the neuropil. Pale astrocytic cytoplasm, As, with conspicuous glyco-gen particles is widely distributed; it partially clothes the neuron and sometimes contains dense bodies of myeloid or other configuration. A dendrite makes synaptic contacts within a glomerulus, G. Major dendrite, D, of degenerating neuron lies at top of figure. Three-day survival (×12,500.) (*Inset*) Dark dendrite contains multivesiculated body, MV, and ribosomal granules, r. Three-day animal. (×35,000.)

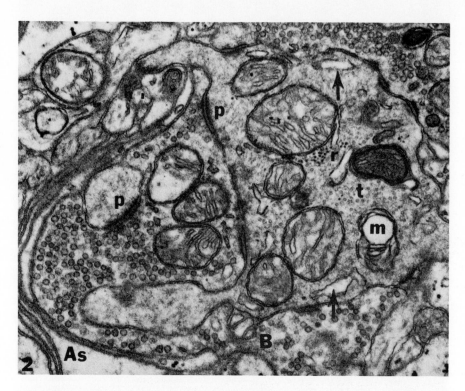

FIG. 2. Rat thalamus. A dark dendrite of intermediate electron density has discernible microtubules, t, ribosomes, r, smooth profiles of endoplasmic reticulum (two marked by *arrows*) and a vacuolated, degenerating mitochondrion, m. Above the latter a dense mitochondrion having a dark envelope is surrounded by a double membrane. Postsynaptic membrane densities, as at p, are still visible. Note slips of clear astrocytic cytoplasm at left of figure, As, and attenuated appearance of bouton, B, at lower margin of figure where synaptic vesicles appear dispersed. Three-day survival. (×40,000.)

gested shrinkage (e.g., Fig. 5). Electron-dense dendrites were enveloped early by microglia (Fig. 6) and astrocytes (Figs. 1 and 7); when engulfed they frequently lacked a limiting membrane in whole or in part (Figs. 6 and 7). Identifiable axonal termini and synaptic membranous specializations were not associated with engulfed dense dendritic detritus. Rarely did mitochondria exhibit clear zones in the matrix between cristae (Fig. 8). Identification of extremely dense profiles as dendrites was assisted by the persistence of identifiable, albeit distorted, mitochondria within them (Fig. 9). Dark dendrites appeared to be directly apposed to neuronal plasma membrane (Fig. 9) more often than did normal dendrites. Noteworthy was the presence of smudged electron-opaque material in some dendrites in which it was concentrated beneath the plasmalemma subjacent to boutons (Fig. 10). Vesicular and vacuolar profiles were frequent in such dendrites. A striking finding was the absence or indistinctness of postsynaptic mem-

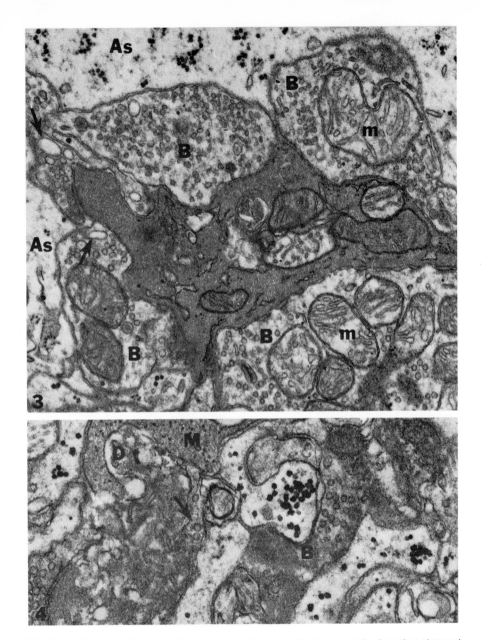

FIG. 3. Rat thalamus. Degenerating dendrite of greater electron opacity than that pictured in Fig. 2 has some electron-opaque mitochondria, visible profiles of smooth ER, and a few free ribosomes. The dendrite is surrounded by boutons, B, some of which have watery or enlarged mitochondria, m. Some synaptic vesicles appear enlarged (as at *arrows*). Synaptic membranous specializations are hardly apparent. Astrocytic cytoplasm at As. Three-day animal. (×35,000.)

FIG. 4. Rat thalamus. Dark dendritic profile, D, appears to merge with collapsed bouton, which retains recognizable synaptic vesicles (*arrow*). Part of another bouton, B, appears electron-dense. Astrocytic and microglial, M, cytoplasm occupies much of the field. Ten-day survival. (×50,000.)

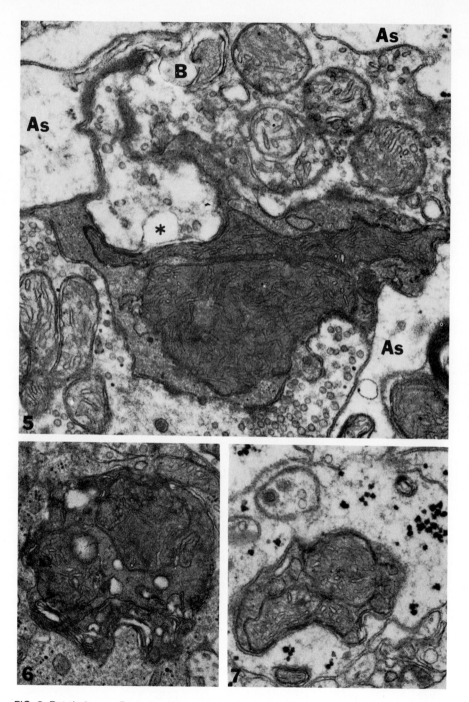

FIG. 5. Rat thalamus. Dark dendrite contains large dense mitochondria having disorganized cristal patterns. Postsynaptic membranous thickenings are lost. Attenuated dendritic profiles project into bouton, B, where synaptic vesicles are few and scattered. Extracellular space (*) may be an artifact or may represent retraction of bouton plasma membrane. Swollen astrocytic cytoplasm, As, is prominent. Three-days postoperatively. (×45,000.)

FIG. 6. Rat thalamus. Dark dendrite within a microgliacyte. Three-day survival. (×40,000.)

FIG. 7. Rat thalamus. Dark dendritic profile surrounded by an astrocyte. Four-days postoperatively. (×36,000.)

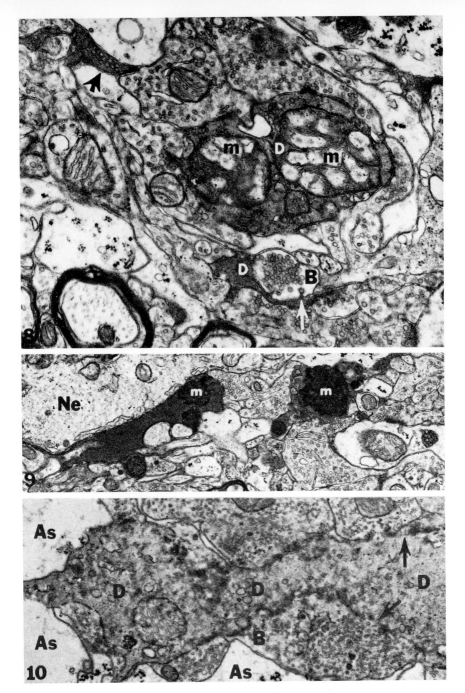

FIG. 8. Rat thalamus. In addition to dark dendritic profiles, D, one of which contains vacuolated mitochondria, m, note dark bouton at upper left (*black arrow*) and another bouton, B, containing centrally aggregated synaptic vesicles and a pinocytotic vesicle (*white arrow*). Matrix density of boutons in the field appears increased. Three-day survival. (×30,000.)

FIG. 9. Rat thalamus. Two dense dendritic profiles occur and one is apposed to neuronal, Ne, plasma membrane. Outlines of abnormal mitochondria, m, are visible. Three-days postoperative. (×17,000.)

FIG. 10. Rat thalamus. Dense degenerating dendrite, D, is surrounded by boutons and astrocytic cytoplasm, As. Plasma membranes are indistinct or broken (e.g., at *arrows*) in places. Irregular densities occur along length of dendritic margin. Cytoplasm of one bouton, B, appears to meld into that of degenerating dendrite. Three-day survival. (×17,-000.)

branous thickenings in very dark dendrites (Fig. 3–5, 8). To a lesser extent, associated presynaptic membranous specializations were lost or blurred. Coated vesicles with electron-opaque content occasionally projected from the altered dendrites into adjacent boutons (Fig. 8). A trilaminar appearance of dendritic plasma membranes and synaptic clefts (Kruger and Hamori, 1970) was not recognized. Electron-dense dendrites were particularly, but not solely, associated with synaptic glomeruli.

Electron-lucent (pale) dendrites: In the 3-day survivals, some dendrites, otherwise unremarkable, had an especially lucent cytoplasm and rather large vacuoles measuring up to 800 nm in width. Later these vacuoles sometimes had a maximum width of 1 μm and more. Four to 5 days after corticectomy pale neurons (Barron et al., 1973) were frequent and cell bodies contained glycogen granules. The latter occurred rarely in 3-day survivals and not at all in those examined earlier. Glycogen granules were unusually numerous in the degenerating nerve cell from a 4-day survival illustrated in Fig. 11, where they extended into a primary dendrite. Lucent dendritic profiles having a paucity of organelles and foci of cytoplasmic clearing occurred in neuropil at this stage, and some contained a few glycogen granules (Fig. 12). By 5 days large aggregates of glycogen granules appeared in some pale dendrites (Fig. 13) and persisted in 10-day animals. Not all lucent dendritic profiles exhibited glycogen, however (Figs. 14 and 15). Pale dendrites in general, and in particular those containing glycogen, were readily distinguished from astrocytes by, among other features, their well-preserved postsynaptic membranous thickenings (Figs. 12–14), although these were lost when investment by phagocytes (usually microglia but also astrocytes) was complete (Fig. 15). Presynaptic membrane thickenings persisted on pale dendrites but appeared thinner or less distinct than in the normal. Lucent dendritic profiles were most numerous 5 and 10 days after corticectomy. As with dense dendrites, pale dendritic profiles did not have a restricted location and were found within synaptic glomeruli. On only one occasion was a vacuolated membranous protrusion, possibly derived from a bouton, observed in a dendritic profile (Matthews, 1973).

By 10 days postsurgery the affected thalamus contained few normal-appearing dendrites.

Boutons: From the lack of firm evidence for occurrence of presynaptic dendrites[1] in normal tissue (see above), all boutons may be assumed to be axonic termini. The fate of terminal axons synapsing on degenerating central neurons has puzzled some investigators (see Discussion). This, plus the fact that they give rise (although rarely) to dense profiles, makes mention of axonic changes pertinent. Bouton alterations occurred sporadically in 3 to 10-day survivals and were concentrated about degenerating neuronal

---

[1] Only two bouton–bouton synapses were found and these, which appeared to be axoaxonic, occurred in atrophic thalamus at 10 days. No conclusions were drawn from this observation.

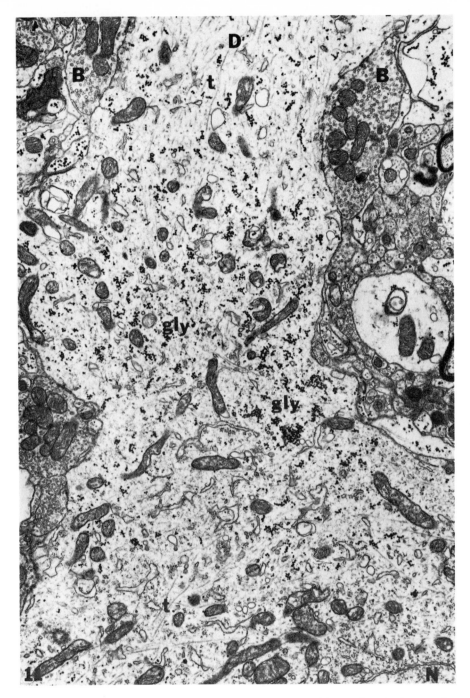

FIG. 11. Rat thalamus. Reacting neuron from 4-day survival has pale cytoplasm and a paucity of ER and other organelles but contains many glycogen granules, gly, and microtubules, t. Nucleus at N. Boutons, B, make synaptic contacts. Glycogen particles extend into major dendrite, D, at top of field. (×14,000.)

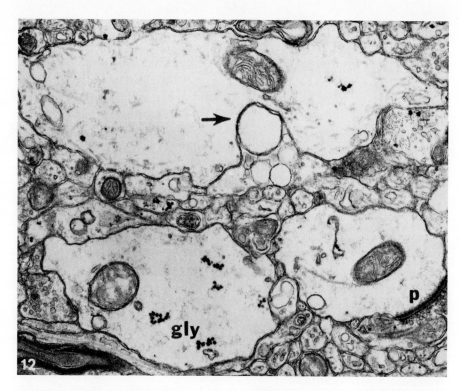

FIG. 12. Rat thalamus. The field contains three pale dendritic profiles. Postsynaptic membranous specialization is well maintained in profile at lower right, p. Note glycogen particles, gly, and protrusion (*arrow*) into uppermost dendrite of membranous profile containing vacuoles and vesicles. Four days. (×24,000.)

cytoplasm. A few boutons adjacent to dark dendrites seemed to have more than ordinarily irregular or attenuated profiles and a paucity of synaptic vesicles proximate to synaptic sites (Fig. 2) or a scarcity of vesicles where attenuated dendritic profiles projected into the bouton (Fig. 5). Loss of definition of presynaptic membranous specializations adjacent to degenerating dendrites has been mentioned. Occasional boutons exhibited enlarged mitochondria or enlarged vesicles (Fig. 3) (Cuenod, Sandri, and Akert, 1970) that could measure 200 nm in their widest dimension. Others displayed cytoplasmic opacification (Figs. 4 and 8) or appeared to meld into the degenerating dendritic profiles (Figs. 4 and 10). Electron-opaque boutons were distinguished from degenerating dendrites by, among other differences, a lack of the distorted mitochondria so characteristic of dark dendrites. More frequently than in the normal, vesicles appeared to aggregate centrally, and even to coalesce (Fig. 8). Only one bouton with apparent neurofilamentous hyperplasia was seen. Limiting membranes were sometimes broken (see, e.g., Fig. 10). In 10-day material, isolated boutons

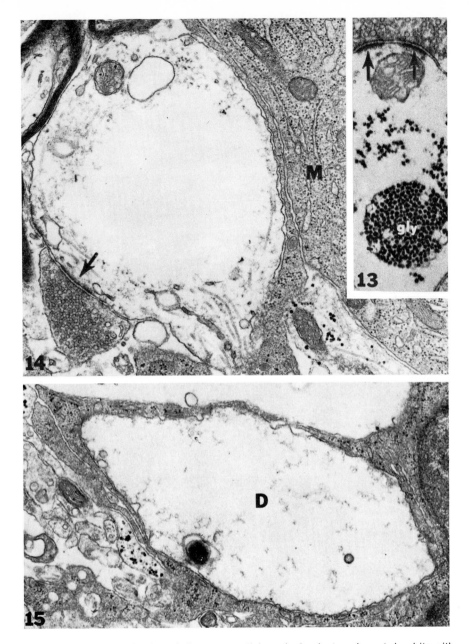

FIG. 13. Rat thalamus. Packet of glycogen particles, gly, in electron-lucent dendrite with normal-appearing synaptic contact at top of figure. Five days. (×30,000.)

FIG. 14. Rat thalamus. Pale dendrite with large focus of cytoplasmic clearing, microtubules and tubulovesicular profiles has normal-appearing synaptic complex (*arrow*). Microgliacyte at M. Ten days. (×25,250.)

FIG. 15. Rat thalamus. Watery dendrite, D, devoid of organelles and synaptic membranous thickenings is surrounded by microgliacyte. Ten days postoperative. (×25,000.)

lacking presynaptic membrane thickenings but packed with vesicles and having an intact plasma membrane sometimes were wholly engulfed within microglia or astrocytes. These phagocyte-enveloped boutons appeared to be related to cytoplasmic spaces that were entirely or partly membrane-bound, lacked vesicles, had the dimensions of boutons, and likewise were located within phagocytes. The foregoing notwithstanding, bouton altera-tions were less conspicuous, even in 10-day survivals, than were dendritic changes. "Stripping" of boutons from degenerating dendrites by glial processes (Blinzinger and Kreutzberg, 1968) was not observed.

Feline Red Nucleus

Only dendritic changes need be mentioned. These paralleled alterations in perikarya of the parent neurons as they underwent axon reaction (Barron et al., 1975). Neurofilamentous hyperplasia (Fig. 16) and proliferation of smooth ER (Fig. 17) were the outstanding changes 14 to 65 days after contralateral cervical rubrospinal tractotomy. Electron-dense dendrites were not identified, although they may occur rarely, as electron-dense opaque degenerating neurons were occasionally seen (Barron et al., 1975) as were dense neuronal fragments within phagocytes. Rubral dendrites showed neither exaggerated electron-lucency nor glycogen accumulation.

DISCUSSION

Rat Thalamus

Electron-Dense Dendrites

In the material studied in this laboratory dark dendrites were limited to degenerating rat thalamus. Dark profiles did not occur in any control tissue (Cohen and Pappas, 1969). Dark dendrites did not accompany the neuronal necrosis that occurs during retrograde atrophy of lateral geniculate body (Barron and Doolin, 1968) and red nucleus (Barron et al., 1975) of the cat, although we do not deny the possibility of their occasional occurrence in the latter situation. Degenerating electron-dense dendritic profiles have been identified by others during retrograde thalamic atrophy (Lund, 1969; Campos-Ortega, Hayhow, and De V. Cluver, 1970; Wong-Riley, 1972; Barron et al., 1973; Ralston and Chow, 1973) and were first described in degeneration of kitten lateral cervical nucleus (Grant and Westman, 1969). Although neuronal perikarya exhibiting various degrees of cytoplasmic darkening are frequent in lateral nucleus of rat thalamus at 3 to 4 days after operation, the number of dense dendritic profiles is even greater. Doubtless this discrepancy is explicable by reference to the ramification of the den-dritic tree, which forms many branches at a distance from degenerating

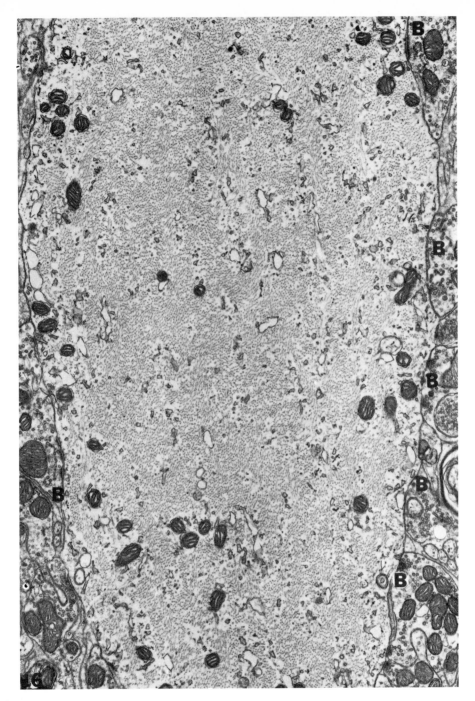

FIG. 16. Cat red nucleus. Major dendrite surrounded by boutons, B, is packed with neurofilaments. There are many smooth profiles of ER. Fourteen days after cervical rubrospinal tractotomy. (×20,000.)

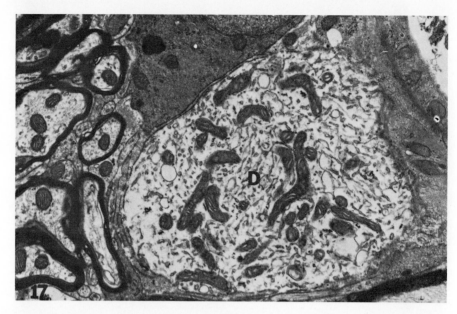

FIG. 17. Cat red nucleus. Dendrite, D, containing numerous smooth profiles of ER. Fourteen days after rubrospinal tractotomy. (×20,000.)

neurons (Grant and Westman, 1969). The data presented herein leave little doubt that electron-dense dendrites occur *pari passu* with and arise from parent cell bodies affected by a similar cytoplasmic alteration. Together with the other reports cited, our findings cast suspicion on Lund's (1969) statement that dense dendritic profiles appear in rat lateral geniculate nucleus at 3 days, whereas cell bodies become electron-opaque about 1 month after corticectomy. Possibly supportive of Lund's findings, however, is the report that dark dendrites may appear during transneuronal degeneration of pyriform cortex without similar change affecting main stem dendrites and parent cell somata (Pinching and Powell, 1971).

Development of electron-opaque dendrites in neuropil cannot be taken as an indication of a purely retrograde axonal reaction. Similar dendritic changes accompany transneuronal degeneration (Pinching and Powell, 1971), radiation injury (Kruger and Hamori, 1970), and hyperbaric oxygen exposure (Balentine, *this volume*). The appearance of subplasmalemmal osmiophilic substance in dark dendrites during retrograde atrophy (Fig. 10) seems to have a parallel in the dendritic alterations accompanying X-irradiation (Kruger and Hamori, 1970) and trans-synaptic degeneration (Wisniewski, Ghetti, and Horoupian, 1972).

The hope implicit in Grant's early observations (Grant and Westman, 1969; Grant, 1970) that dark dendrites might be useful in neuroanatomic research as a reliable index of a truly retrograde response to experimental lesions is not sustainable. Foregoing remarks notwithstanding the development of electron-opaque dendrites in rat lateral thalamic nucleus after corticectomy may well be a truly retrograde phenomenon. The rapidity of the degenerative reaction is unlike the delayed appearance and slow progress of transneuronal changes in adult animals of this species. Thus, Pinching and Powell (1971), studying transneuronal degeneration of the olfactory system, first observed dense degeneration of dendrites 200 days after destruction of the nasal olfactory mucosa. Furthermore, dark dendritic degeneration in lateral cervical nucleus of kittens is a purely retrograde reaction (Grant and Westman, 1969).

Some investigators have been unimpressed by any change in boutons and synaptic membranous specializations associated with electron-dense dendritic profiles of degenerating thalamus (Campos-Ortega et al., 1970; Wong-Riley, 1972; Ralston and Chow, 1973). Others have seen bouton and membranous alterations similar to those reported in this chapter. However, in retrograde axonal degeneration uncomplicated by deafferentation, alterations in presynaptic structures are minimal or absent (Grant, 1970; Raisman, 1973). In any case, the observations reported here clearly show that synaptic membrane thickenings are generally lost with dense dendritic degeneration, but that they may be retained at an intermediate, earlier stage of cytoplasmic darkening. Increased cytoplasmic density in dendrites appears to *precede* loss of associated synaptic structures, and it is difficult to attach to this loss a role in the genesis of neuronal dissolution (Pinching and Powell, 1971). Pale dendrites also lose postsynaptic membrane thickenings, and their associated presynaptic membranes alter, but less obviously and over a slower time course.

We have not observed a change in the unit membrane structure of dark dendrites (Kruger and Hamori, 1970); Wisniewski et al., 1972), nor were associated synaptic clefts and presynaptic structures distinguishable when these elements had been engulfed or phagocytosed by glial cells. This negative finding contrasts with other reports on anterograde degeneration of terminals in cat striate cortex in which pre- and postsynaptic elements were each distinguishable in phagocytic glia (Ghetti and Wisniewski, 1972; Wisniewski et al., 1972). All investigators have noted mitochondrial aberrations in dark dendrites that aid in their differentiation from other tissue elements.

The cause of cytoplasmic darkening is unknown. It cannot be caused solely by shrinkage. In companion light-microscopic studies of thalamic degeneration accompanying unilateral corticectomy in rat, Thionine stains showed marked chromatolysis in neuronal perikarya at 3 days postoperatively. The areas of chromatolytic perikarya equaled those of the contralateral thalamus, however, despite an approximately 25% atrophy of the nuclei of the degenerating neurons (Barron, *unpublished observations*).

Following axon section, dendrites of degenerating neurons of young kittens may be silver-impregnable by the Nauta method (Grant, 1965; Grant and Aldskogius, 1967; Grant and Westman, 1969). Whether the silver-impregnated dendrites correspond to the electron-opaque dendrites seen in these animals is unknown (Grant, 1970). Silver impregnability of electron-dense dendrites might complicate interpretation of neuroanatomic studies using Nauta-type methods.

Electron-Lucent Dendrites

In 1968 Barron and Doolin, reporting on fine structural features of retro-grade atrophy of cat lateral geniculate body, described "grossly disordered" pale dendrites the "contents [of which] consisted entirely of smooth, electron-lucent vesicles and vacuoles." Many such structures occurred in 42- and 70-day postoperative survivals. Similar "watery" dendrites appear in rat thalamus after corticectomy (Barron et al., 1973). Others have ob-served degenerating pale dendrites during retrograde atrophy of thalamus (Horoupian Ghetti, and Wisniewski, 1973; Matthews, 1973; Ralston and Chow, 1973). Although Wong-Riley (1972) found only electron-dense degenerating dendrites in lateral geniculate of squirrel monkey after cortical ablation, Horoupian et al. (1973) illustrated vacuolated lucent degenerating dendrites in the same nucleus of rhesus monkey after ablation of the occipi-tal lobe. Exaggerated electron-lucency of dendrites containing vacuolar profiles is reported also for transneuronal degeneration (Pinching and Powell, 1971; Ghetti, Horoupian, and Wisniewski, 1972). As there were two distinct populations of degenerating nerve cells in our material, one electron-dense and one electron-lucent, it is tempting to speculate that their projection fields and/or sources of input are different. Could electron-lucent cells normally receive a cortical input important to their viability, and might their degeneration after corticectomy indicate participation of a trans-neuronal effect in the ultimate dissolution of the cell? This speculation seems unlikely if only from what has been said above concerning the slow onset and progression of transneuronal degeneration in rat. Furthermore, dark degeneration may mark trans-synaptic atrophy (Pinching and Powell, 1971). It may be noteworthy, however, that lucent dendritic degeneration has not been reported with retrograde axonal degeneration of central (Lieberman, 1971) neurons uncomplicated by deafferentation (Grant and Westman, 1969; Raisman, 1973).

Accumulations of glycogen were confined to lucent dendrites. Their significance is unknown but may reflect a change in glycogen metabolism consequent to the profound changes in enzymatic activities that may ac-company axon reaction (Barron and Doolin, 1969). Glycogen accumulation occurs in central and peripheral neurons during axon reaction (Barron et al., 1973) and in swollen dendrites in cobalt-induced necrosis of rat cerebral cortex (Fischer and Blinzinger, 1968).

Cat Red Nucleus

The alterations in rubral dendrites that accompany axon reaction resemble those of rat thalamus only in that they mirror concurrent abnormalities in the parent somata (Barron et al., 1975). Whether neurofilamentous hyperplasia reflects slowed intradendritic transport (Kreutzberg, Schubert, Toth, and Rieske, 1973) is unknown, but it would be an interesting question to investigate. The proliferation of smooth ER in perikarya and dendrites of reacting rubral neurons resembles the accumulation of tubulovesicular profiles described in dendrites of rhesus lateral geniculate nucleus during transneuronal degeneration (Ghetti et al., 1972). Furthermore, neurofilamentous hyperplasia may constitute a major abnormality in neurons undergoing trans-synaptic degeneration (reviewed in Barron et al., 1975).

General Remarks

The dendritic alterations described do not seem to have significance in and of themselves. They reflect the severity and necrotizing nature of axon reaction in central neurons (Barron et al., 1973). The vulnerability of dendrites of vertebrate central and peripheral neurons to axotomy stands in sharp contrast to the morphologic stability of dendrites of axotomized insect nerve cells (Tweedle, Pitman, and Cohen, 1973).

In closing, the author, a morphologist, wishes to voice dismay that so many of the ultrastructural features of axon reaction bear similarity to those of transneuronal degeneration, even when the high resolving power of an electron microscope is brought to bear on the examination of two apparently disparate phenomena!

SUMMARY

Retrograde atrophy of rat thalamus is marked by the appearance of profound alterations in dendrites. Concurrently, similar changes occur in parent cell somata. Electron-dense and abnormally electron-lucent dendritic profiles appear and are removed over different time courses. The morphologic features of the abnormal dendrites are detailed.

Electron-dense and electron-lucent dendritic profiles are not observed in cat red nucleus after rubrospinal tractotomy. Rather, neurofilamentous hyperplasia and proliferation of smooth endoplasmic reticulum appear in affected dendrites and are identical to changes observable at the same time in the reacting parent nerve cells.

The literature is reviewed and discussion is developed on the similarities of perikaryal and dendritic changes that occur in axon reaction and transneuronal degeneration.

ACKNOWLEDGMENTS

Dr. Eugene D. Means collaborated in the collection of this material. This work was done under Project MRIS 0822-01, Veterans Administration Hospital, Albany, New York 12208 and was supported by the National Institute of Health Grants NS-08735 and NS-05038.

REFERENCES

Barron, K. D., and Doolin, P. F. (1968): Ultrastructural observations on retrograde atrophy of lateral geniculate body. II. The environs of the neuronal soma. *J. Neuropathol. Exp. Neurol.,* 27:401–420.

Barron, K. D., and Doolin, P. F. (1969): Neuronal responses to axon injury. In: *Motor Neuron Diseases,* edited by F. H. Norris and L. Kurland, pp. 301–318. Grune & Stratton, New York.

Barron, K. D., Means, E. D., and Larsen, E. (1973): Ultrastructure of retrograde degeneration in thalamus of rat. 1. Neuronal somata and dendrites. *J. Neuropathol. Exp. Neurol.,* 32: 218–244.

Barron, K. D., Means, E. D., Feng, T., and Harris, H. (1974): Ultrastructure of retrograde degeneration in thalamus of rat. 2. Changes in vascular elements and transvascular migration of leukocytes. *Exp. Mol. Pathol.,* 20:344–362.

Barron, K. D., Dentinger, M. P., Nelson, L. R., and Mincy, J. E. (1975): Ultrastructure of axonal reaction in red nucleus of cat. *J. Neuropathol. Exp. Neurol. (In press.)*

Blinzinger, K., and Kreutzberg, G. (1968): Displacement of synaptic terminals from regenerating motoneurons by microglial cells. *Z. Zellforsch. Mikrosk. Anat.,* 85:145–157.

Campos-Ortega, J. A., Hayhow, W. R., and De V. Cluver, P. F. (1970): The descending projections from the cortical visual fields of *Macaca mulatta* with particular reference to the question of a cortico-lateral geniculate pathway. *Brain Behav. Evol.,* 3:368–414.

Cohen, E. B., and Pappas, G. D. (1969): Dark profiles in the apparently normal central nervous system: A problem in the electron microscopic identification of an early anterograde axon degeneration. *J. Comp. Neurol.,* 136:375–396.

Cuenod, M., Sandri, C., and Akert, K. (1970): Enlarged synaptic vesicles as an early sign of secondary degeneration in the optic nerve terminals of the pigeon. *J. Cell Sci.,* 6:605–613.

Fischer, J., and Blinzinger, K. (1968): Vorkommen von glykogen in geschwollenen dendriten bei experimenteller kobaltnekrose des rattengehirns. *Virchows Arch. (Zellpathol.,)* 1:201–210.

Ghetti, B., Horoupian, D. S., and Wisniewski, H. M. (1972): Transsynaptic response of the lateral geniculate nucleus and the pattern of degeneration of the nerve terminals in the Rhesus monkey after eye enucleation. *Brain Res.,* 45:31–48.

Ghetti, B., and Wisniewski, H. M. (1972): On degeneration of terminals in the cat striate cortex. *Brain Res.,* 44:630–635.

Grant, G. (1965): Degenerative changes in dendrites following axonal transection. *Experientia,* 21:1–4.

Grant, G., and Aldskogius, H. (1967): Silver impregnation of degenerating dendrites, cells and axons central to axonal transection. I. A Nauta study on the hypoglossal nerve in kittens. *Exp. Brain Res.,* 3:150–162.

Grant, G., and Westman, J. (1969): The lateral cervical nucleus in the cat. IV. A light and electron microscopic study after midbrain lesions with demonstration of indirect Wallerian degeneration at the ultrastructural level. *Exp. Brain Res.,* 7:51–67.

Grant, G. (1970): Neuronal changes central to the site of axon transection. A method for the identification of retrograde changes in perikarya, dendrites and axons by silver impregnation. In: *Contemporary Research Methods in Neuroanatomy,* edited by W. J. H. Nauta and S. O. E. Ebbesson, pp. 173–183. Springer-Verlag, New York.

Horoupian, D., Ghetti, B., and Wisniewski, H. (1973): Retrograde transneuronal degeneration of optic fibers and their terminals in lateral geniculate nucleus of rhesus monkey. *Brain Res.,* 49:257–275.

Kreutzberg, G. W., Schubert, P., Toth, L., and Rieske, E. (1973): Intradendritic transport to postsynaptic sites. *Brain Res., 62*:399–404.

Kruger, L., and Hamori, J. (1970): An electron microscopic study of dendritic degeneration in the cerebral cortex resulting from laminar lesions. *Exp. Brain Res., 10*:1–16.

Lieberman, A. R. (1971): The axon reaction: A review of the principal features of perikaryal responses to axon injury. *Int. Rev. Neurobiol., 14*:49–124.

Lund, R. D. (1969): Fine structural changes within the dorsal lateral geniculate body of the rat following lesions of the visual cortex. *Anat. Rec., 163*:220 (Abstr.).

Matthews, M. A. (1973): Death of the central neuron: An electron microscopic study of thalamic retrograde degeneration following cortical ablation. *J. Neurocytol., 2*:265–288.

Pinching, A. J., and Powell, T. P. S. (1971): Ultrastructural features of transneuronal cell degeneration in the olfactory system. *J. Cell Sci., 8*:253–287.

Raisman, G. (1973): An ultrastructural study of the effects of hypophysectomy on the supraoptic nucleus of the rat. *J. Comp. Neurol., 147*:181–208.

Ralston, H. J., and Chow, K. L. (1973): Synaptic reorganization in the degenerating lateral geniculate nucleus of the rabbit. *J. Comp. Neurol., 147*:321–350.

Spacek, J., and Lieberman, A. R. (1974): Ultrastructure and three-dimensional organization of synaptic glomeruli in rat somatosensory thalamus. *J. Anat., 117*:487–516.

Tweedle, C. D., Pitman, R. M., and Cohen, M. J. (1973): Dendritic stability of insect central neurons subjected to axotomy and de-afferentation. *Brain Res., 60*:471–476.

Wisniewski, H. M., Ghetti, B., and Horoupian, D. S. (1972): The fate of synaptic membranes of degenerating optic nerve terminals, and their role in the mechanism of trans-synaptic changes. *J. Neurocytol., 1*:297–310.

Wong-Riley, M. T. T. (1972): Changes in the dorsal lateral geniculate nucleus of the squirrel monkey after unilateral ablation of the visual cortex. *J. Comp. Neurol., 146*:519–548.

Advances in Neurology, Vol. 12, edited by
G. W. Kreutzberg, Raven Press, New York
© 1975.

Acute and Long-Term Transneuronal Response of Dendrites of Lateral Geniculate Neurons Following Transection of the Primary Visual Afferent Pathway

Bernardino Ghetti, Dikran S. Horoupian, and
Henryk M. Wiśniewski

*Department of Pathology (Neuropathology), Albert Einstein College of Medicine, Bronx,
New York 10461*

Since the early studies on transneuronal degeneration and atrophy (Minkowski, 1920) in the central nervous system (CNS), the attention of the investigators has been devoted to the perikaryonal alterations and to the estimate of the numerical loss of nerve cells (see review by Cowan, 1970). Only in recent years has it become apparent that the injury of deafferentation is shared by both the perikaryon and dendrites. Some of the most interesting data concerning alterations of the dendritic tree have become available since the Golgi method has been more systematically used to study neuronal populations deprived of their afferent input. Therefore, in the newborn animal, within different areas of the CNS subjected to deafferentation, it has been possible to visualize a decrease in number of dendritic spines (Globus and Scheibel, 1967) as well as alterations in the orientation of dendrites (Smith, 1974).

However, morphologic data concerning the fine structural changes of dendritic processes of neurons deprived of their afferent input are still fragmentary and by and large come from short-term observations. The majority of the investigations in different regions of the central nervous system, following transection of their primary or secondary afferent pathway, were concerned with the ultraarchitecture of a given nucleus as well as with the pattern of anterograde degeneration of the axon terminals. Only in a few cases was the observation of pathologic changes extended beyond the axon terminal undergoing Wallerian degeneration (Walberg, 1963; McMahan, 1967; Westman, 1969; Gentschev and Sotelo, 1973).

Most of the ultrastructural data on long-term deafferentation come from immature animals. Some of these studies have given new insight on the alternative routes of development and organization of the neuropil in areas deafferentated at different stages of maturation (Lund and Lund, 1971), whereas other studies have shown some of the pathologic alterations of the neuron and its processes (Pinching and Powell, 1971; Berger, 1973).

The purpose of this investigation is to describe the dendritic changes in the adult rhesus monkey lateral geniculate nucleus (LGN) soon after and at the late-stage postenucleation of the eye. Attention will also be paid to the mechanism of removal of the presynaptic axon terminals of the optic nerve and to the extensive atrophy of the neuropil in the chronic animals.

MATERIALS AND METHODS

Anterograde transneuronal degeneration was studied in eight adult rhesus monkeys. One served as a control; five had bilateral simultaneous enucleation; one had bilateral enucleation at different time intervals (10 and 12 days before perfusion); and in one, only the left eye was removed. The animals with bilateral simultaneous enucleation were allowed to survive for 4, 7, 14, 36, and 170 days. The animal with only one eye removed was sacrificed after 7 days.

Following heparinization and combined Sarnylan® and Nembutal® anesthesia, the animals were perfused through the heart with 4% paraformaldehyde at room temperature, followed by 5% glutaraldehyde in phosphate buffer at pH 7.3. The perfusion was carried out for 15 min under a controlled pressure of 120 mm Hg. Immediately following each perfusion, the LGN was sectioned coronally into 1-mm-thick slices. These were then postfixed in Dalton's chrome osmium, dehydrated, and embedded in Epon 812.

One-μm-thick sections were taken from the rostral and caudal portions of the nucleus, as well as from its middle third (where the laminas are distinct), and were stained with toluidine blue. From the LGN blocks, representative pieces of each layer were cut with a razor blade and re-embedded in Epon. Thin sections were taken and stained with uranyl acetate and lead citrate. Electron microscopy was carried out on a Siemans Elmi-skop IA.

RESULTS

The Neuropil in the Normal LGN

Before presenting our data, we would like to define the criteria we used to identify the profiles of LGN. The classification of the elements of the neuropil was made on the basis of studies published by the following investigators: Colonnier and Guillery (1964), Glees, Meller, and Eschner (1966), Campos-Ortega, Glees, and Neuhoff (1968), Guillery and Colonnier (1970), Kanagasuntheram, Krishnamurti, Ahmed, Wong, and Chan (1971), Le Vay (1971), Ghetti, Horoupian, and Wiśniewski (1972), Wiśniewski, Ghetti, and Horoupian (1972), Wong-Riley (1972 a,b,c), Horoupian, Ghetti, and Wiśniewski (1973), Kanagasuntheram, Krishnamurti, and Wong (1973), Pasik, Pasik, Hámori, and Szentágothai (1973).

In the LGN neuropil the following profiles were recognized: RLP and RSD axon terminals, F processes, and dendrites.

RLP Axon Terminals

The optic nerve terminals (ONT) have been called RLP axons [round vesicles (R), large synaptic knobs (L), pale mitochondria (P)]. They are 5 to 7 μm in diameter, occasionally larger, and contain loosely packed round vesicles and pale mitochondria. In addition, these axon terminals may show profiles of smooth endoplasmic reticulum and neurofilaments. The ONT are presynaptic to dendrites of principal (P) cells and to F processes, less frequently to the perikaryon of P cells. The ONT disappear almost completely from the neuropil 14 days after eye enucleation (Ghetti et al., 1972).

RSD Axon Terminals

They are so-called because they have round vesicles (R); the terminals are small (S) (1 to 2 μm in diameter), and the mitochondria, when present, are dark (D) with closely spaced cristae. They are presynaptic to dendrites and to F processes. Despite the fact that endings of this group could well belong to more than a single population, some of them have been proved to be axons of cortical origin in squirrel monkey (Wong-Riley, 1972c). Direct and conclusive experimental ultrastructural data on the origin of such axons in *Macaca mulatta* have not been published. Campos-Ortega, Hayhow, and de V. Cluver (1970) did not find any ultrastructural evidence of a cortico-geniculate projection following occipital lobectomy in *Macaca mulatta,* whereas in the study by Horoupian et al. (1973), dark degenerating axon terminals were occasionally seen 5 and 14 days following occipital lobectomy. Morphologic results demonstrating the cortical origin of the RSD axon endings have been obtained by Hámori (*personal communication*). Furthermore, according to Pasik et al. (1973), and in our own experience (*unpublished observations*), the RSD disappeared following removal of occipital cortex. These profiles were recognizable at all times in this investigation.

F Processes

They measure 1 to 4 μm in diameter and contain a proportion of flattened vesicles. In our material the latter were very few. The F processes are seen in postsynaptic position to RLP and RSD axon terminals and presynaptic to dendrites, to the perikaryon of principal cells and interneurons, and to other F processes. In our study it was possible to confirm the distinction into two types of F processes as reported by Le Vay (1971). In the first type, the profile contains synaptic vesicles distributed evenly, and occasional mitochondria. In the second type, the vesicles are seen only in one part of the profile close to a synaptic contact, whereas the rest of the profile is occupied by microtubules, mitochondria, and ribosomes. The latter type of process has characteristics of presynaptic dendrites. There is evidence (Le Vay, 1971; Pasik et al., 1973) that the F profiles are processes of the Golgi type II interneurons. In support of the view of their interneuronal origin is the fact that they remain in postsynaptic position to RLP axons for many months after occipital lobectomy, i.e., a long time after disappearance of principal neurons (Pasik et al., 1973; Horoupian, Ghetti, and Wiśniewski, *unpublished observations*). The F processes were recognizable at all times in the experimental study reported here.

Dendrites

The primary dendrites of P cells are 2 to 7 μm in diameter and contain numerous cytoplasmic organelles. The mitochondria are large and similar to those observed in the perikaryon. The secondary dendrites branch off the primary dendrites. They are smaller in caliber and less rich in cytoplasmic organelles. Dendrites of P cells are postsynaptic to RLP and RSD axon terminals as well as to F processes. The dendrites of interneurons are narrow and contain small mitochondria and abundant cytoplasmic organelles. They are postsynaptic to any other axonal terminal and to F processes. A clear distinction between dendrites of P cells and of interneurons was not always possible in this study. Although the mitochondria of P neurons are larger than those of interneurons, there are numerous ambiguous profiles that cannot be identified with certainty.

Response of LGN Neuropil to Deafferentation

The first pathologic changes in the dendrites of deafferentated LGN were observed on the seventh and tenth postoperative day when the terminals of the transected optic nerve showed advanced filamentous proliferation (Figs. 1 and 2) and the beginning of dark transformation. During this initial stage, dendrites were seen deformed by glial processes and on occasion they showed widening of the postsynaptic density. However, most characteristic were the dendritic profiles with watery appearance and those containing tubulovesicular structures. Deformation of dendrites probably took place as a consequence of the fact that the ONT on the seventh and tenth day postenucleation had undergone a conspicuous filamentous hypertrophy (Fig. 1) and many had reached up to 15 μm in diameter, i.e., two times their normal width; because ONT were not dissociated at the synaptic junction, as response to this degenerative change of the axons of retinal origin, the glial processes invested both axon and the contacting postsynaptic dendrite often causing the latter to have an irregular outline (Fig. 2). Such alterations ap-

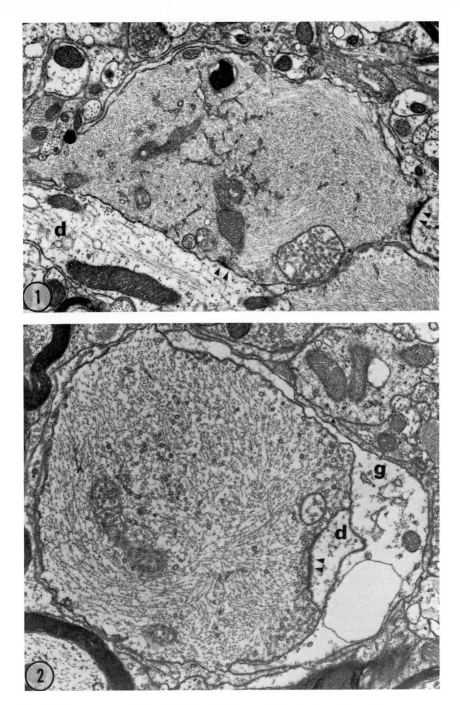

FIG. 1. Optic nerve terminal within the first layer of LGN displays filamentous degeneration, 7 days after enucleation. Two synaptic contacts (*arrow heads*) are recognizable.
The dendrite, d, of the principal cell, seen on the left, is normal. (×13,500.)
FIG. 2. Optic nerve terminal of the sixth layer, displaying filamentous degeneration, 10
days after enucleation. A synaptic contact (*arrow heads*) with an unidentifiable dendrite,
d, is recognizable. The glial process, g, invests both presynaptic and postsynaptic profiles.
Note the irregular outline of the dendrite, d. (×14,800.)

peared first where the ONT were forming sporadic contacts with dendrites. However, on the 10th day, all the elements within the synaptic island also, i.e., dendrites of P neurons, F processes, and retinal axon terminals appeared deformed and often invested by the glial profiles. At the same postoperative interval, many medium-sized dendrites in postsynaptic contacts with darkened ONT showed a discrete widening of the postsynaptic density. As mentioned above, many dendrites which in a given plane of section appeared in synaptic relation either with ONT or with RSD axons or F processes had an electron-lucent watery appearance. These round, swollen profiles contained structureless floccular material, multivesicular bodies, few or no mitochondria, and no microtubules. Glycogen-like particles occasionally were observed within the boundaries of the dendritic profile. Sometimes processes interpreted as dendritic appendages of principal neurons contained tubulo-saccular and vesicular structures. On occasion, the same profiles showed a definite increase in neurofilaments. Dendrites affected with these changes were not very numerous at this stage. However, in the animal that had bilateral enucleation, they were found more often. Among the other profiles of the neuropil, RSD axons and F processes did not show significant changes.

Between 10 and 12 days following eye enucleation (Figs. 3–5 and 7–10), the dendritic changes were more widespread, advanced, and showed a greater spectrum of pathology. At this time interval, there were dendrites that appeared to take an active part in the final process of removal of the electron-dense debris of fragmented axon terminals of retinal origin. There were also many dendrites still showing persistence of the synaptic specialization, attached together with remnants of degenerating ONT. These fragments and the synaptic membranes were invaginated within the boundaries of the dendrites and frequently appeared deeply intussuscepted into the latter profile (Figs. 3 and 5). Appearances suggesting the total engulfment of the electron-dense fragment and the synaptic specialization by the dendrite were also observed. In situations in which F processes showed persistence of synaptic specialization attached together with remnants of ONT, the latter was never seen invaginated within the boundaries of the vesicle-containing profiles. Neither dissociation of the synaptic specialization between ONT and any other profile nor "free" postsynaptic thickening lying opposite myelin or glial processes were observed. The pre- and postsynaptic membranes always appeared to be in close apposition to each other. Therefore, during the process of removal of the debris of the ONT, pictures were seen where a portion of postsynaptic dendritic cytoplasm or F process was pinched off and engulfed together with synaptic membranes and the electron-dense remnant of the degenerated axon (see Fig. 5). At this stage, the glial processes previously seen encircling the light filamentous ONT and dendrites had increased in number and size (Fig. 4). When large dendrites in synaptic contact with altered ONT were seen invested by glial processes,

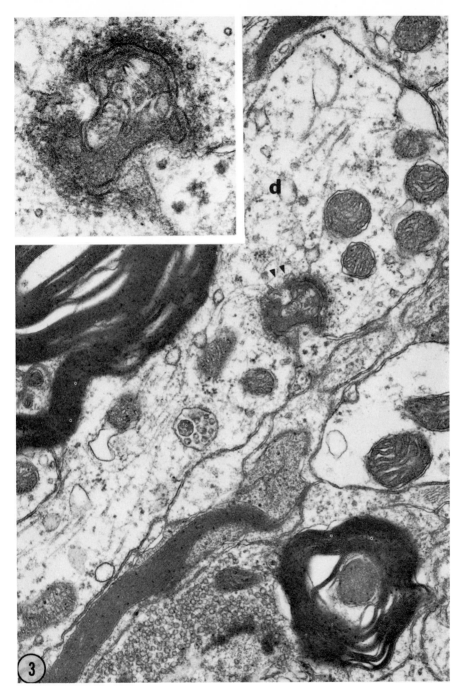

FIG. 3. Dendrite, d, with almost completely engulfed fragment of degenerating optic nerve terminal (*arrow heads; insert*). Third layer, 12 days after enucleation. (×26,700.) (Inset): Synaptic membranes and postsynaptic density of the degenerating fragment are still recognizable. (×65,100).

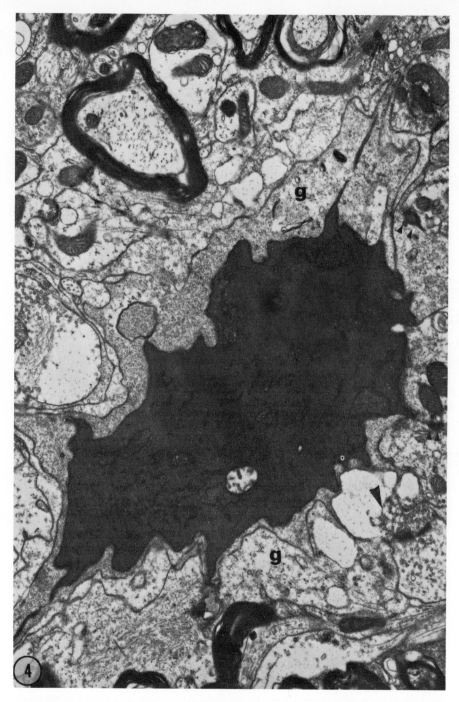

FIG. 4. Optic nerve terminal in late stage of degeneration, has undergone dark transformation. The profile has an irregular outline, and is almost completely surrounded by glial cytoplasm, g. Note the detached fragments of synaptic membranes (*small arrow heads*), and the disrupted and unidentifiable axon terminal (*large arrow head*). Fourth layer, 10 days after enucleation. (×13,200.)

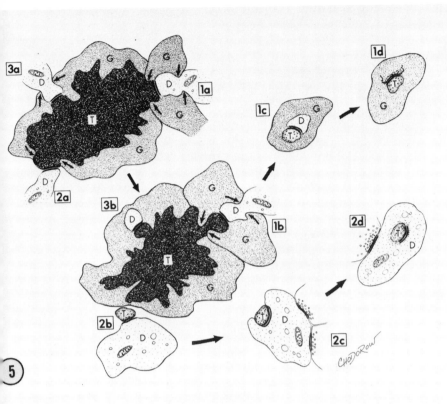

FIG. 5. The drawing recapitulates the final stages of degeneration and phagocytosis of the optic nerve terminal. In the upper left portion, a terminal, T, with irregular outline is invested by glial cytoplasm, G, except for the areas in which synaptic junctions with postsynaptic dendrites, D, are present. The irregular outline of the terminal is a prelude to its fragmentation. In area 1a, the fragmentation seems to take place on the presynaptic as well as on the postsynaptic side (*arrows*). In 2a, a tendency to nipping off is more evident on the presynaptic side (*arrows*). In 3a, the nipping off is more evident on the postsynaptic side. The center area, 1b, shows that the portions of pre- and postsynaptic terminal are not yet pinched off (*arrows*). Subsequently pinching off and total engulfment within glial cytoplasm takes place (1c and 1d). In area 2b, the portion of presynaptic terminal is pinched off from the large profile, T, and remains attached to the dendrite, D, being progressively invaginated (2c) and engulfed (2d) within the latter profile. In 3b, the postsynaptic dendrite remains engulfed within the glia, G, along with the large portion of terminal, T. Dissociation of synaptic junctions does not take place.

often it was difficult to follow the continuity of the dendritic plasma membrane. In some instances, it appeared that the membrane was indeed disrupted. As was mentioned previously, in these profiles, synaptic specializations were still recognizable. However, they often showed focal disruption, and, although occasionally they appeared displaced from their original position, they were still apposed to each other (Fig. 4).

In the monkey sacrificed 14 days after enucleation, dendrites with engulfed synaptic specializations were rarely found. However, large electron-dense profiles with irregular outlines, seen also at the 10th and 12th days after enucleation, were still encountered. They were the remnants of the axons of retinal origin stripped of the synaptic specializations.

These irregular profiles were surrounded and/or engulfed by the phagocytes. Often, more than one cell was taking part in the removal of the remnants of a single axon terminal. Areas previously occupied by normal neuropil now showed profiles twice as large as their original size accompanied by proliferation of glial elements. As a consequence of this hypertrophy and hyperplasia, dendritic and axonal profiles situated at the periphery of such areas showed irregular outlines (Fig. 4). Often the plasma membrane of these terminals was disrupted and the cytoplasm vacuolated. Some dendrites and F processes appeared swollen and watery, with marked reduction of cytoplasmic organelles. In particular, F processes showed fewer synaptic vesicles. It was not established whether synaptic specialization between profiles other than ONT were dissociated. It was interesting to note that dendrites postsynaptic to profiles tentatively identified as F processes also showed disruption of their plasma membrane occasionally. Despite the fact that synaptic junctions were preserved, the plasma membrane next to the synapse showed deep indentation and irregular outline. However, remodeling of the interneuritic connections did not appear to take place in these areas. It was difficult to determine whether new contacts of the type observed in control were established; however, no type of connection other than those seen in normal animals was observed. Dendrites postsynaptic to both the soma of an interneuron and to degenerating axons of retinal origin were on occasion encountered (Fig. 6); after disappearance of ONT they remained postsynaptic to the soma of the interneuron (Fig. 7).

The neuropil elements, situated away from areas where phagocytosis of debris of ONT was taking place also showed pathologic features. The number of watery dendrites was remarkably increased and the depletion of their cytoplasmic organelles was more evident (Fig. 8). The dendrites with tubulovesicular structures were also more numerous (Figs. 9 and 10). They showed a wide range of morphologic features. Some of them contained only few vesicular membrane-bound structures near the center (Fig. 9), the rest of the profile being occupied by neurofilaments and rare neurotubules. Other dendrites were also filled with these vesicular elements (Fig. 10). When present in large numbers such structures were round, ovoid, or tubular. On occasion they appeared as flattened sacs or as a single tortuous membrane. Their size varied from 600 to 2,000 Å and occasionally they gave way to larger vacuoles. Almost invariably, these structures were embedded within an amorphous electron-dense material the origin of which could not be de-

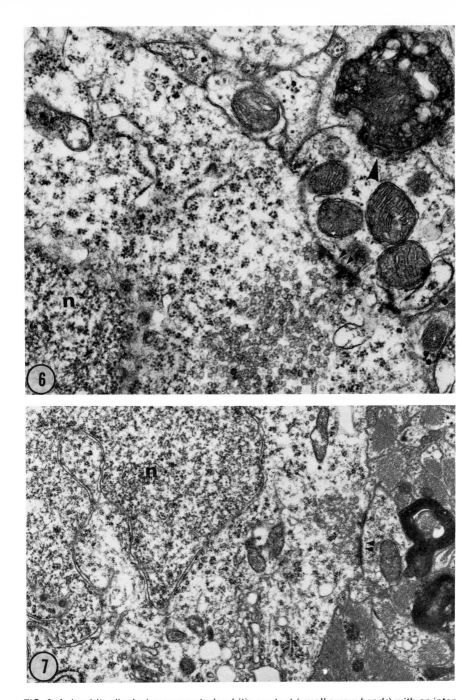

FIG. 6. A dendrite displaying a somatodendritic contact (*small arrow heads*) with an inter-neuron, and an axodendritic contact (*large arrow head*) with a degenerating optic nerve terminal, 10 days after enucleation. n, Nucleus of interneuron. (×27,900.)

FIG. 7. A dendrite postsynaptic to the perikaryon of an interneuron 170 days after enuclea-tion. n, Nucleus of interneuron. (×16,900.)

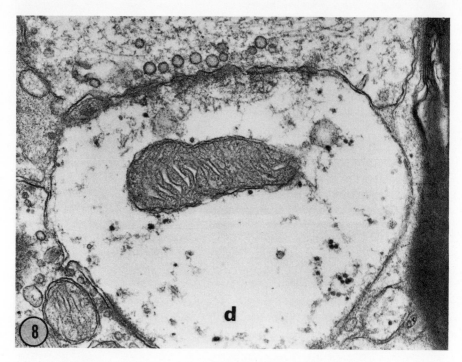

FIG. 8. A dendrite, d, shows moderate depletion of cytoplasmic organelles. Note the very few neurotubules and the sparse floccular material. Ten days after enucleation. (×52,400.)

termined (Figs. 9 and 10). In the animal sacrificed 1 month following enucleation, many profiles were seen entirely surrounded by glial processes. They were F processes and, on occasion, RSD presynaptic to dendrites. There were appearances suggesting the total engulfment of some of these profiles.

Following disappearance of debris of the ONT the glial processes continued to occupy large areas of the neuropil. The removal of the myelinated portion of the axons of retinal origin was slow and continued for months following eye enucleation, causing further scarring within and between the layers of LGN. However, in areas less severely involved by the process of scarring numerous axon terminals characterized by crowding of their synaptic vesicles were observed. Watery dendrites and dendrites with tubulo-vesicular profiles were also common findings. The latter, when encountered, did not seem to trigger a glial reaction. In fact, these profiles were not seen encircled or engulfed by glial processes. One month after enucleation, the neuropil was still rich in neuronal processes and dendritic shafts, and appendages were frequently seen. Six months after bilateral enucleation, the organization of the neuropil appeared completely disrupted and a tight network of astroglial processes had replaced most of the neuronal processes

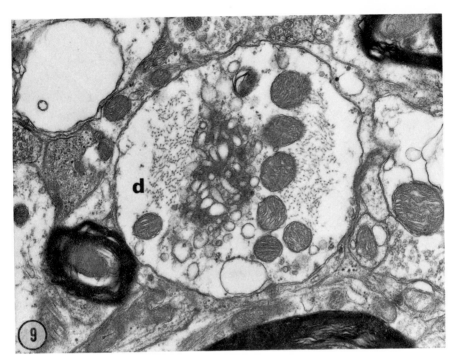

FIG. 9. A dendrite, d, with tubulovesicular profiles, 10 days after enucleation. Note the amorphous osmiophilic material associated with the vesicular structures. The rest of the profile shows increased numbers of filaments. (×21,100.)

(Fig. 11). At this stage, the identification of neurites was difficult because of the disruption of interneuritic relationships and the alteration in appearance of individual profiles undergoing changes secondary to deafferentation. However, watery, vacuolated dendritic profiles containing few or no mito-chondria and some granular and/or membranous material were readily rec-ognizable (Fig. 12) between the processes of fibrous astrocytes. Dendrites with deeply indented plasma membrane were commonly observed (Fig. 13). These were mostly dendrites of medium and small size. Dendritic shafts as seen in control LGN and in the first weeks after enucleation were rare. The remaining dendrites often contained vacuoles and vesicular profiles sometimes surrounded by electron dense amorphous material similar to that observed after shorter survival (Figs. 14 and 15).

On occasion, electron-dense shrunken dark dendrites were seen in the neuropil (Fig. 16). The dark appearance of these profiles was caused by the tight clustering of neurotubules and to the overall increased electron density of the cytoplasm. Not infrequently, despite the already advanced degenera-tive changes, the affected dendrites were still in postsynaptic position (Fig. 16).

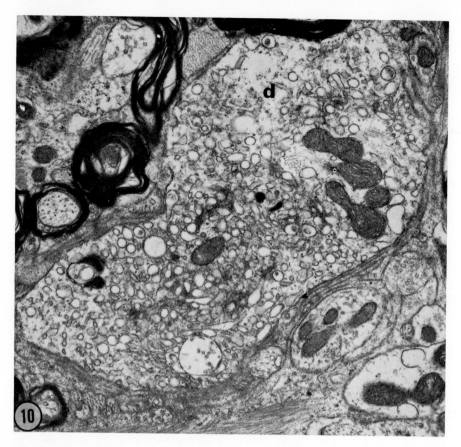

FIG. 10. A large dendrite, d, of a principal neuron is filled with tubulovesicular and sacular structures. Third layer, 12 days after enucleation. (×13,800.)

Among the remnants, small dendrites were often seen postsynaptic to small profiles measuring 1 to 2 μm, which contained numerous crowded synaptic vesicles and were interpreted as RSD. The synaptic membranes and cleft were often well preserved. Dendrites were also found postsynaptic to F processes. Furthermore, dendrites postsynaptic to the soma of interneurons were still present 6 months following eye enucleation (Fig. 7). In addition to the decrease in number of dendrites, F processes were also encountered much more rarely in the neuropil, and the remaining ones were watery and electron-lucent.

Anterograde Transneuronal Response of LGN Neurons

Four days after bilateral enucleation, some of the neurons of the LGN showed slight distention of the Golgi apparatus and minimal dilatation of

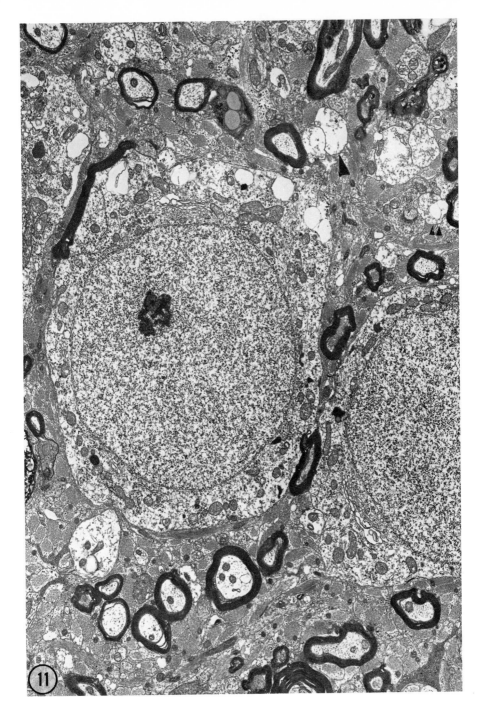

FIG. 11. Neurons surrounded by a meshwork of fibrous astrocytic processes, 170 days after enucleation. Note the presence of some watery profiles in the neuropil (*arrow heads*). (×7,000.)

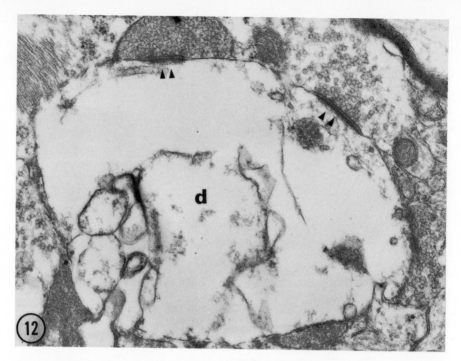

FIG. 12. A watery dendrite, d, depleted of cytoplasmic organelles and containing floccular and membranaceous material, 170 days after enucleation. Synaptic contacts are recognizable (*arrow heads*). However, the plasma membrane shows indentations and disruption. (×31,200.)

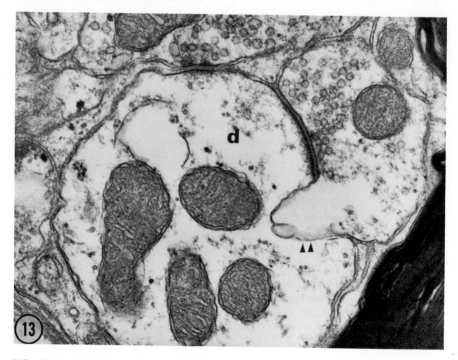

FIG. 13. A dendrite, d, 170 days after enucleation, showing a deep indentation of its plasma membrane (*arrow heads*) next to the synaptic specialization. (×46,500.)

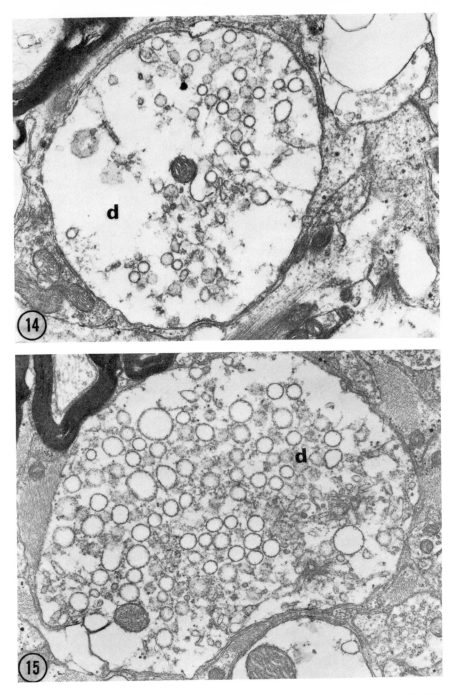

FIG. 14. A dendrite, d, partially filled with tubulovesicular structures giving way to vacuoles, 170 days after enucleation. Note that no cytoplasmic organelles are recognizable besides the mitochondrion. (×22,900.)

FIG. 15. A dendrite, d, filled with membrane, round vacuoles, and tubulovesicular profiles, 170 days after enucleation. (×19,700.)

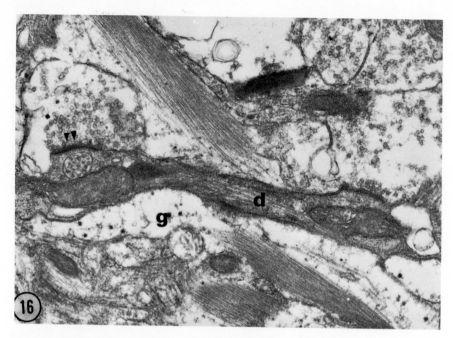

FIG. 16. An electron-dark dendrite, d, surrounded by glial processes, g, 170 days after enucleation. Note that a synaptic specialization (*arrow heads*) is still recognizable; however, the plasma membrane adjacent to it is disrupted. (×42,500.)

the endoplasmic reticulum (ER). Seven days after bilateral enucleation, the distention of the ER and the Golgi system gave way to vacuoles. Cytoplasmic vacuolation was very pronounced in the interneurons causing the perikaryon of these cells to appear fenestrated. In the principal neurons, the vacuoles were mainly distributed at the periphery of the cell. The mitochondria were somewhat reduced in number, and many appeared swollen or had a washed-out appearance. The undistended segments of the rough ER were poorly garnished with ribosomes that had been shed as free particles in the cytoplasm.

In the interval between 10 and 36 days, these perikaryonal changes were more pronounced and widespread. At 170 days the nerve cells were seen embedded in a dense network of astrocytic processes. Both the nuclei and the perikaryonal cytoplasm appeared to be reduced in size, the rim of the cytoplasm surrounding the nucleus being thinner than in control. The rough ER in many neurons was partially replenished with ribosomal particles. However, the nucleus of many of the principal cells, especially in layer 1 and 2, was still located eccentrically. Nucleoli appeared smaller in size and not infrequently were seen closer to the nuclear membrane. Several dark nerve cells were observed. They showed an overall increase in electron density of cytoplasmic organelles and matrix with blurring of the outline of

all membrane-bound systems; however, appearances suggesting neuro-
nophagia were not observed.

DISCUSSION

The present study has shown that dendritic changes first appeared 7 days
following enucleation. Some of the affected profiles were electron lucent,
containing floccular material and few cytoplasmic organelles. Other dendrites were filled with tubulovesicular and saccular structures. Such changes
were first observed when ONT were already in an advanced stage of filamentous degeneration, and they persisted for months following disappearance of the ONT. The latter underwent phagocytosis between 10 and
14 days after enucleation. The dendrites took part in the removal of both
synaptic specialization and the fragment of ONT still attached to it. Owing
to the strong adhesions of the synaptic membranes, portions of dendrites
with the fragments of degenerated axonal endings appeared to be engulfed
by the phagocytes. Six months after enucleation, in addition to dendrites
characterized by electron-lucent cytoplasm and by tubulovesicular profiles,
dark dendrites were often encountered. At this time the neuropil displayed
remarkable reduction in the number of neuronal processes. Dendrites of P
cells and F processes seemed to be most affected while the RSD axons continued to be numerous 6 months after enucleation. The most frequent type
of connection observed was axodendritic with RSD axons in presynaptic
position, in contrast to what was observed in the LGN several months
after cortical ablation when the most frequent profiles seen were ONT
presynaptic to F processes (Pasik et al., 1973; Horoupian, Ghetti, and
Wiśniewski, *unpublished observations*). At no time interval in the present
study did we observe new types of synaptic connections. It has been observed (Le Vay, 1971) that somatodendritic synapsis appear in the LGN
45 days after enucleation. In our material such contacts were observed at
all time intervals, following the appearance of degenerating ONT. In addition, somato dendritic contacts are a normal feature also in the squirrel
monkey LGN (Wong-Riley, 1972*a*).

The role of dendrites in the removal of degenerating terminal bouton was
first observed by Walberg (1963). He noticed that in the olivary nucleus of
adult cat the dendrites postsynaptic to degenerating terminals apparently
disposed of the synaptic adhesions by invaginations of the postsynaptic
membranes into their cytoplasm. A similar phenomenon was described
during the study of development of the basket axon synapses by Larramendi
(1969) who observed invaginations of pre- and postsynaptic membranes
into the postsynaptic soma of the Purkinje cell. The role of dendrites in
engulfing larger fragments of degenerating material was also reported by
Conradi (1969) in the spinal cord, and by Wiśniewski et al. (1972) and by
Ghetti and Wiśniewski (1972*b*) in the LGN. More recent studies have

shown that this mechanism takes place in other nuclei of adult CNS, as recently reported by Gentschev and Sotelo (1973) in the ventral cochlear nucleus of the rat and by Rustioni and Sotelo (1974) in the nucleus gracilis of the cat.

The second and most frequent mechanism of debris removal was with the active participation of phagocytic cells. In these instances, fragments of dendrites and F processes were engulfed together with the presynaptic element or portion of it. This mechanism of removal of pre- and postsynaptic elements by the glial cytoplasm was first described by Colonnier (1964) in undercut cortex. In deafferentated structures it was shown in the granular layer of frog cerebellum following transection of the spinocerebellar tracts (Sotelo, 1969), in the visual cortex following destruction of LGN (Ghetti and Wiśniewski, 1972a) and in LGN following enucleation (Ghetti et al., 1972; Ghetti and Wiśniewski, 1972b; Wiśniewski et al., 1972).

From the interpretation of our data, it appears that the dendrites are damaged during removal of axonal debris, i.e., with the introduction within their cytoplasm of foreign material and with a partial amputation. However, it should be emphasized that during this period and later, formation of new types of contacts was not observed. This means that, in LGN, in addition to the physical trauma the postsynaptic structures also lost a physiologic input, but did not have to deal with an aberrant function that could follow if synaptic contacts of a new type were established.

Watery dendrites and dendrites with tubulovesicular structures were seen at every time interval after enucleation, starting from the seventh day. Large degenerating profiles with tubulovesicular structures were first reported by Glees, Hasan, and Tischner (1967) in LGN of *Macaca mulatta* after enucleation, and were interpreted as neurons undergoing transsynaptic degeneration. Le Vay (1971) has also described similar dendritic changes in LGN of *Macaca,* and according to his data they were still present in the monkey sacrificed 29 months after enucleation. It is interesting that despite the extensive vacuolization shown by P cells and interneurons we did not observe any neuron with such tubulovesicular structures. Furthermore, it should be noted that clearly postsynaptic dendrites containing aggregates of amorphous or membranous material in the center of the profiles, and very similar to those observed by us, have been shown by Wong-Riley (1972c) in the LGN of squirrel monkey 5 days after cortical ablation. The pathogenesis of these pathologic dendrites is unclear. Le Vay (1971) has hypothesized that these are dendrites that have broken off from their parent cells during a process of dendritic withdrawal, thereby implying a process of anterograde degeneration. Data on anterograde dendritic degeneration appear to be lacking. However, in a study of dendritic degeneration in layers of the rat cerebral cortex above laminar lesions induced by ionizing particles, Kruger and Hámori (1970) have described the degenerating dendrites as being characterized by a dense cytoplasmic matrix, disruption of mitochondria, irregular outline, and marked alterations of the plasmalemma. Engulfment of such degenerating profiles within glial cytoplasm was also a common feature.

It is conceivable that the morphologic appearance of dendritic damage in transneuronal degeneration takes place more slowly than one might expect after dendritic transection; this seems to be confirmed also by the fact that in the model described by Kruger and Hámori (1970) the glial reaction was very prompt around the degenerating ONT, but did not seem to take place around the dendrites containing tubulovesicular profiles. Therefore, one could speculate that the dendrites with tubulovesicular structures are neuronal processes that remain for some time in a dystrophic state.

In deafferentated LGN, the watery dendrites were the most common among profiles displaying pathologic features, especially after endings of retinal origin had been removed. Characteristic for these dendrites was the reduction or absence of cytoplasmic organelles and the occasional presence of glycogen-like particles. Similar dendritic changes have recently been described by Berger (1973) in a study of the olfactory bulb of the immature rabbit following deafferentation. In our material such alterations lead to appearances suggesting a dissolution of the profile. It should be noted that, not only the dendrites of P neurons, but also the processes of interneurons displayed this type of change. Whether watery appearance is the result of increased membrane permeability followed by swelling of the cytoplasm or whether a release of hydrolytic enzymes causes a clearing of the cytoplasm have to be investigated further.

In the long-term animal, electron-dense degenerating dendrites were also observed, and they were thought to be processes of neurons undergoing the electron-dark type of degeneration. Despite the fact that the most frequent alterations seen in perikarya during transsynaptic degeneration were vacuolization and watery appearance of the cytoplasm, electron-dark neurons also appeared in the animal sacrificed in the sixth month after enucleation. Dark neurons have been described in diverse pathologic and experimental situations (Campos-Ortega et al., 1970; Garey and Powell, 1971; Brown and Brierley, 1972; Barron, Means, and Larsen, 1973; Wiśniewski, Ghetti, and Terry, 1973). They have been reported in transneuronal degeneration by Pinching and Powell (1971) and by Fuentes and Marty (1973).

It has been shown that in the CNS, two types of degenerative changes may be observed (Gentschev and Sotelo, 1973; O'Neal and Westrum, 1973). One type characterized by the well-known electron-dense pattern probably corresponds to the coagulative necrosis; the other, characterized by the clear and swollen degenerative changes, probably corresponds to the liquefactive necrosis (Gentschev and Sotelo, 1973). These two types of degeneration have been well documented in the axon (Cook and Wiśniewski, 1973; Cook, Ghetti, and Wiśniewski, 1974) and axon terminals (Gentschev and Sotelo, 1973); however, they also occur at the level of the perikaryon (Herndon, 1968; Campos-Ortega et al., 1970; Barron et al., 1973; Sipe, Vick, Schulman, and Fernandes, 1973). Therefore, it is possible that the dark and the watery dendrites observed in our study are expressions of the two degenerative patterns.

In addition to the morphologic changes in dendrites and F processes in the animal killed 6 months after enucleation of the eye, the neuropil was occupied in large part by a glial scar. It is known that a gradual loss of neurons takes place in the primate LGN. However, according to Matthews, Cowan, and Powell (1960), there is a statistically insignificant decrease in neuronal number at 4 months after enucleation, while the loss is between 4 and 22% in the magnocellular layers, and 14 to 16% in the parvocellular layers after a 1-year interval (Matthews, 1964).

We did not evaluate numerical loss of neurons or elements of the neuropil; however, the loss of dendrites within the neuropil was of such degree that it could not be interpreted as only secondary to cell death. It was rather believed that the dendritic tree was undergoing degenerative changes, and reduction before an appreciable decrease in number of cells could be observed.

ACKNOWLEDGMENTS

The authors thank Dr. Robert D. Terry for his continued support and constructive criticism. This investigation was supported in part by Grants NS-02255 and NS-05275 from the National Institutes of Health, and by a grant from the Alfred P. Sloan Foundation. The excellent technical assistance of Carol Fitzgerald, Jack Godrich, Larry Gonzales, Sidney Gravney, Loyda Nolasco, and Roselyne Schwartz is gratefully acknowledged.

REFERENCES

Barron, K. D., Means, E. D., and Larsen, E. (1973): Ultrastructure of retrograde degeneration in thalamus of rat. I. Neuronal somata and dendrites. *J. Neuropathol. Exp. Neurol.*, 32:218–244.

Berger, B. (1973): Dégénérescence transsynaptique dans le bulbe olfactif du lapin après désafférentation périphérique. *Acta Neuropathol. (Berl.)*, 24:128–152.

Brown, A. W., and Brierley, J. B. (1972): Anoxic-ischaemic cell change in rat brain. Light microscopic and fine-structural observations. *J. Neurol. Sci.*, 16:59–84.

Campos-Ortega, J. A., Glees, P., and Neuhoff, V. (1968): Ultrastructural analysis of individual layers in the lateral geniculate body of the monkey. *Z. Zellforsch. Mikrosk. Anat.*, 87:82–100.

Campos-Ortega, J. A., Hayhow, W. R., and de V. Cluver, P. F. (1970): The descending projections from the cortical visual fields of Macaca mulatta with particular reference to the question of a cortico-lateral geniculate pathway. *Brain Behav. Evol.*, 3:368–414.

Colonnier, M. (1964): Experimental degeneration in the cerebral cortex. *J. Anat.*, 98:47–53.

Colonnier, M., and Guillery, R. W. (1964): Synaptic organization in the lateral geniculate nucleus of monkey. *Z. Zellforsch. Mikrosk. Anat.*, 62:333–355.

Conradi, S. (1969): Ultrastructure of dorsal root boutons on lumbosacral motoneurons of the adult cat, as revealed by dorsal root section. *Acta Physiol. Scand. (Suppl.)*, 332:85–115.

Cook, R. D., Ghetti, B., and Wiśniewski, H. M. (1974): The pattern of Wallerian degeneration in the optic nerve of newborn kittens: an ultrastructural study. *Brain Res.,* 75:261–275.

Cook, R. D., and Wiśniewski, H. M. (1973): The role of oligodendroglia and astroglia in Wallerian degeneration of the optic nerve. *Brain Res.,* 61:191–206.

Cowan, W. M. (1970): Anterograde and retrograde transneuronal degeneration in the central and peripheral nervous system. In: *Contemporary Research Methods in Neuroanatomy,* edited by W. J. H. Nauta and S. O. E. Ebbesson. Springer-Verlag, New York.

Fuentes, C., and Marty, R. (1973): Dégénérescence neuronique dans l'écorce cérébrale, consécutive à la destruction d'un noyau de relais thalamique. *J. Neurol. Sci.,* 20:303–312.

Garey, L. J., and Powell, T. P. S. (1971): An experimental study of the termination of the lateral geniculo-cortical pathway in the cat and monkey. *Proc. R. Soc. Lond. (Biol.),* 179: 41–63.

Gentschev, T., and Sotelo, C. (1973): Degenerative patterns in the ventral cochlear nucleus of the rat after primary deafferentation. An ultrastructural study. *Brain Res.,* 62:37–60.

Ghetti, B., Horoupian, D. S., and Wiśniewski, H. M. (1972): Transsynaptic response of the lateral geniculate nucleus and the pattern of degeneration of the nerve terminals in the rhesus monkey after eye enucleation. *Brain Res.,* 45:31–48.

Ghetti, B., and Wiśniewski, H. M. (1972a): On degeneration of terminals in the cat striate cortex. *Brain Res.,* 44:630–635.

Ghetti, B., and Wiśniewski, H. M. (1972b): Fate of synaptic membranes during degeneration of optic nerve terminals in the lateral geniculate nucleus. *J. Cell Biol.,* 55:84a.

Glees, P., Hasan, M., and Tischner, K. (1967): Ultrastructural features of transneuronal atrophy in monkey geniculate neurons. *Acta Neuropathol. (Berl.),* 7:361–366.

Glees, P., Meller, K., and Eschner, J. (1966): Terminal degeneration in the lateral geniculate body of the monkey: An electron microscope study. *Z. Zellforsch. Mikrosk. Anat.,* 71:29–40.

Globus, A., and Scheibel, A. B. (1967): Synaptic loci on visual cortical neurons of the rabbit: the specific afferent radiation. *Exp. Neurol.,* 18:116–131.

Guillery, R. W., and Colonnier, M. (1970): Synaptic patterns in the dorsal lateral geniculate nucleus of the monkey. *Z. Zellforsch. Mikrosk. Anat.,* 103:90–108.

Herndon, R. M. (1968): Thiophen induced granule cell necrosis in the rat cerebellum. An electron microscopic study. *Exp. Brain Res.,* 6:49–68.

Horoupian, D. S., Ghetti, B., and Wiśniewski, H. M. (1973): Retrograde transneuronal degeneration of optic fibers and their terminals in the lateral geniculate nucleus of rhesus monkey. *Brain Res.,* 49:257–275.

Kanagasuntheram, R., Krishnamurti, A., Ahmed, M. M., Wong, W. C., and Chan, H. L. (1971): Degenerative changes in the optic terminals in the lateral geniculate nucleus of the monkey. *Acta Anat. (Basel),* 80:58–67.

Kanagasuntheram, R., Krishnamurti, A., and Wong, W. C. (1973): The termination of optic fibres in the lateral geniculate nucleus of some primates. An ultrastructural study. *Acta Anat. (Basel),* 84:76–84.

Kruger, L., and Hámori, J. (1970): An electron microscopic study of dendritic degeneration in the cerebral cortex resulting from laminar lesions. *Exp. Brain Res.,* 10:1–16.

Larramendi, L. M. H. (1969): Analysis of synaptogenesis in the cerebellum of the mouse. In: *Neurobiology of Cerebellar Evolution and Development,* edited by R. Llinás. American Medical Association, Chicago, Illinois.

Le Vay, S. (1971): On the neurons and synapses of the lateral geniculate nucleus of the monkey, and the effects of eye enucleation. *Z. Zellforsch. Mikrosk. Anat.,* 113:396–419.

Lund, R. D., and Lund, J. S. (1971): Synaptic adjustment after deafferentation of the superior colliculus of the rat. *Science,* 171:804–807.

Matthews, M. R. (1964): Further observations on transneuronal degeneration in the lateral geniculate nucleus of the macaque monkey. *J. Anat.,* 98:255–263.

Matthews, M. R., Cowan, W. M., and Powell, T. P. S. (1960): Transneuronal cell degeneration in the lateral geniculate nucleus of the macaque monkey. *J. Anat.,* 94:145–169.

McMahan, O. J. (1967): Fine structure of synapses in the dorsal nucleus of the lateral geniculate body of normal and blinded rats. *Z. Zellforsch. Mikrosk. Anat.,* 76:116–146.

Minkowski, M. (1920): Über den Verlauf, die Endigung und Zentrale Repräsentation von gekreuzten und ungekreuzten Sehnervenfasern bei einigen Säugetieren und beim Menschen. *Schweiz. Arch. Neurol. Psychiatr.,* 6:201–252; 7:268–303.

O'Neal, J. T., and Westrum, L. E. (1973): The fine structural synaptic organization of the cat lateral cuneate nucleus. A study of sequential alterations in degeneration. *Brain Res.*, 51: 97–124.

Pasik, P., Pasik, T., Hámori, J., and Szentágothai, J. (1973): Golgi Type II interneurons in the neuronal circuit of the monkey lateral geniculate nucleus. *Exp. Brain Res.*, 17:18–34.

Pinching, A. J., and Powell, T. P. S. (1971): Ultrastructural features of transneuronal cell degeneration in the olfactory system. *J. Cell Sci.*, 8:253–287.

Rustioni, A., and Sotelo, C. (1974): Some effects of chronic deafferentation on the ultrastructure of the nucleus gracilis of the cat. *Brain Res.*, 73:527–533.

Sipe, J. C., Vick, N. A., Schulman, S., and Fernandes, C. (1973): Plasmocid encephalopathy in the rhesus monkey: a study of selective vulnerability. *J. Neuropathol. Exp. Neurol.*, 32:446–457.

Smith, D. E. (1974): The effect of deafferentation on the postnatal development of Clarke's nucleus in the kitten: A Golgi study. *Brain Res.*, 74:119–130.

Sotelo, C. (1969): Ultrastructural aspects of the cerebellar cortex of the frog. In: *Neurobiology of Cerebellar Evolution and Development,* edited by R. Llinás. American Medical Association, Chicago, Illinois.

Walberg, F. (1963): Role of normal dendrites in removal of degenerating terminal boutons. *Exp. Neurol.*, 8:112–124.

Westman, J. (1969): The lateral cervical nucleus in the cat. III. An electron microscopical study after transection of spinal afferents. *Exp. Brain Res.*, 7:32–50.

Wiśniewski, H. M., Ghetti, B., and Horoupian, D. S. (1972): The fate of synaptic membranes of degenerating optic nerve terminals, and their role in the mechanism of trans-synaptic changes. *J. Neurocytol.*, 1:297–310.

Wiśniewski, H. M., Ghetti, B., and Terry, R. D. (1973): Neuritic (senile) plaques and filamentous changes in aged rhesus monkeys. *J. Neuropathol. Exp. Neurol.*, 32:566–584.

Wong-Riley, M. T. T. (1972a): Neuronal and synaptic organization of the normal dorsal lateral geniculate nucleus of the squirrel monkey, Saimiri sciureus. *J. Comp. Neurol.*, 144: 25–60.

Wong-Riley, M. T. T. (1972b): Terminal degeneration and glial reactions in the lateral geniculate nucleus of the squirrel monkey after eye removal. *J. Comp. Neurol.*, 144:61–92.

Wong-Riley, M. T. T. (1972c): Changes in the dorsal lateral geniculate nucleus of the squirrel monkey after unilateral ablation of the visual cortex. *J. Comp. Neurol.*, 146:519–548.

Advances in Neurology, Vol. 12, edited by
G. W. Kreutzberg, Raven Press, New York
© 1975.

Denervation and Neuronal Interdependence

Samuel Gelfan[*]

New York Medical College, Valhalla, New York 10595

It has already been demonstrated that severely denervated spinal neurons — survivors of temporary lumbosacral ischemia — are altered neurons, both functionally and morphologically. The increased excitability is the most obvious neurophysiologic modification, manifested in the chronic preparation by the "spastic" behavior of α-motoneurons, whose spontaneous discharges maintain the hind limbs in continuous pillar-like extension (Gelfan, 1966). The morphologic alterations consist, first, of the denervation itself. With the loss of some two-thirds of the lumbosacral interneurons during the ischemic episode (Gelfan and Tarlov, 1963), the receptive surface of the surviving neurons in such preparations is denuded of about two-thirds of its normal synaptic covering (Gelfan and Rapisarda, 1964; Gelfan, Field, and Pappas, 1974), and is exposed to an environment altered by the replacement of the missing neurons and their extensions by intercellular fluid (Gelfan et al., 1974). The loss of most of their synaptic connections with other neurons is compounded in the surviving neurons by the loss of nearly two-thirds of their dendritic trees; that is, a major reduction of the normal dendritic receptive surface area (Gelfan, Kao, and Ling, 1972). In addition, the specialized receptor sites, the identifiable postsynaptic thickenings which had apposed the now missing synaptic terminals, are also missing from the denuded surfaces of surviving cell bodies and their truncated dendrites (Gelfan et al., 1974). This structural alteration at the ultramicroscopic level has also been observed in cortical neurons whose afferent input had been surgically interrupted (Gray and Hamlyn, 1962; Colonnier, 1964). Similarly, dendritic tree size reductions have been observed in supraspinal centers, where it has been possible to denervate their neurons adequately by surgical interruption of known major or principal afferent pathways to such centers (Le Gros Clark, 1957; Jones and Thomas, 1962; Matthews and Powell, 1962; White and Westrum, 1964; Globus and Scheibel, 1967; Valverde, 1968). A reduction in branching, as well as depletion of dendritic spines, has been reported for the dendrites on surviving neurons within alumina-induced epileptogenic foci in sensorimotor cortices of adult monkeys (Westrum, White, and Ward, 1964).

The alteration of the neurophysiologic properties of the surviving lumbo-

---

[*] Deceased, March 16, 1975.

sacral neurons was attributed to denervation in our first paper on the hind-limb rigidity preparation (Gelfan and Tarlov, 1959). From this work on severely denervated spinal neurons emerged the concept of neuronal inter-dependence (Gelfan, 1964), which postulated that the physiologic character-istics, physical constants of each neuron, are homeostatically maintained and controlled by trophic factors furnished transneuronally by the many synaptic connections with other neurons. This neuroneuronal dependence is comparable to the dependence of skeletal muscle upon the input from its motor nerve, without which the muscle undergoes profound morphologic, biochemical, and physiologic alterations (Gutmann, 1962, 1964; Gutmann and Hník, 1963; Guth, 1968; Drachman, 1974). In the case of the neurons, not only is there a multiple source of trophic factors, but there is an inter-dependence among the neurons for such factors, as there is for the exchange of signals, "information," provided by the vast intercommunicating network. The reduction of the dendritic tree size, as well as the ultramicroscopic structural modifications in denervated neurons, and very likely changes at the molecular level, constitute the morphologic concomitants of the func-tional alterations. The postulate that a critical minimum of neurotrophic input is indispensable for the viability of the more distal portion of the den-dritic tree is an extension of the neuronal interdependence concept (Gelfan et al., 1972)—the proposal that the integrity of the thickenings as a post-synaptic structural specialization is dependent upon neurotrophic factors (Gelfan et al., 1974) also fits into the general concept. The amputation of the more distal part of the dendritic tree is not fatal to the rest of the neuron. The neuron is only "crippled." It is crippled not only by the loss of a large fraction of the contacts with other neurons through the loss of a major frac-tion of the dendritic tree, but also by the severe reduction in number of synaptic contacts on the remaining portion of the neuron. The remaining neuron survives but it is no longer the same neuron; it is transformed, altered structurally and electrophysiologically, and its behavior is con-sequently altered. Such a neuron does not and can no longer fit into an overall integrating scheme of which it was a component before denerva-tion.

It may be added, in view of the title of this volume, that the pathology of the dendritic tree, the pathology of the whole neuron, indeed of the entire lumbosacral cord in animals with experimental hind-limb rigidity, is the pathology of denervation.

PRE- AND POSTSYNAPTIC RELATIONSHIPS

Volume of Terminals

The axon terminals are the immediate and only source of the neuro-trophic materials exchanged between neurons, and the range of synaptic

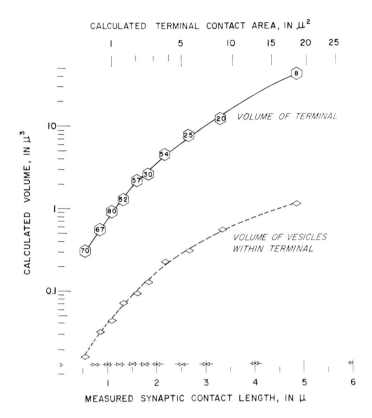

CALCULATED TERMINAL CONTACT AREA, IN μ^2

VOLUME OF TERMINAL

VOLUME OF VESICLES
WITHIN TERMINAL

CALCULATED VOLUME, IN μ^3

MEASURED SYNAPTIC CONTACT LENGTH, IN μ

FIG. 1. (Upper) Mean volumes of categories of terminals distributed according to their mean measured synaptic contact lengths. Total sample of terminals from L_7 spinal segment of normal dog and one dog with experimental hind-limb rigidity of 14 days duration, segregated into ten categories the contact length ranges of which are given by the distances between each pair of arrows on the lower abscissa. The sample size in each category is given by the numbers within the symbols. (See footnote 2 for calculation of volumes for each of the terminals in the sample.) The terminal contact area (upper abscissa) equals π (contact length)^2/4; mean for entire sample = 2.326 μm^2. (Bottom) Mean volumes of total number of vesicles within the terminals in each of the same size categories as in upper curve. Volume of each vesicle, treated as sphere with mean diameter of 0.04 μm, = $\pi D^3/6$; this volume times computed vesicle number per terminal (see legend for Fig. 2) equals the volume occupied by vesicles within each terminal. Mean volume of vesicles per terminal for entire sample is 0.122484572 μm^3, 4% of the mean of the terminal volumes. Scaling of ordinate is logarithmic. (Based on computations of accumulated data in addition to those already reported by Gelfan et al., 1974.)

size must reflect to some degree a range of synaptic release, including a quantal range of the neurotrophic factors made available to the postsynaptic surface. On the basis of measured contact lengths, the size ranges from a fraction of a micron to about 6 or 7 μm in lumbosacral neurons (Conradi, 1969a; McLaughlin, 1972; Gelfan et al., 1974), exclusive of those in Clarke's nucleus. When the calculated volumes of the terminals are compared, and thereby their contents, the synaptic size range becomes impressively larger. The volume of the presynaptic envelope, containing cytoplasm, vesicles, and other organelles, increases exponentially with increase in synaptic contact length, or diameter of the bag. The mean calculated size of terminals with contact lengths of 4 μm and over, expressed in μm^3, is more than 100 times greater than the mean value of the terminals with contact lengths of less than 0.75 μm (Fig. 1). Almost one-half of the terminals in the total sample from all areas of the L_7 spinal gray are in the 1- to 2-μm contact length range. The calculated individual volumes of these knobs range from 0.6 to 4.7 μm^3 and the calculated contact areas (upper abscissa in Fig. 1) range from 0.9 to 3 μm^2. The volumes of terminals with contact lengths above 3-μm range from 9.1 to 75.6 μm^3 and their calculated contact areas range from 8 to 23.4 μm^2. The size parameter, expressed as volume, thus provides a measure of the total space occupied by each terminal and a more appropriate basis for establishing the size range. The calculated contact area is also a more useful measure of pre- and postsynaptic surface relationships at the synaptic complex.

Vesicle and Cytoplasm Content of Terminals

The fraction of the synaptic volume occupied by the vesicles is surprisingly small (Fig. 1). This is consistently true for all of the terminal size categories. Actually, as the bottom curve of Fig. 1 indicates, there is a progressive decrease of the vesicle fraction with increasing size of terminals above the average. This is because of the small inverse relationship between vesicle density/μm^3 of terminal volume and size of terminal (Fig. 3). Assuming that the rest of the organelles in the terminal occupy on the average about the same volume as the vesicles, the mean ratio of cytoplasm volume to total volume of vesicles for the entire sample of terminals is 23:1. In spite of this preponderance of cytoplasm over the vesicle component of the terminal,[1] the total number of vesicles per terminal in the largest of the synaptic knobs is nevertheless impressively large. The calculated number of vesicles in each of the terminals in the entire sample is plotted in Fig. 2, showing the degree of variation and the total range. The vesicles in the largest of the terminal size category may occupy only a little more than 1% of the mean total terminal volume, but their mean number in these terminals is nevertheless more than 31,000. This number per terminal is also nearly 15 times the mean for the terminals in the 1 to 2 μm contact length range, which comprises nearly one-half of the entire sample.

The density of vesicles in axodendritic terminals, in both the dorsal and

---

[1] The role of the cytoplasm within the terminal, in addition to the role of the vesicles, in the synthesis, storage, and release of transmitters, "macromolecules," enzymes, etc., is emphasized in the special issue of *Brain Research* [62: (2) (1973)] on the *Dynamic Aspects of the Synapse*.

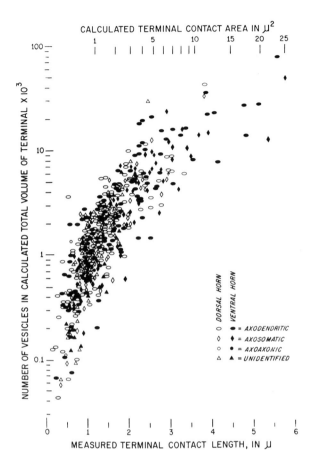

FIG. 2. The number of vesicles in each terminal of the entire sample as in Fig. 1 scattered according to the measured synaptic contact length. Contact area in upper abscissa as in Fig. 1. The vesicle number equals vesicle density/μm^3 in each terminal times volume of terminal (footnote 2). Density/μm^3 obtained from counted

$$\frac{\text{Number of vesicles in each profile in EMG}}{\text{profile volume in } \mu m^3}$$

Profile volume equals measured area of profile in $\mu m^2 \times 0.05 \ \mu m$ (thickness of section). Scaling on ordinate is logarithmic. (Scatter diagram constructed from accumulated data of Gelfan et al., 1974.)

ventral horns, is greater than in axosomatic ones. The difference is small but is consistently true for almost all terminal size categories (bottom curve in Fig. 3). This difference is also maintained within the inverse relationship between density of vesicles and size of terminals. As a consequence of this difference in density the total number of vesicles within the axodendritic terminals is greater than in the axosomatic ones (upper curve, Fig. 3).

Distribution of Different-Sized and Different-Shaped Terminals
within Lumbosacral Gray

The entire terminal size spectrum was not observed in all areas of L_7 spinal gray. With the exception of five terminals, all the rest in the sample with contact lengths between 3.000 and 3.999 μm were from the ventral horns; all the terminals with contact lengths of 4 μm and above were observed only in the ventral horns (Gelfan et al., 1974). The largest terminal observed in the dorsal horns had a calculated volume of 14.5 μm^3, all the terminals with volumes greater than this, and ranging to 75 μm^3 were observed only in the ventral horns. Hence, there is a morphologic distinction, in size and content, between the terminals in the two parts of the spinal gray. These observations also indicate that most, if not all, of the axon and axon collaterals of neurons from supraspinal centers, exteroreceptors, and the intrinsic system, with a mean terminal volume at least 10 times greater than the mean for the rest of synaptic knob population, project only to the ventral horns. Terminals with the largest contact length have been identified, presumably, on α-motoneurons (Conradi, 1969a; McLaughlin, 1972), but it has not been established that such terminals do not contact other neurons in the ventral horns. The average synaptic density on lumbosacral neuron population, as determined by light microscopy, also differs somewhat in different locations of the spinal gray, with the highest densities observed on ventral horn neurons (Gelfan and Rapisarda, 1964).

There is also a suggestion of a possible shape difference between the terminals of the two parts of the spinal gray. The assumption that the measured lengths of the synaptic knob profiles observed in the electron micrographs were equal to their diameters, when the measured cross-sectional areas of the profiles are considered as those of circles ($A = \pi D^2/4$), proved to be valid for the terminals with the highest contact length frequency, 1 to 1.5 μm (Gelfan et al., 1974). The mean ratio of the contact length to such a calculated diameter for the terminals in this size category was 1.01. This may also be observed in Fig. 4, in which the mean ratios are plotted against the mean contact lengths of the terminals, segregated according to location in the spinal gray as well as length categories.[2] For the terminals with contact lengths less than 1 μm, the ratios of less than 1 are identical for the samples from the dorsal and ventral horns. But the course

---

[2] The diameters, as derived from converting the measured cross-sectional areas into those of circles, $D = \sqrt{A \times 4/\pi}$, are thus larger than predicted for the knobs with contact lengths below the average and smaller for those with contact lengths above the average. The volumes of the synaptic knobs were originally calculated from $V = \pi D^3/6$, using the derived diameter for D. All the knob volumes in this report are based on a recalculation considering the terminals with contact lengths larger than the calculated diameters as oblate spheroids, $V = \pi a^2 b/6$, and those with contact lengths smaller than the calculated diameters as prolate spheroids, $V = \pi ab^2/6$, where a is the measured contact length and b is the calculated diameter, in microns. The mean of the volumes thus derived for all the terminals in the sample is 3.001 μm^3.

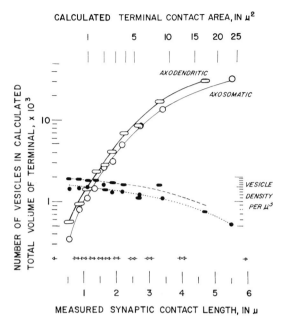

CALCULATED TERMINAL CONTACT AREA, IN μ^2

FIG. 3. (Upper) Data represented in Fig. 2 segregated to provide mean vesicle number per axosomatic and axodendritic terminals within categories of same sample as in Fig. 1, distributed according to mean measured synaptic contact length in each category. Contact ranges within categories given by distances between each pair of arrows on lower abscissa. Upper abscissa as in Fig. 1. (Bottom) Mean vesicle densities (see legend for Fig. 2) for axodendritic and axosomatic terminals in same categories as in upper curves, with same symbols. Scaling on left and right ordinates is logarithmic. (Based on computations of accumulated data in addition to those already reported by Gelfan et al., 1974.)

of the increasing ratios for the terminals with contact lengths greater than 1.5 μm is not the same in the two locations. The samples are small but the divergence of the two ratio curves increases consistently with increasing terminal size, pointing to a sufficient difference between the shapes of the larger terminals in the two halves of the spinal gray as to effect the mean values of the ratios.

Pre- and Postsynaptic, Axodendritic, and Axosomatic Volume Relationships

It is known that the total surface area of the dendritic tree is greater than that of the perkaryon. This is true for the neuronal population of the entire spinal gray of lumbosacral segments (Gelfan, Kao, and Ruchkin, 1970), as well as for the ventral horn population containing most of the larger neurons (Aitken and Bridger, 1961). Applying the mean $\pi/2$ correction factor derived for estimating the true length of the dendrites in the population as a

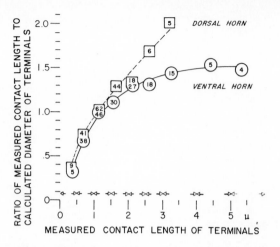

FIG. 4. Means of ratios of measured synaptic contact length to diameter of dorsal and ventral horn terminals in same sample as in Fig. 1, plotted against mean of contact lengths whose category ranges are indicated by pairs of arrows on abscissa. Terminal diameter derived from treating the measured cross-sectional area of terminal profile as that of circle, $D = \sqrt{A \times 4/\pi}$ (Based on computations of accumulated data in addition to those already reported by Gelfan et al., 1974.)

whole (Gelfan et al., 1970), the calculated mean surface area of the small neurons, which outnumber the large ones 24:1 (Gelfan and Tarlov, 1963), is some four times as great as the perikaryonal, and about three times as great in the large neurons (Table 1). With an essentially uniform average synaptic density for the entire receptive surface of spinal neurons of at least one synaptic knob per 5 μm^2 of surface (Gelfan and Rapisarda, 1964; Conradi, 1969a), this means an equivalently greater synaptic population on the dendritic portion of the receptive surface (Gelfan et al., 1970, 1972). But the mean volume of the dendritic tree is only slightly larger than the cell body one of the small neurons, and considerably smaller in the case of the large neurons (Table 1). Therefore, the mean synaptic density per post-synaptic unit volume, instead of per surface area, is some four times as great for the dendritic tree as for its cell body in the small neurons and about 5.5 times as great for the large ones. This greater per volume mean synaptic density for the dendritic tree cannot be uniform for the entire tree — With a uniform surface density, the volume density would be inversely proportional to the dendrite diameter.

The greater synaptic density per dendrite volume than per cell body volume becomes more relevant when the volumes of both the pre- and postsynaptic components are considered. The ratio of the total volume of all the terminals, of average size, to the volume of the average-sized dendritic tree to which the terminals synaptically adhere, is considerably

TABLE 1. *Pre- and postsynaptic parameters of lumbosacral neurons*

		Surface area $(\mu m^2)^a$	Mean number of terminals[b]	Volume $(\mu m^3)^c$	Pre- to postsynaptic volume ratio[d]
Average large neuron	Cell body	7,250	1,450	57,906	0.075
	Dendritic tree	24,000	4,800	34,839	0.413
Average small neuron	Cell body	1,018	204	3,054	0.200
	Dendritic tree	4,500	900	3,449	0.783
Ten-μm-long dendrite segment	Diameter (10 μm)	314	62.8	785	0.240
	Diameter (2 μm)	62.8	12.56	31.4	1.200
	Diameter (1 μm)	31.4	6.28	7.85	2.400

[a] Cell body: πD^2, using the mean diameter of 49 μm for the large and 18 μm for the small neurons, derived from treating the directly measured cross-sectional areas, of more than 50,000 neurons from all areas of L_7 spinal gray of three dogs, as circles (Gelfan and Tarlov, 1963). Dendritic tree: $\pi r \sqrt{r^2 + h^2}$, treating the sum of all measured dendrite lengths (h) in tree, times $\pi/2$ average length correction, as a cone, with the determined mean primary dendrite diameters of large and small neurons, times 0.5, serving as radii (r) of the cone base (Gelfan et al., 1970). Ten-μm-long dendrite segment: $2\pi rh$, treating segment as cylinder.

[b] Synaptic density of 20 knobs per 100 μm^2 of receptive surface area (Gelfan and Rapisarda, 1964) times mean surface areas of each of cell body, dendritic tree, and 10-μm-long dendrite segment.

[c] $\pi D^3/6$ for cell bodies, treated as sphere; $(\pi/3)r^2h$ for dendritic tree, treated as cone; $= \pi r^2h$ for 10-μm-long dendrite segments, treated as cylinder.

[d] $\dfrac{(2) \times 3 \; \mu m^3 \; \text{(mean terminal volume; see footnote 2)}}{\text{volume of postsynaptic component}}$

greater than the terminal/cell body volume ratio (Table 1). With a constant synaptic release rate per terminal, the materials transneuronally transferred would be diluted postsynaptically to some five-fold greater extent in the cell body, on the average, than in the dendroplasm. What is more, such dilution in the dendroplasm must decrease with progressive tapering of dendrite segments with increasing distances from cell body. About 12.5 μm^3 of the volume of a 10-μm-diameter dendrite segment, on the average, is "serviced" by one terminal. One-tenth of this volume in a 1-μm-diameter segment is serviced by one terminal, with a mean volume of 3-μm^3, which is more than twice as great as this postsynaptic volume (Table 1). Any preemption of the neurotrophic material by the postsynaptic membrane should not alter the variability of the contributory proportion between postsynaptic cytoplasm and presynaptic material toward the maintenance of membrane integrity and functional properties more or less according to the pre- and postsynaptic volume relationship indicated in Table 1.

GRADATIONS OF DEPENDENCY UPON NEUROTROPHIC FACTORS

The implication from the above considerations of a gradient dependent upon neurotrophic factors was foreshadowed by the report on the dendritic tree size of denervated spinal neurons (Gelfan et al., 1972). It was observed that the more slender dendrites, the segments of the dendritic tree located more than 100 μm from the cell body, were the ones missing from the surviving denervated neurons (Fig. 5). It was therefore concluded that "the dependency of distal segments on the neurotrophic factors may thus increase, with increasing distances from cell body, as a consequence of the decreasing availability of the materials provided by the dendroplasmic flow from cell body" (Gelfan et al., 1972). It is the very viability of the more distal radiations of the dendritic tree in this case that is dependent upon neurotrophic factors. It was therefore proposed "that some minimal amount of 'trophic' factor, or factors, provided transneuronally by the synaptic endings, is indispensable for the dendrites and their branches; that this dependence upon trophic transmission is a continuous one in the same sense as is the dependence upon molecular O_2; and that those portions of the dendritic tree whose supply of the trophic factor is reduced below the minimal level by denervation promptly succumb and are sloughed."

The mean synaptic density on the perikarya of surviving neurons in the hind-limb rigidity preparation is reduced to a considerably greater extent than on the surviving more proximal portion of the dendritic tree (Gelfan and Rapisarda, 1964). The possibility that even the proximal part of the tree is more dependent upon neurotrophic factors than the cell body would be consistent with the difference in the pre- to postsynaptic volume ratios between these two components of the neuron, including the greater total connectivity of the dendritic tree with other neurons (Table 1). Apparently, the size of the dendritic tree in cortical neurons of maturing

---

FIG. 5. Summary of effects of severe denervation on size of dendritic tree, based on means of measured parameters of entire unselected sample of 360 neurons from L_7 segments of three normal dogs and of entire unselected sample of 300 neurons from L_5 to L_7 segments of three dogs with experimental hind-limb rigidity of 14 to 28 days duration, in Golgi-Kopsch preparations. Mean sizes of small and large neuron samples schematically represented in single plane within concentric circles separated by 20 μm. Means of measured perikaryon cross-sectional areas compressed into circles. Fractions of mean numbers of primary dendrites, with and without branches, and mean number of branches per neuron compensated for by appropriate increase or decrease in mean lengths. Lengths of all components, diameter of perikarya and primary dendrites according to magnification scale. The side panels represent the mean dendritic tree sizes as single extensions, segmented into p dendrites without branches (1), with branches (2) and branches (3), including the mean number of each of these per neuron. The lengths in the side panels are also according to the magnification scale in the center of diagram but the diameters are further magnified approximately four times. (From Gelfan et al., 1972.)

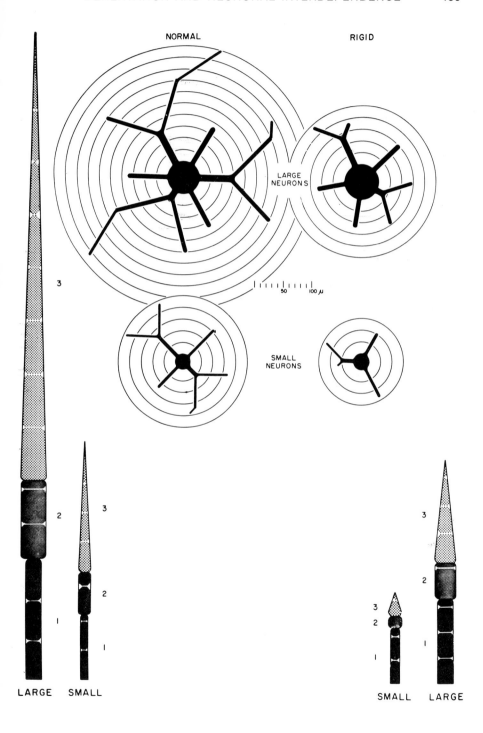

animals can also be influenced by "use" (rearing complexity) and "disuse" (sensory deprivation), that is, by the size of the total synaptic input (Greenough, Volkmar, and Juraska, 1973; and references therein).

In contrast, the axons and axon terminals in severely denervated neurons appear to be least or not at all dependent upon neurotrophic materials from other neurons. To be sure, there is an almost complete absence of the largest terminals on the receptive surfaces of surviving neurons in the L_7 population of dogs with hind-limb rigidity. But this is attributed to a higher mortality rate during the ischemic episode of those neurons in the intrinsic system whose axons have the largest-sized terminals. The means of the terminal parameters of the surviving axons within the narrowed size range, however, are the same as those of the neurons from the normal animals (Gelfan et al., 1974).[3] The axonal extensions of surviving neurons, in contrast to their cell bodies and dendritic extensions, also do not seem to suffer functional alterations (Gelfan, 1966). Whereas about 50% of the neuronal receptive surface of spinal neurons is covered by terminals from other neurons, the axon, the output channel of the neuron for both impulses and trophic materials to other neurons, is itself not "innervated"; except on the axon hillock of adult cat spinal neurons (Conradi, 1969b; Saito, 1972) and occasional axoaxonal junction.[4] The morphologic integrity and functional characteristics of the axonal extension normally appear to depend essentially upon the axoplasmic flow from its cell body, and this transport system seems to be least or not at all affected by severe denervation of the rest of the neuron.[5]

CONCLUSION: THE FUNCTIONAL ROLE OF NEUROTROPHIC FACTORS

The conclusion that denervation is responsible for the truncation of the more distal portion of the dendritic tree in the hind-limb rigidity preparation, as stated at the beginning of this chapter, constitutes an extension of the concept of neuronal interdependence. In this case the materials furnished by the terminals, together with those of the dendroplasm, are metabolically indispensable. It is postulated that the continuous supply of these metabolic requirements by the terminals becomes critical for the slender dendritic extensions because of the large increase in the pre- to postsynaptic volume ratio with dendrite attenuation. It is held, however, that the role of neurotrophic factors in the maintenance of membrane integrity for appropriate and normal responses of both cell body and dendrites is also a continuous

---

[3] The samples of terminals upon which the computations for Figs. 1 through 4 are based, therefore, are from L_7 segments of both the normal dog and the dog with experimental hind-limb rigidity.

[4] In the sample of terminals whose postsynaptic contact surfaces were identified, only slightly more than 3% were axoaxonal, with the largest contact length not exceeding 1.75 μm.

[5] It has also been known for some time that the electrophysiologic characteristics of axons normally differ from those of cell bodies and their dendrites.

one. It had already been noted that the stabilizing influence of neurotrophic factors upon postsynaptic structures "is not an unimportant aspect of the totality of integrative processes" (Gelfan, 1963). This may now be amplified.

The constancy and orderliness of performance, rather than randomness, under any given set of conditions and the unity of function are guaranteed by the precision and constancy of response of each neuron in the vast and intact intercommunication network. For such precision there must be practically an invariance in the sequence of electrochemical events involved in excitation and inhibition, an invariance in the physical constants of the participating components. It is proposed that the maintenance of such constancy of the physicochemical parameters, the local homeostasis, depends in each neuron upon the neurotrophic factors continuously supplied transneuronally by the neurons with which it is in contact. A reduction in the supply of these neurotrophic factors, as by partial denervation, will modify the neurophysiologic characteristics. That is, such characteristics are not fixed and unalterable. This lability is no doubt a factor in the so-called "plasticity" of the nervous system. The altered characteristics will influence, modify the behavior of the affected neurons and with more severe denervation the behavior becomes abnormal; abnormal because such behavior no longer fits into the overall integration plan.

In the case of the dendrites, in which the electrophysiologic activities consist so much of electrotonic propagation, decremental conduction, graded responses, interaction between and summation of synaptic inputs, the final output by the primary dendrite to the cell body, after all the local processing of signals, should be particularly dependent upon the local homeostatic control. Without such control, there could be neither constancy nor predictability of performance.

The magnitude of the neuronal receptive surface, the synaptic density, and the size of the neuronal population provide some indication of the scope of neuronal interdependence and its role in the functional organization of the central nervous system.

ACKNOWLEDGMENTS

The data upon which the computations were carried out were accumulated in the past years with the support of Research Grants NS 04417 from the National Institutes of Health, Bethesda, Maryland. The author is also grateful for computer assistance by the staff of the Biomedical Information Processing Center of this institution.

REFERENCES

Aitken, J. T., and Bridger, J. E. (1961): Neuron size and population density in lumbosacral region of the cat's spinal cord. *J. Anat.*, 95:38–53.

Colonnier, M. (1964): Experimental degeneration in the cerebral cortex. *J. Anat.*, 98:47–54.
Conradi, S. (1969*a*): Ultrastructure and distribution of neuronal and glial elements on the motoneuron surface in the lumbosacral spinal cord of the adult cat. *Acta Physiol. Scand. (Suppl.)*,
332:5–48.
Conradi, S. (1969*b*): Observations on the ultrastructure of the axon hillock and initial segment
of lumbosacral motoneurons in the cat. *Acta Physiol. Scand. (Suppl.)*, 332:65–84.
Drachman, D. B., editor (1974): *Trophic Functions of the Neuron. Ann. NY Acad. Sci.*, 228.
Gelfan, S. (1963): Neurone and synapse population in the spinal cord: Indication of role in total
integration. *Nature*, 198:162–163.
Gelfan, S. (1964): Neuronal interdependence. In: *Organization in the Spinal Cord, Vol. 11:
Progress in Brain Research*, edited by J. C. Eccles and J. P. Schadé. Elsevier, Amsterdam.
Gelfan, S. (1966): Altered spinal motoneurons in dogs with experimental hind-limb rigidity.
J. Neurophysiol., 29:583–611.
Gelfan, S., Field, T. H., and Pappas, G. D. (1974): The receptive surface and axonal terminals
in severely denervated neurons within lumbosacral cord of the dog. *Exp. Neurol.*, 43:162–
191.
Gelfan, S., Kao, G., and Ling, H. (1972): The dendritic tree of spinal neurons in dogs with
experimental hind-limb rigidity. *J. Comp. Neurol.*, 146:143–174.
Gelfan, S., Kao, G., and Ruchkin, D. S. (1970): The dendritic tree of spinal neurons. *J. Comp.
Neurol.*, 139:385–412.
Gelfan, S., and Rapisarda, A. F. (1964): Synaptic density on spinal neurons of normal dogs and
dogs with experimental hind-limb rigidity. *J. Comp. Neurol.*, 123:73–96.
Gelfan, S., and Tarlov, I. M. (1959): Interneurons and rigidity of spinal origin. *J. Physiol.
(Lond.)*, 146:594–717.
Gelfan, S., and Tarlov, I. M. (1963): Altered neuron population in L_7 segment of dogs with
experimental hind-limb rigidity. *Am. J. Physiol.*, 205:606–616.
Globus, A., and Scheibel, A. B. (1967): Synaptic loci on parietal cortical neurons: terminations
of corpus callosum fibers. *Science*, 156:1127–1129.
Gray, E. G., and Hamlyn, L. H. (1962): Electron microscopy of experimental degeneration in
the avian optic tectum. *J. Anat.*, 96:309–316.
Greenough, W. T., Volkmar, F. R., and Juraska, J. M. (1973): Effects of rearing complexity on
dendritic branching in frontolateral and temporal cortex of the rat. *Exp. Neurol.*, 41:371–378.
Guth, L. (1968): "Trophic" influence of nerve on muscle. *Physiol. Rev.*, 48:645–687.
Gutmann, E., editor. (1962): *The Denervated Muscle.* Czechoslovak Academy of Sciences,
Prague.
Gutmann, E. (1964): Neurotrophic relations in the regeneration process. In: *Mechanisms of
Neural Regeneration, Vol. 13: Progress in Brain Research*, edited by M. Singer and J. P.
Schadé. Elsevier, Amsterdam.
Gutmann, E., and Hník, P., editors. (1963): *The Effect of Use and Disuse on Neuromuscular
Functions.* Czechoslovak Academy of Sciences, Prague.
Jones, W. H., and Thomas, D. B. (1962): Changes in the dendritic organization of neurons in
the cerebral cortex following deafferentation. *J. Anat.*, 96:375–381.
Le Gros Clark, W. E. (1957): Inquiries into the anatomical basis of olfactory discrimination.
Proc. R. Soc. Lond. (Biol.), 146:299–319.
Matthews, M. R., and Powell, T. P. S. (1962): Some observations on transneuronal cell de-
generation in the olfactory bulb of the rabbit. *J. Anat.*, 96:89–102.
McLaughlin, B. J. (1972): The fine structure of neurons and synapses in the motor nuclei of the
rat spinal cord. *J. Comp. Neurol.*, 144:429–460.
Saito, K. (1972): The initial segment of DSCT (dorsal spino-cerebellar tract) neurons in the
cat. *J. Electron Microsc. (Tokyo)*, 21:325–326.
Valverde, F. (1968): Structural changes in the aria striata of the mouse after enucleation. *Exp.
Brain Res.*, 5:274–292.
Westrum, L. E., White, L. E., Jr., and Ward, A. A., Jr. (1964): Morphology of the experimental
focus. *J. Neurosurg.*, 21:1033–1046.
White, L. E., Jr., and Westrum, L. E. (1964): Dendritic spine changes in prepyriform cortex
following olfactory bulb lesions — rat, Golgi method. *Anat. Rec.*, 148:410.

Advances in Neurology, Vol. 12, edited by
G. W. Kreutzberg, Raven Press, New York
© 1975.

Dendrites and Neuroglia Following Hemisection of Rat Spinal Cord: Effects of Puromycin

Jerald J. Bernstein,* Michael R. Wells, and Mary E. Bernstein

*Department of Neuroscience and Ophthalmology, University of Florida, College of Medicine, Gainesville, Florida 32610, and *Department of Pathology, Hadassah Medical School, Jerusalem, Israel*

Hemisection of the mammalian spinal cord results in hemiplegia with a concomitant alteration in the spinal cord just proximal to the hemisection. This lesion results in recombination of the intramedullary neuronal synaptic complement (Bernstein, Gelderd, and Bernstein, 1974) and an alteration in dendritic (Bernstein, 1970; Bernstein and Bernstein, 1971, 1973; M. E. Bernstein and Bernstein, 1973), and perikaryal morphology (Cragg, 1970; Bernstein and Bernstein, 1973) in the spinal cord just proximal to the lesion. Following spinal cord hemisection there is a progressive formation of varicosities on the dendrite, starting at the periphery, which eventually involves the entire dendrite (Bernstein and Bernstein, 1971, 1973; M. E. Bernstein and Bernstein, 1973). The dendritic varicosities form after partial deafferentation of intramedullary neurons and have been shown to act as postsynaptic sites for regenerating axons or as axonal sprouts or both (Bernstein and Bernstein, 1971, 1973). However, the mechanism of varicosity formation is not known.

Varicosity formation may be related to alterations of dendritic neuroplasmic flow rate following deafferentation, since deafferentation results in decreases in neuronal RNA synthesis (Kupfer, 1966) and thus protein synthesis. Recent findings have shown that there is a neuroplasmic flow rate in dendrites of about 3 mm/hr following iontophoretic injection of radioactive amino acids into neurons (Schubert, Lux, and Kreutzberg, 1971; Kreutzberg, Schubert, Toth, and Rieske, 1973). The neuroplasmic transport rate into motoneuron dendrites can be decreased by the application of colchicine (Schubert, Kreutzberg, and Lux, 1972). The dendritic neuroplasmic flow can be altered by drugs that decrease axoplasmic flow resulting in the loss of neurotubules.

The production of new protein within limited periods of time has been shown to be an important factor in the inhibition of the onset of supersensitivity in muscle (Grampp, Harris, and Thesleff, 1971, 1972). Inhibition of protein synthesis in muscle results in the failure of denervated muscle to attain the physiologic criteria for supersensitivity. Because muscles that are denervated are receptive to reinnervation at the original sole plate (Guth, 1962), there appears to be a correlation between supersensitivity, ability to receive innervation, and the production of new protein soon after denervation. Since dendritic varicosities have been shown to act as postsynaptic sites for regenerating axons or axonal sprouts or both (Bernstein and Bernstein, 1971, 1973), the continued growth of intramedullary axons may be enhanced by the removal of potential postsynaptic sites proximal to the lesion by suppression of dendritic varicosity formation. The following experiments were undertaken to study the effect of protein inhibition (puromycin) on varicosity formation on dendrites and on the neuroglial reaction following spinal cord hemisection in the rat.

PROCEDURE

Sixty-four male, adult, Long-Evans hooded rats weighing approximately 225 g were used in this series of experiments. All operations were performed using chloral hydrate anesthesia (5 mg/kg). In addition to normals, animals were utilized 5, 7, 10, 14, 30, 45, 60, and 90 days postoperatively.

The spinal cords of a group of animals were hemisected with a scalpel following laminectomy at the T2 vertebra. Care was taken to avoid the dorsal and ventral roots. The musculature and skin were then sutured. Experimental animals had the spinal cord hemisected and a Gelfoam sponge saturated with a 1-mM solution of puromycin dihydrochloride (Sigma) dissolved in sterile water placed in the lesion site. A series of carrier control animals was prepared in which Gelfoam saturated with only sterile distilled water was placed in the site of hemisection. These animals were utilized to assess the effects of the Gelfoam and water alone.

On each designated postoperative day, the spinal cords of two normal, two hemisected, two Gelfoam water implants, two Gelfoam puromycin implants were prepared for Golgi impregnation or electron microscopy. The spinal cord, 0 to 5 mm proximal to the lesion, was studied.

ALTERATION FOLLOWING HEMISECTION ALONE AND HEMISECTION, GELFOAM, WATER IMPLANTATION

Histology of the Dendrite

The dendritic alterations to be described from the Golgi-impregnated material were similar following hemisection alone or hemisection, Gelfoam, distilled water implant (carrier control), and will be described simultaneously. Five days after lesion, the motoneurons in the first 5 mm appeared essentially normal (Fig. 1A). The dendritic shaft was widest at the primary dendrite and tapered through the various bifurcations to the peripheral

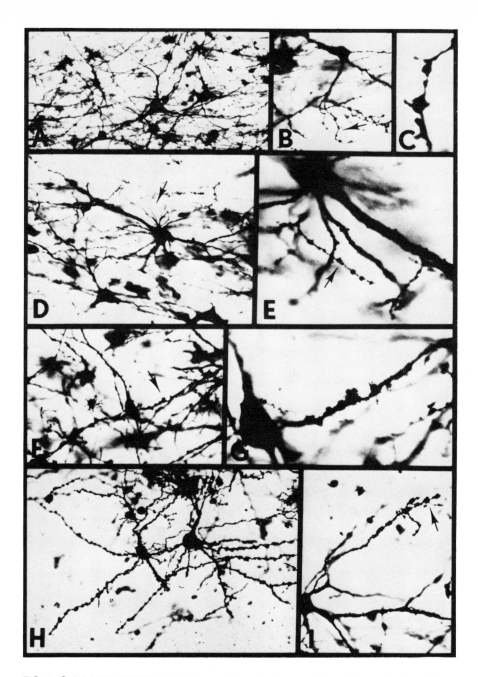

FIG. 1. Golgi-impregnated motoneurons following hemisection of the spinal cord alone or following distilled water, Gelfoam implantation (A–H). (A) At 5 days postoperative the motoneuron appears normal. (B,C) At 10 days varicosities were observed on peripheral dendrites. (D,E) At 14 to 15 days the numbers of varicosities increase along the dendritic shaft. There is a concomitant loss of the terminal dendrite. (F,G) By 30 days entire dendrites could be varicose, whereas other dendrites of the same neuron were not involved. (H) At 90 days all dendrites were varicose, the dendritic field was reduced and fewer branches were seen on dendrites. (I) Beginning at 60 to 90 days after hemisection and puromycin implantation there were occasional dendritic varicosities on some terminal dendrites of motoneurons.

dendrite. The dendritic shaft had few dendritic spines and was more or less cylindrical.

After 10 days postoperative, varicosities were observed on the terminal dendrites (Fig. 1B,C). These varicosities were joined by areas of dendrite that were cylindrical and of various diameters. The varicosities were irregular in outline and often had short processes extending from their borders. There was also a concomitant loss of the fine terminal dendritic processes.

At 14 days, increased numbers of varicosities were observed on the peripheral dendrite with increased dendritic involvement (Fig. 1D,E). At this time occasional varicosities were observed on secondary dendrites. The dendritic field was further reduced by the additional loss of fine terminal dendrites.

At 30 days postoperative there was a further reduction in the dendritic field of the neurons by the loss of fine terminal dendrites. Entire dendrites were varicose (Fig. 1F,G). The process of varicosity formation did not occur on all dendrites since there were dendrites that were free of varicosities (Fig. 1F). Usually dendrites that formed varicosities were oriented toward the lesion or a degenerating tract.

At 60 to 90 days after hemisection, the varicosity formation process was completed. The large majority of dendrites observed had varicosities along their entire length (Fig. 1H). The dendritic field was severely reduced and dendrites were frequently unbranched.

Ultrastructure of the Dendrite

At 5 to 14 days the organelles of the dendrite appeared essentially normal; however, the numbers of mitochondria and vacuoles appeared to be slightly increased. There were also areas of expanded smooth endoplasmic reticulum. Postsynaptic membrane specializations were observed which abutted expanded extracellular space or were opposing a neuroglial process. From 5 to 14 days these postsynaptic membrane specializations decreased in number and were difficult to locate. During this time period there was an increase in the number of dendritic subsurface cisterns that peaked at 30 to 45 days. The dendritic membrane adjacent to the cistern abutted enlarged extracellular space or was in apposition to a neuroglial cell process. At 30 days the numbers of varicosities had increased. The varicosities contained the organelles normally associated with dendrites. The neurofilaments, neurotubules, and mitochondria in the varicosities appeared normal. However, there appeared to be increased numbers of vacuoles and areas of expanded smooth endoplasmic reticulum associated with the varicosities. Normal boutons were observed to make synaptic complexes in the indentations of the surface of the varicosity. The remaining portion of the varicosity could be adjacent to enlarged extracellular space or in apposition to a neuroglial process (Fig. 2B) and could not be innervated. There were no dif-

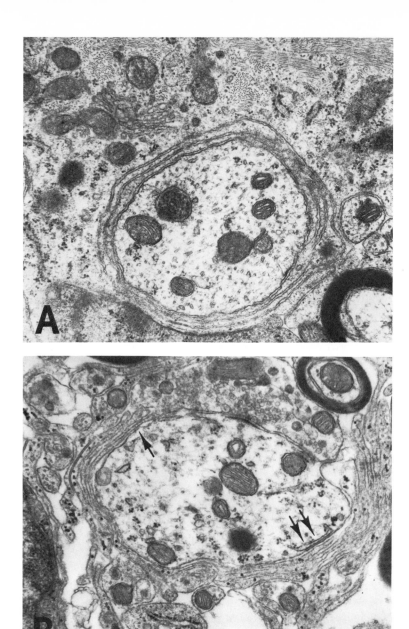

FIG. 2. (A) Dendrite of ventral horn neuron encapsulated by a single neuroglial cell process (30 days after hemisection and Gelfoam saturated with sterile distilled water implantation). The encapsulating cell could be identified as an astrocyte. (×30,000.) (B) Dendrite of ventral horn neuron encapsulated by several neuroglial cell processes. Some processes were observed between the bouton and the dendrite, and others passed lateral to the bouton. The arrows indicate dendritic subsurface cisterns 45 days after hemisection. (×28,000.)

ferences in the ultrastructure of the dendrite or varicosities from 30 to 90 days postoperative.

Neuroglia

The Golgi-impregnated material revealed the classic picture of reactive neuroglial cells with gliosis and phagocytosis. However, the ultrastructural analysis over days postoperative was informative. At 5 to 14 days, the dendrite was surrounded by neuronal degeneration products. The classic types of degenerating boutons were observed along the dendritic shaft (light, dense, and some fibrillar). Increased extracellular space was prominent within the first 2.0 mm, and decreased to limited zones of degeneration or degenerating boutons 2.0 to 2.5 mm rostral to the lesion. At 7 to 10 days postoperative, neuroglial projections were observed along the dendritic shaft or varicosity. The neuroglial projections often surrounded the dendrite and were observed to have terminal processes that were overlying normal boutons or were inserted between a bouton and dendrite. At 30 to 90 days postoperative, the neuroglial processes were observed to form multilaminate projections on the dendritic shaft (Figs. 2A,B and 3A,B). These laminae usually had projections from more than a single neuroglial process. When it was possible to ascertain the cell of origin (Fig. 2A) the laminating cell was found to be an astrocyte.

The membranes of the neuroglial cell processes were usually distinct and were separated by a space approximately 100 to 250 Å. The projections could entirely surround a dendrite (Fig. 2A), partially surround a dendrite (Fig. 3B), surround a dendrite and a bouton, have projections inserted between the bouton and the dendrite, and/or wrap more than one dendrite (Fig. 2B). The number of laminae varied and could not be predicted. In general, there appeared to be a relationship between the number of laminae and the amount of extracellular space, the greater the space, the larger the number of laminae. The number of neuroglial laminae was most extensive at 0 to 2.0 mm proximal to the lesion where extracellular space was maximal. At 2.0 mm proximal to the lesion as many as eight neuroglial wraps were observed, whereas two to three wraps were most common 3.0 to 5.0 mm proximal to the lesion. Multilaminate neuroglial projections were often observed overlying dendritic subsurface cisterns (Figs. 2B and 3B). Adjacent membranes of multilaminate neuroglial cell projections could form intercellular attachments composed of pentalaminate (Barron, Chiang, Daniels, and Doolin, 1971) or quintuple-layered units (Peters, 1962) (Fig. 3A). The pentalaminate membrane units could be derived from neuroglial projections from the same or different neuroglia. The length and position of a pentalaminate membrane unit was not consistent. Not all dendrites observed had neuroglial projections and dendritic shafts and varicosities without neuroglial cell projections were observed.

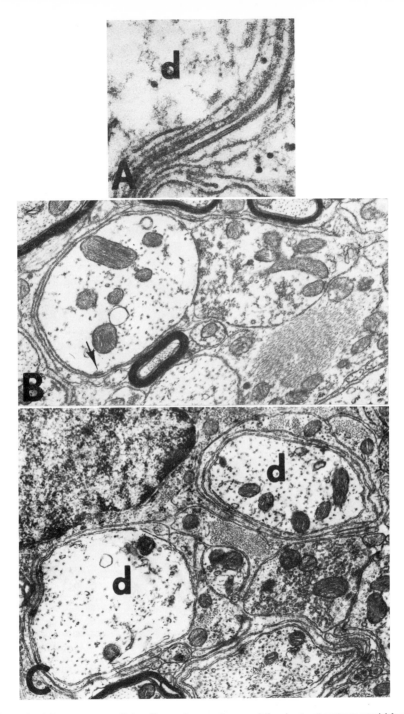

FIG. 3. (A) Adjacent neuroglial cell membranes in a multilaminate structure could form a pentalaminate or quintuple membrane unit 45 days after hemisection. (×72,000.) (B) Dendrites were also partially encapsulated and the neuroglial cell process could overlie a dendrite and a bouton. Arrow indicates a dendritic subsurface cistern 60 days after hemisection. (×15,000.) (C) Thirty days after hemisection and Gelfoam impregnated with puromycin implantation characteristic multilaminate projections of neuroglial cell processes were observed on dendrites. (×24,000.)

ALTERATIONS FOLLOWING GELFOAM, WATER, PUROMYCIN IMPLANTATION

Histology of the Dendrite

Five to 7 days after puromycin administration, the neurons within the first millimeter of the lesion were all necrotic. Neurons 2.0 to 5.0 mm from the lesion site were necrotic or appeared normal. At 7 days (Golgi-impregnated material) the dendrites of neurons that were not necrotic appeared normal from the primary shaft to the terminal portions of the dendrite. The dendrite was comparable to Fig. 1A. These findings were consistent up to 60 days postoperative. At 60 days, no neurons or dendrites were observed 1.0 mm from the site of lesion. Three to 5.0 mm from the lesion those neurons present appeared normal. At 60 days motoneuron dendrites were observed with terminal dendritic varicosities. The varicosities were few in number (one to three varicosities), were irregular in shape, and were joined by cylindrical portions of dendrite of varying length and diameter. The dendritic varicosity formation had stabilized and did not progressively involve more of the dendritic shaft between 60 and 90 days postoperative (Fig. 1I). There was no discernible difference between varicosity formation with puromycin at 60 to 90 days (Fig. 1I) and varicosity formation at the earliest stages (10 days, Fig. 1B,C) without puromycin administration. A summary of the various dendritic alterations are presented in Fig. 4.

Ultrastructure of the Dendrite following Puromycin Administration

Five to 7 days after puromycin treatment, the neurons in the first millimeter rostral to the lesion were necrotic. The nuclear and cytoplasmic membranes were fragmented. Mitochondria were greatly expanded and the membranes of the organelles were fragmented. Two to 5.0 mm rostral to the lesion, the neurons appeared normal, although there were occasional necrotic neurons. The dendritic neurotubules and neurofilaments appeared in normal proportions. However, the numbers of mitochondria and vacuoles appeared slightly elevated. Postsynaptic membrane specializations were observed which abutted extracellular space or were overlayed by a neuroglial cell process. Profiles of degenerating boutons and membraneous material were observed in the extracellular space. The cellular debris decreased according to the distance from the lesion. At 14 to 45 days the dendritic organelles appeared normal in ultrastructure and numbers. At 14 days, there were few postsynaptic membrane specializations that were not in a synaptic complex. By 30 days, the postsynaptic membrane specializations opposing enlarged extracellular space or neuroglia were rare. From 14 to 30 days there was an increase in the number of dendritic subsurface cisterns that peaked at 30 to 45 days and returned to normal levels by 60 days. The

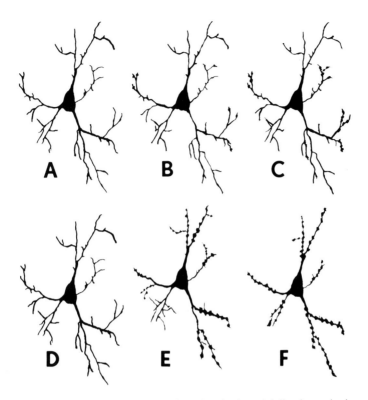

FIG. 4. Schematic of neuronal dendritic alteration in the rat following spinal cord hemi-section and puromycin administration (A–C), spinal cord hemisection alone or with hemisection and water, Gelfoam implantation (D–F). At 7 days after puromycin administration (A) the neurons appeared normal; at 60 days (B) there were a few terminal dendritic varicosities on occasional dendrites; and by 90 days (C) the numbers of dendritic varicosities stabilized. There was only a slight decrease in the dendritic field. In contrast, following hemisection alone or hemisection, Gelfoam, water implantation, the number of dendritic varicosities increased over days postoperative: (D) 5 days; (E) 30 days; (F) 90 days; there was an extensive and progressive loss of dendritic field.

dendrites were partially denervated, as normal synaptic complexes were observed over all postoperative days. At 60 days, varicosities were formed on the terminal dendrites but were difficult to locate in electron microscopy. When identified, the varicosities were of irregular shape, had increased numbers of vacuoles and areas of expanded smooth endoplasmic reticulum. The varicosities formed at 60 days with puromycin treatment were morphologically indistinguishable from varicosities seen in control animals.

Neuroglial Reaction after Puromycin Treatment

The Golgi-impregnated material revealed the classic picture of reactive neuroglial cells with gliosis and phagocytosis. The neuroglial cell types observed were indistinguishable from normal and controls. However, there was increased gliosis in the first millimeter rostral to the site of lesion caused by the complete loss of neurons by 30 days postoperative.

Ultrastructurally at 5 to 14 days the dendrites of the neurons 2.0 to 5.0 mm proximal to the site of hemisection were surrounded by degeneration products. The amount of degeneration products decreased passing proximally from the lesion. At 7 to 10 days postoperative, neuroglial projections were observed in apposition to dendrites. The neuroglial cell processes could entirely or partially surround a dendrite and include a normal bouton innervating the dendrite. At 30 to 90 days postoperative the neuroglial cell processes were observed to form multilaminate projections on dendritic varicosities or on the dendritic shaft. Three to 5.0 mm proximal to the lesion two to three neuroglial laminae were most frequently observed. The laminae could be formed from one neuroglial cell process or could have processes derived from two or more neuroglial cells. The multilaminate projections were often found to overlie a dendritic subsurface cistern. Areas of dendrite were also observed to be free of neuroglial cell processes. When the origin of the neuroglial cell projection could be established, it was found to be an astrocyte (Fig. 3C). The membranes of apposing neuroglial cell projections could form pentalaminate (Barron et al., 1971) or a quintuple membrane unit (Peters, 1962). A comparison of the neuroglial cell reaction of hemisected, carrier control, and puromycin-treated animals showed similar neuroglial cell reactions with reactive neuroglia responding to the lesion and cell necrosis (mechanically or drug induced) by proliferation, phagocytosis, and the encapsulation of neuronal dendritic processes. Puromycin did not appear to affect the neuroglial reaction to mechanical spinal cord injury.

NEURONAL RESISTANCE TO VARICOSITY FORMATION
AFTER HEMISECTION AND PUROMYCIN TREATMENT

These data show that puromycin treatment of neurons following spinal cord hemisection in the rat results in resistance to varicosity formation on dendrites, whereas puromycin does not affect the neuroglial reaction. These results are interesting in the context of the action of puromycin and the time period in which it is active. Puromycin is a bacteriostatic antibiotic that inhibits protein synthesis by disrupting translation of protein at the ribosome with the resultant formation of inappropriate puromycyl peptides rather than the normal protein constituent, as well as a variety of other metabolic effects (Barondes, 1970). The action of puromycin is relatively short as protein synthesis is resumed by 27 hr after direct application of the drug to the brain (Gambetti, Gonatas, and Flexner, 1968a,b; Barondes, 1970). The only ultrastructural change is the swelling of neuronal perikaryal mitochondria. This effect lasts for 36 hr after which time mitochondrial morphology returns to normal (Gambetti et al., 1968*a*,*b*). Thus 27 to 36 hr after direct application of puromycin to the brain in dosages sufficient to result in memory deficits, protein production and normal ultrastructural morphology are restored in neurons. The resistance to the formation of dendritic varicosities after puromycin treatment appears to be correlated with the production of new protein during a critical period of approximately 27 to 36 hr after the hemisection and drug application.

Following spinal cord hemisection the intramedullary neurons within 5 mm proximal of the lesion are partially deafferented (Bernstein et al., 1974). There is a decrease in RNA synthesis (Kupfer, 1966) with a concomitant decrease in protein production (Barondes, 1970) and the formation of dendritic varicosities (Bernstein and Bernstein, 1971, 1973) among other events such as neuronal membrane hypersensitivity. Because neurons are resistant to varicosity formation after puromycin treatment, there is a correlation between protein production and varicosity formation. The decreased protein synthesis following deafferentation of neurons may affect the rate of neuroplasmic transport into the dendrite (Schubert et al., 1971, 1972; Kreutzberg et al., 1973) and result in morphologic alteration perhaps caused by (1) decreased flow; (2) pulsating flow resulting from differential production of protein; (3) or sol–gel changes in dendritic protoplasm resulting in differential compressability caused by altered flow rates in the dendrite. Neuroplasmic flow rate into dendrites can be decreased by alteration of the transport mechanism through the application of colchicine in acute preparations (Schubert et al., 1972). However, it is not known if colchicine would reduce varicosity formation in chronically deafferented neurons thus relating availability of protoplasmic constituents with varicosities.

A signal for varicosity formation appears to be in part new protein production. Is the new protein production critical or is the production of different proteins critical? The neuroglial reaction apparently was not affected by the delay in protein synthesis as the puromycin-hemisected and hemisected neuroglial reactions were morphologically indistinguishable, although these cells had protein inhibition presumably in the same time period as neurons. This could be an indication that not only new but perhaps different protein must be produced by the neuron during a critical period of 27 to 36 hr after deafferentation for varicosity formation. When normal protein production resumes, sufficient protein is synthesized to allow a neuroglial reaction indistinguishable from that in animals hemisected alone, but varicosity formation on neuronal dendrites is extremely limited. This indicates that proteins different from those normally produced in the neuron are not produced in amounts sufficient to involve the entire dendritic complement in varicosity formation after puromycin treatment. Following protein inhibition some neurons do not appear to produce sufficient protein to sustain the neurons because of the necrotic neurons observed. However, those neurons that do show very limited varicosity formation appeared normal.

Puromycin treatment following hemisection of spinal cord resulted in the resistance of varicosity formation on intramedullary ventral horn neurons proximal to the site of lesion and thus effectively reduced part of the neuronal apparatus that attracts regenerating axons and sprouts (Bernstein and Bernstein, 1971, 1973). This mechanism may play an effective role in the attempts to regenerate growing axons in lesioned mammalian spinal cord by reducing the numbers of postsynaptic sites and resulting in the growth of central nervous axons into the distal spinal cord.

SUMMARY

Within 60 to 90 days of spinal cord hemisection or hemisection, Gelfoam, water implantation in the lesion site, ventral horn neurons 0 to 5 mm proximal to the site of lesion form varicosities along the dendrite. The varicosities form on peripheral dendrites at 10 days and progressively involve the entire dendritic shaft by 60 to 90 days. Following spinal cord hemisection and Gelfoam puromycin implantation the neurons in the ventral horn are resistant to varicosity formation. Sixty days after hemisection puromycin-treated neurons form a few varicosities on occasional peripheral dendrites with no further involvement of the dendrite by 90 days postlesion. The neuroglial reaction to hemisection is not altered by puromycin treatment. The correlation of inhibition of protein synthesis and resistance to dendritic varicosity formation is discussed.

ACKNOWLEDGMENTS

This work was supported by a grant (NS 06164) from the National Institute of Neurological Diseases and Stroke of the National Institutes of Health. The authors thank Ms. C. Lucas and G. Hunter for the histology.

REFERENCES

Barondes, S. H. (1970): Cerebral protein synthesis inhibitors block long-term memory. *Int. Rev. Neurobiol.,* 12:177–205.
Barron, K. D., Chiang, T. Y., Daniels, A. C., and Doolin, P. F. (1971): Subcellular accompaniment of axon reaction in cervical motoneurons of the cat. In: *Progress in Neuropathology,* edited by H. M. Z. Zimmerman, Vol. 1, pp. 255–280. Grune & Stratton, New York.
Bernstein, J. J. (1970): The relation of collateral sprouting to CNS regeneration. In: *The Enigma of Central Nervous System Regeneration,* edited by L. Guth and W. Windle, *Exp. Neurol. Suppl.,* 5:9–18.
Bernstein, J. J., and Bernstein, M. E. (1971): Axonal regeneration and formation of synapses proximal to the site of lesion following hemisection of the rat spinal cord. *Exp. Neurol.* 30:336–351.
Bernstein, J. J., and Bernstein, M. E. (1973): Neuronal alteration and reinnervation following axonal regeneration and sprouting in the mammalian spinal cord. *Brain Behav. Evol.* 8:135–161.

Bernstein, J. J., Gelderd, J., and Bernstein, M. E. (1974): Alteration of neuronal synaptic compliment during regeneration and axonal sprouting of rat spinal cord. *Exp. Neurol.,* 44:470–482.

Bernstein, M. E., and Bernstein, J. J. (1973): Regeneration of axons and synaptic complex formation rostral to the site of hemisection in the spinal cord of the monkey. *Int. J. Neurosci.,* 5:15–26.

Cragg, B. G. (1970): What is the signal for chromatolysis? *Brain Res.,* 23:1–21.

Gambetti, P., Gonatas, N. K., and Flexner, L. B. (1968a): Puromycin: Action on neuronal mitochondria. *Science,* 161:900–902.

Gambetti, P., Gonatas, N. K. and Flexner, L. B. (1968b): The fine structure of puromycin induced changes in mouse entorhinal cortex. *J. Cell. Biol.,* 36:379–390.

Grampp, W., Harris, J., and Thesleff, S. (1971): Inhibition of denervation changes in mammalian skeletal muscle by actinomycin-D. *J. Physiol. (Lond.),* 217:47P-48P.

Grampp, W., Harris, J., and Thesleff, S. (1972): Inhibition of denervation changes in skeletal muscle by blockers of protein synthesis. *J. Physiol. (Lond.),* 221:743–754.

Guth, L. (1962): Neuromuscular function after regeneration of interrupted nerve fibers into partially denervated muscle. *Exp. Neurol.,* 6:129–141.

Kreutzberg, G. W., Schubert, P., Toth, L., and Rieske, E. (1973): Intradendritic transport to postsynaptic sites. *Brain Res.,* 62:399–404.

Kupfer, C. (1966): Ribonucleic acid content and metabolic activity of lateral geniculate nucleus in monkey following afferent denervation. *J. Neurochem.,* 14:257–263.

Peters, A. (1962): Plasma membrane contacts in the central nervous system. *J. Anat.,* 96:237–248.

Schubert, P., Lux, H. D., and Kreutzberg, G. W. (1971): Single cell isotope injection technique, a tool for studying axonal and dendritic transport. *Acta Neuropathol. (Berl.),* 5:179–186.

Schubert, P., Kreutzberg, G. W., and Lux, H. D. (1972). Neuroplasmic transport in dendrites: Effect of colchicine on morphology and physiology of motoneurons in the cat. *Brain Res.,* 47:331–343.

Advances in Neurology, Vol. 12, edited by
G. W. Kreutzberg, Raven Press, New York
© 1975.

Quantitative Study on Dendrites and Dendritic Spines in Alzheimer's Disease and Senile Dementia

P. Mehraein, M. Yamada, and E. Tarnowska-Dziduszko

Max Planck Institute for Psychiatry, D-8000, Munich 40, Federal Republic of Germany

The classic morphologic changes found in cases of Alzheimer's disease and senile dementia are nerve cell loss, argyrophilic plaques, and neurofibrillar tangles. The dendritic tree also appears to be involved in this process, as was indicated by a recent electron-microscopic investigation of brain biopsies (Wisniewski and Terry, 1973). The investigation described in this chapter attempts to find light-microscopic support for such an involvement. Using the Golgi technique, quantitative aspects of dendritic morphology are studied in cases of senile dementia and Alzheimer's disease. This chapter shows that the extent of the dendritic tree as well as the density of spines are clearly reduced when compared to normal control cases.

METHODS AND MATERIALS

By means of a modified Golgi method developed by Kelemen and Yamada in our laboratory, it is possible to obtain a reliable demonstration of dendrites and dendritic spines in autopsy material stored in Formalin over an extended period of time. The essential steps of the method are as follows. The Formalin-fixed tissue blocks were incubated in a solution containing 3% potassium bichromate (150 ml), 96% ethylene alcohol (50 ml), and concentrated acetic acid (50 ml) for 24 hr at 37°C, and for 4 more days at room temperature after changing the solution twice. The tissue blocks were then kept for 5 days at room temperature in a 3% potassium bichromate solution. Following a thorough rinsing for 1 day in tap water and three washings in distilled water, the blocks were impregnated for $\frac{1}{2}$ to 1 hr in a 0.5% $AgNO_3$ solution, for a further 4 days at room temperature in a 1% $AgNO_3$ solution, three times briefly washed in distilled water, and again impregnated for 4 to 5 days in a 2% $AgNO_3$ solution. Following a thorough rinsing in distilled water (to prevent the formation of nonspecific precipitates) the tissue blocks were embedded in paraffin and 50 to 100-μm sections were prepared.

Using this method we carried out quantitative investigations on the apical dendrites from 20 cases with senile dementia, 15 cases with Alzheimer's disease, and 30 control brains. The test material was divided into two groups based upon the patient's age at the time of the first clinical manifestation of the disease; a diagnosis of senile dementia was made if the patient was 65 or more years of age. In each specimen a sample was selected from the cingulate gyrus and the hippocampus of the same brain section.

RESULTS AND DISCUSSION

The distribution of the spines along apical dendrites of the pyramidal cells of the fifth and third cortical layers was compared with that obtained in controls. In well-impregnated cells, the apical dendrite was subdivided into 50-μm segments starting from the soma. Generally, 7 to 11 segments (a to k) were studied so that a total length of 350 to 550 μm was evaluated. We investigated 30 to 50 cells per brain in each of the above-mentioned regions. The first curve obtained from the control brains shows the average spine density as a function of the distance from the cell body (Fig. 1). The control curve demonstrates that the number of spines increases sharply with increasing distance from the cell body after which the number plateaus. In some cells in which counting was possible over a longer distance (600 to 900 μm), a slight decrease in spine density was discernible after a distance of 500 to 600 μm. This near-logarithmic increase of the spine density confirms the observations of Valverde (1967) in mouse visual cortex and of Marin-Padilla (1967) in human auditory cortex. The second and third curves show the average values obtained from Alzheimer disease and senile dementia brains in comparison with the control curve.

In all segments a decrease in spine density in comparison to the control segments was observed (Fig. 1). The two groups were statistically compared by calculating the average values for single segments and by applying the Krustkal-Wallis test. For each of the segments c to i rejection levels were below 1%. Therefore, the statistical significance test shows a clear-cut decrease in spines for both diseases in the single segments as well as along the entire dendrite. A remarkable discrepancy between Alzheimer's disease and senile dementia was also noted, the spine density being smaller in the former than in the latter. Of further interest were changes in the spine distribution in the different segments. The spine decrease in segments near the soma was almost the same in both groups, yet the distal segments were less affected in the senile dementia group (Fig. 1). The statistical analysis revealed no significant difference between the two groups for segments c to e, but a significant difference at the 1% level was ascertained for segments g to i.

These results show that Alzheimer's disease and senile dementia are associated with a partial spine loss from the cortical pyramidal cells, at least as far as the cortex of the cingulate gyrus and Ammonshorn is concerned.

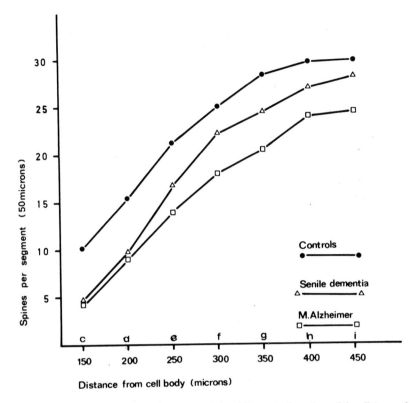

FIG. 1. Average density of spines in the apical dendrites as a function of the distance from the cell body. ●, Control brains; △, senile dementia, and □, Alzheimer's disease.

This "deafferentation" of the cortical cells is probably the primary morphologic change underlying the clinical picture of these diseases.

Evaluation of our material suggests a decrease in the number of dendrites and in the extent of the dendritic arborization in Alzheimer's disease and senile dementia. To verify this impression, we investigated Purkinje cells with our modified Golgi staining method. Although Purkinje cells are thought to be largely unaffected by these diseases, they are well suited to investigation because of their location and size. We studied two blocks, one each from the vermis and the posterior lobe, in 14 brains with Alzheimer's disease and senile dementia and in an equal number of control brains. The mean age was 65.3 years for the test group and 69.5 years for the control group. The clinical duration of the disease ranged from 1 to 20 years. All Purkinje cells sectioned along the plane of greatest dendritic spread were photographed. The photographs were enlarged and divided into 17 regions concentric to the nucleus.

For each cell the following parameters were determined.

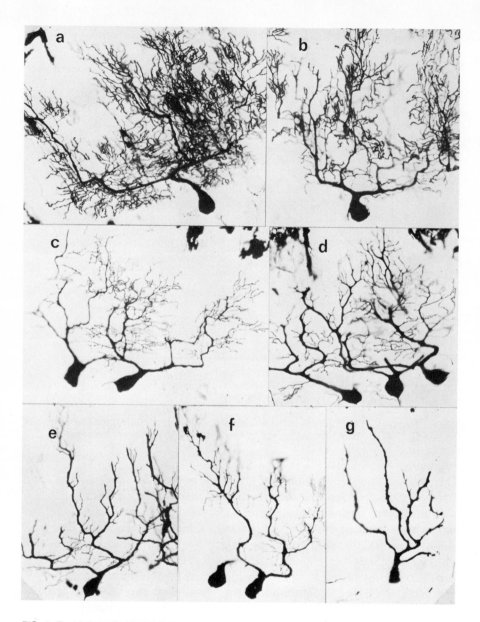

FIG. 2. Purkinje cells (Golgi staining) in normal cells (a,b); and showing a decrease of the dendritic arborization and extent in affected cells (c–g).

1. The sum of dendritic penetration into all regions (X_1)
2. The maximal dendritic penetration (X_2)
3. The smallest radius in which all dendrites were contained (X_3)

In each specimen arithmetic mean values were determined for each of the above-mentioned parameters. These mean values were calculated separately for the vermis and the posterior lobe. Combined mean values were calculated for the Alzheimer and senile dementia groups and compared with those of the control group. Brains from which only five or less cells were evaluated were not included. The statistical analysis was carried out with the Wilcox-Mann-Whitney test.

The mean value of density and extent of the dendrites (X_1) was 58.6 for the dorsal vermis of the test group compared with 105.0 for that of the control group. This indicates that dendrite density for the average test cell was reduced about one-half in comparison to those for the average control cell. Likewise, the mean value for the maximal zone penetration was about one-third smaller compared to the control mean value. In the posterior lobe the investigation led to a similar conclusion, but the difference between test and control group was smaller and the standard deviations were somewhat larger. In this region the largest difference was in the mean value for density of dendrites in the test group (56.9) versus that in the control group (91).

The mathematical treatment of these studies on Purkinje cells revealed a significant difference for density and extent per cell (X_1) for the dorsal vermis (0.1% level) and for the posterior lobe (2.5% level). The maximal arborization of dendrites (X_2) also revealed a significant difference between test and control groups — vermis: 0.1% level; hemisphere: 5% level. The dendritic lengths were significantly different at the 0.5% level in the vermis but were only at a 10% level in the posterior lobe. In conclusion, one can say that the statistical investigation has confirmed the impression gained from the study of the Golgi preparations. Comparison of the values showed the Purkinje cells to be heavily affected in the test group, their dendrites being shorter and reduced in number (Fig. 2). The involvement of these cells was found to be more extensive in the vermis than in the posterior lobe.

Generally, Purkinje cells are not considered to be affected in Alzheimer's disease. As shown in this material, changes in the dendrites also occur in Purkinje cells. This can be taken as an indication that Alzheimer's disease and senile dementia affect nerve cells throughout the central nervous system. This involvement consists essentially in a reduction of dendrite number and extent. Similar changes in dendrites can be produced, for example, by the experimental block of the dendritic transport in nerve cells (Schubert, Kreutzberg, and Lux, 1972). It may be assumed that such disturbances in the dendritic transport mechanism play a large role in Alzheimer's disease and in senile dementia.

REFERENCES

Marin-Padilla, M. (1967): Number and distribution of the apical dendritic spines of the layer V pyramidal cells in man. *J. Comp. Neurol.,* 131:475–490.

Schubert, P., Kreutzberg, G. W., and Lux, H. D. (1972): Neuroplasmic transport in dendrites: Effect of colchicine on morphology of motoneurones in the cat. *Brain Res.,* 47:331–343.

Valverde, F. (1967): Apical dendritic spines of the visual cortex and light deprivation in the mouse. *Exp. Brain Res.,* 3:337–352.

Wisniewski, H., and Terry, R. (1973): Morphology of the aging brain, human and animal. In: *Neurological Aspects of Mutation and Aging,* edited by D. H. Ford, pp. 167–186. Elsevier, Amsterdam.

Advances in Neurology, Vol. 12, edited by
G. W. Kreutzberg, Raven Press, New York
© 1975.

Virions and Virus-Associated Structures Within Dendrites in an Experimental Flavovirus Encephalomyelitis

K. Blinzinger, S. Luh, and A. P. Anzil

Electron Microscopy Unit, Department of Neuropathology, Max Planck Psychiatric Institute, Munich, Federal Republic of Germany

In viral encephalomyelitides, local spread of the infectious process is probably based on passive virus transfer along the intercellular gaps of the neuropil (Blinzinger and Müller, 1971) and/or on virus transport by infected mobile cells (Simon, Peters, Blinzinger, Magrath, and Boulger, 1970). Generalized virus dissemination throughout the neuraxis requires different mechanisms. One such mechanism could be a sequential infection of nerve cells the perikarya which are far apart from each other and which nonetheless are in contact with each other by means of their processes (for literature, see Johnson and Mims, 1968). In this chapter we present some pertinent findings and we discuss them in relationship to such a hypothetical mechanism.

MATERIALS AND METHODS

Thirty adult Swiss albino mice weighing approximately 20 g were inoculated intracerebrally with 17 D vaccine strain of yellow fever virus. Each received 0.02 to 0.03 ml of a freshly prepared suspension of the lyophilized agent in saline, diluted according to the manufacturer's prescription for human vaccination (Pasteur Institute, Paris). The animals developed hind-leg paralysis and other signs of central nervous system involvement between the 7th and 10th day postinoculation. Ten mice in a moribund stage were selected for pathomorphologic studies. They were sacrificed by whole-body perfusion through the ascending aorta with a 4% glutaraldehyde solution adjusted with phosphate buffer at pH 7.2 to 7.4. Specimens from both cerebral cortex and lumbar spinal cord were postfixed with osmium tetroxide and embedded in Epon 812. Examination of ultrathin sections stained with uranyl acetate and lead citrate was carried out with a Zeiss EM 9A electron microscope at magnifications of ×1,900 to ×41,000.

OBSERVATIONS

Ultrastructural details of the encephalomyelitic process evoked in mice by inoculation with yellow fever virus have already been described (Blinzinger, 1972, 1975). The following is an account of our observations concerning dendrite involvement. Numerous nerve cells contained newly formed virions as well as vesicular and rod-like formations characteristic of flavovirus infections (for literature, see Blinzinger, 1975). Progeny particles and the structures closely associated with them occurred not only within neuronal perikarya but also, though less frequently, in dendrites of different caliber including terminal ramifications and spines (Figs. 1 to 4). Intradendritic viral material was encountered more regularly in the spinal than in the cortical neuropil. Sometimes large complexes of free and membrane-bound viral collections, ribosomes, and mitochondria occupied a considerable portion of the dendritic profiles (Figs. 1 and 2).

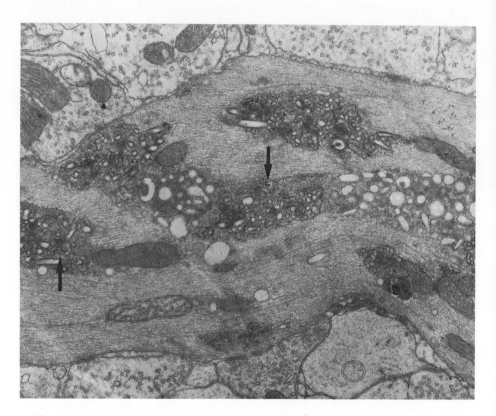

FIG. 1. Stem dendrite of a spinal motoneuron containing large collections of viral materials of varied appearance. Some virus particles (*arrows*) become recognizable at this magnification. Diminution of neurotubules goes along with filamentous overgrowth. (×18,000.)

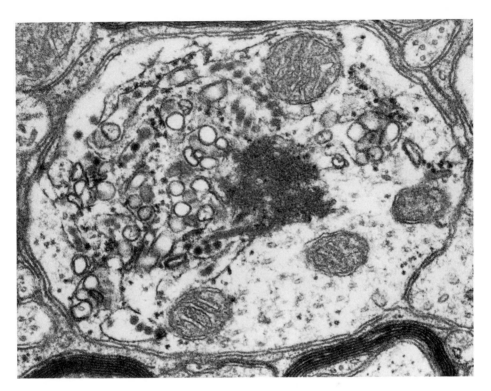

FIG. 2. Medium-sized dendrite packed with virions, vesicles, rod-like structures, mitochondria, ribosomes, and an electron-opaque, finely granular substance. (×54,000.)

Vacuoles containing virions and/or virus-associated structures occurred very often close to and sometimes in immediate contact with the dendritic plasmalemma (Fig. 3). A few virus-laden vacuoles appeared to be about to fuse with postsynaptic membranes (Fig. 4). Actual discharge of vacuole

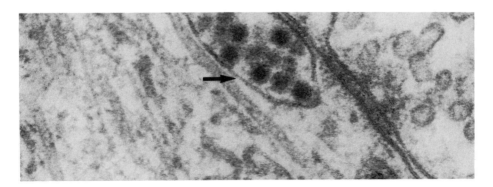

FIG. 3. Axodendritic synapse: cytoplasmic vacuole filled with virus particles (*arrow*) lying close to the postsynaptic segment of the dendrite membrane. (×123,000.)

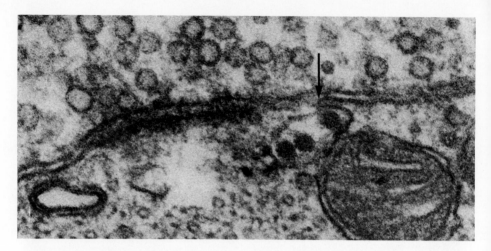

FIG. 4. Axodendritic synapse: a virus-laden vacuole appears to be about to open into synaptic cleft. Point at which vacuole membrane and postsynaptic dendrite membrane are continuous indicated by arrow. (×123,000.)

content into a synaptic cleft was never seen. In contrast, virus particles were sometimes present within distended intercellular gaps adjacent to synaptic clefts. Normal constituents of the affected dendrites appeared for the most part to be essentially unaltered. A small number of apical dendrites of spinal motoneurons exhibited reduction of the neurotubular system and filamentous hypertrophy (Fig. 1). Some dendritic terminals crowded with viral material were shrunken and condensed. Unequivocal evidence of virions inside axons was found very rarely. However, because of the close resemblance of virus particles and dense-cored synaptic vesicles, it was always difficult and often impossible to identify positively a given profile as belonging to the infectious agent or to the host. The distinct vesicular and rod-like elements spatially related to progeny particles in perikarya and dendrites, were never observed in axons.

DISCUSSION

The frequent observation of virions and virus-associated structures inside dendrites in our material raises the following possibilities: (1) either virus morphogenesis takes place within nerve cell bodies and to some extent also in dendrites, or (2) virus particles and structures spatially related with them are formed in neuronal somata and transported to the most peripheral parts of the dendritic tree; or (3) both possibilities are equally true.

The first explanation certainly holds true for the perikarya and cannot be dismissed for the dendrites, at least for the larger ones in which the biochemical and structural equipment required for establishing so-called virus factories is most probably also available (see Bell, Field, and Narang, 1971). However, the occurrence of viral material in the smallest telodendritic ramifications and the demonstration of a colchicine-sensitive somatofugal transport of several macromolecular substances within dendrites (Schubert, Kreutzberg, and Lux, 1972; Kreutzberg, Schubert, Tóth, and Rieske, 1973) forces us to give due consideration also to the second and third explanations. In this context it can be recorded that Sriurairatna, Bhamarapravati, and Phalavadhtana (1973) saw virions in dendrites of mice infected with another flavovirus, namely Dengue-2 virus. However, these authors interpreted their finding as indicative of viral propagation through the dendrites but failed to mention the possibility of intradendritic virus synthesis. Be that as it may, presence of virus particles in numerous dendritic ramifications will most likely facilitate the transmission of the agent from one neuron to many others (see Baringer and Griffith, 1970).

The present study provides no conclusive evidence about the mechanisms by which cell-to-cell infection at points remote from the perikarya actually occurs. However, some of our findings seem to suggest virus release at postsynaptic dendrite membranes by a process of "reverse pinocytosis" (Demsey, Steere, Brandt, and Veltri, 1974). Further steps along this pathway are speculative. Therefore, subsequent to virus discharge from the postsynaptic sites of a given nerve cell, infection of other neurons may take place by endocytosis of the agent at or near presynaptic axon terminals (Turner and Harris, 1973; Kristensson, Sheppard, and Bornstein, 1974), intraaxonal virus decoating (Gordon, Bensch, Deanin, and Gordon, 1968), and retrograde axoplasmic transport of the liberated nucleic acid to the perinuclear region (LaVail and LaVail, 1972). Completion of virus decoating in the outermost axonal segments could satisfactorily explain why virions are so infrequently encountered within this type of neurite in our material and in other experimental models as well (Baringer and Griffith, 1970; Gonatas, Margolis, and Kilham, 1971). When virus particles are observed in greater numbers inside axons, the agent probably replicates in the nucleus or perikaryon of the parent cells and spreads in an anterograde direction along the axon (Jenson, Rabin, Bentinck, and Melnick, 1969; Kristensson, Ghetti, and Wiśniewski, 1974).

SUMMARY

In experimental yellow fever virus encephalomyelitis of adult albino mice, virions, and virus-associated structures were observed not only inside neuronal perikarya but also within dendrites of varied size. The finding permits the following explanations: (1) either the viral agent is synthesized in the nerve cell bodies and transported intradendritically in a proximodistal direction; or (2) virus morphogenesis takes place in neuronal perikarya and dendrites as well; or (3) both possibilities are equally valid. Some incidental findings were suggestive of virus release at postsynaptic dendrite membranes. They are discussed with reference to a hypothetical long-distance pathway of viral dissemination involving endocytosis of the agent by presynaptic axon terminals, intraaxonal virus decoating, and retrograde axoplasmic transport of the infectious nucleic acid to the cell soma.

REFERENCES

Baringer, J. R., and Griffith, J. F. (1970): Experimental measles virus encephalitis. A light, phase, fluorescence, and electron microscopic study. *Lab. Invest.,* 23:335–346.

Bell, T. M., Field, E. J., and Narang, H. K. (1971): Zika virus infection of the central nervous system of mice. *Arch. Ges. Virusforsch.,* 35:183–193.

Blinzinger, K. (1972): Comparative electron microscopic studies of several experimental group B arbovirus infections of the murine CNS (CEE virus, Zimmern virus, yellow fever virus). *Ann. Inst. Pasteur,* 123:497–519.

Blinzinger, K. (1975): Vergleichende elektronenmikroskopische Untersuchungen bei experimentellen Infektionen mit dem fränkischen Zimmern-Virus (Stramm ZIU VIII-BM) und zwei bekannten Togaviren der Gruppe B. In: *Arboviruserkrankungen des Nervensystems, der Haut und innerer Organe in Europa,* edited by W. K. Müller and G. Schaltenbrand. Thieme, Stuttgart. (*In press.*)

Blinzinger, K., and Müller, W. (1971): The intercellular gaps of the neuropil as possible pathways for virus spread in viral encephalomyelitides. *Acta Neuropathol. (Berl.),* 17:37–43.

Demsey, A., Steere, R. L., Brandt, W. E., and Veltri, B. J. (1974): Morphology and development of dengue-2 virus employing the freeze-fracture and thin-section techniques. *J. Ultrastruct. Res.,* 46:103–116.

Gonatas, N. K., Margolis, G., and Kilham, L. (1971): Reovirus type III encephalitis: observations of virus-cell interactions in neural tissues. II. Electron microscopic studies. *Lab. Invest.,* 24:101–109.

Gordon, M. K., Bensch, K. G., Deanin, G. G., and Gordon, M. W. (1968): Histochemical and biochemical study of synaptic lysosomes. *Nature,* 217:523–527.

Jenson, A. B., Rabin, E. R., Bentinck, D. C., and Melnick, J. L. (1969): Rabiesvirus neuronitis. *J. Virol.,* 3:265–269.

Johnson, R. T., and Mims, C. A. (1968): Pathogenesis of viral infections of the nervous system. *N. Engl. J. Med.,* 278:23–30; 84–92.

Kreutzberg, G. W., Schubert, P., Tóth, L., and Rieske, E. (1973): Intradendritic transport to postsynaptic sites. *Brain Res.,* 62:399–404.

Kristensson, K., Ghetti, B., and Wiśniewski, H. M. (1974*a*): Study on the propagation of Herpes simplex virus (type 2) into the brain after intraocular injection. *Brain Res.,* 69:189–201.

Kristensson, K., Sheppard, R. D., and Bornstein, M. B. (1974*b*): Observations on uptake of Herpes simplex virus in organized cultures of mammalian nervous tissue. *Acta Neuropathol. (Berl.),* 28:37–44.

LaVail, J. F., and LaVail, M. M. (1972): Retrograde axonal transport in the central nervous system. *Science,* 176:1416–1417.

Schubert, P., Kreutzberg, G. W., and Lux, H. D. (1972): Neuroplasmic transport in dendrites: Effect of colchicine on morphology and physiology of motoneurones in the cat. *Brain Res.,* 47:331–343.

Simon, J., Peters, G., Blinzinger, K., Magrath, D., and Boulger, L. (1970): The pathogenic role of the inflammatory reaction in poliomyelitis. Immunofluorescence, electron-microscopic and virological studies with type 3 poliovirus. *Experientia,* 26:1241–1242.

Sriurairatna, S., Bhamarapravati, N., and Phalavadhtana, O. (1973): Dengue virus infection of mice: Morphology and morphogenesis of dengue type-2 virus in suckling mouse neurones. *Infect. Immun.,* 8:1017–1028.

Turner, P. T., and Harris, A. B. (1973): Ultrastructure of synaptic vesicle formation in cerebral cortex. *Nature,* 242:57–59.

Advances in Neurology, Vol. 12, edited by
G. W. Kreutzberg, Raven Press, New York
© 1975.

Pathology of Dendrites in Subacute Spongiform Virus Encephalopathies

Peter W. Lampert, D. Carleton Gajdusek, and
Clarence J. Gibbs, Jr.

*Department of Pathology, University of California at San Diego, La Jolla, California 92037
and National Institute of Neurological Diseases and Stroke, National Institutes of Health,
Bethesda, Maryland 20014*

The term subacute spongiform virus encephalopathies has been applied to a group of transmissible diseases that are characterized by a long incubation time lasting from months to years, a slowly progressive clinical course, and destructive changes restricted to the brain, which consist of vacuolar neuronal degeneration and gliosis without leukocytic infiltrates or any other evidence of an immune response (Gajdusek and Gibbs, 1973; Gibbs and Gajdusek, 1974). Scrapie, kuru, and Creutzfeldt-Jakob disease belong to this group of slowly progressive virus infections of the brain (Lampert, Gajdusek, and Gibbs, 1972). Scrapie occurs naturally in sheep and goats but can be transmitted to many species, notably mice. Kuru and Creutzfeldt-Jakob disease affect man. The infectious etiology of these diseases has been established by their transmission to chimpanzees (Gajdusek, Gibbs, and Alpers, 1966; Gibbs and Gajdusek, 1969). The exact nature of the causative viruses is still debated. The virus, although not visualized by electron microscopy, is closely related to membranes and can be inactivated by membrane-disrupting substances (Gibbs and Gajdusek, 1974). As demonstrated in this report alterations of membranes particularly in dendrites account for the pathognomonic spongiform alterations in the affected brains.

MATERIALS AND METHODS

Scrapie was studied in mice 4 to 5 months after intracerebral injection of scrapie-infected brain suspensions (Lampert, Hooks, Gibbs, and Gajdusek, 1971*b*). Cerebral cortex from chimpanzees afflicted with experimental kuru and Creutzfeldt-Jakob disease also served as material for this study (Lampert, Earle, Gibbs, and Gajdusek, 1969; Lampert, Gajdusek, and Gibbs, 1971*a*).

The brains of the mice were fixed by perfusion, whereas the cerebral cortex of chimpanzees was studied after fixation by immersion. The fixation consisted of 5% phosphate buffered glutaraldehyde and 1% buffered osmium tetroxide. Small blocks were dehydrated by graded alcohols and embedded in Epon or Araldite. Sections were prepared with an LKB ultramicrotome, stained with uranyl acetate and lead citrate and examined with a Siemens Elmiscope 101.

RESULTS

Status spongiosus and gliosis without inflammatory reactions were present in the gray matter of all affected animals (Fig. 1). The degree of the spongiform changes varied, being most marked in the cerebral cortex of chimpanzees afflicted with experimental kuru and least in experimental Creutzfeldt-Jakob disease. The vacuoles were located within the neuropil but rarely in perivascular regions suggesting that perivascular astrocytic foot processes were least responsible for the spongiform changes. This is in striking contrast to vacuolation of nervous tissue caused by autolysis or anoxia. Swollen nerve cells showing chromatolysis were present in severely altered cortex of affected chimpanzees (Fig. 2).

Electron microscopy showed the status spongiosus to correspond mainly to swelling and vacuolation of dendrites and perikaryal cytoplasm of nerve cells and to a lesser degree to the swelling of astrocytic processes adjacent to altered neurons. The affected dendrites or neuronal cytoplasm showed focal clear areas that were devoid of organelles but contained finely granular material. The surface membrane next to such clear cytoplasmic regions often revealed a rupture associated with curled fragments of membranes. Rows of vesicles or fragments of membranes demarcated the clear cytoplasmic portions in other neuronal processes (Fig. 3). Large vacuoles occurred in many dendrites that were identified by the presence of intact synaptic junctions (Fig. 4). These vacuoles were lined and occasionally filled by aggregates of curled fragments of membranes. Higher magnification of these fragments revealed the triple layered structure of unit membranes. When compared to adjacent normal plasma membranes they appeared slightly wider and more osmiophilic (Fig. 5). Other alterations pointing to damaged membranes consisted of fusion of cells and processes. At points of cell fusion, ruptured curled membranes were again prominent.

Apart from the pathognomonic swelling and vacuolation of neurons, there were other less specific pathologic features. Nerve cells contained abundant lipochrome pigment and some cells were filled with aggregates of randomly oriented straight tubules (Lampert et al., 1969, 1971a). There were also occasional dendrites filled with vesicles measuring about 350 Å in width. Degenerating axons filled with clumped disintegrated neurofilaments, mitochondria, and dense bodies were also noted. Myelin sheaths around degenerating axons were well preserved except when phagocytosed by macrophages. In such cells myelin was broken down into layered lamellae and homogenous lipid bodies. Astrocytes displayed a striking increase of glial filaments, ribosomes, mitochondria and glycogen granules, i.e., features seen in proliferated reactive astrocytes.

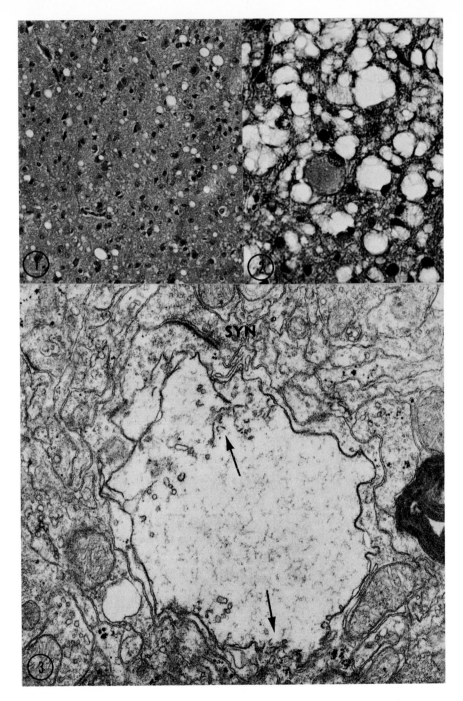

FIG. 1. Status spongiosus and glial proliferation in the cerebral cortex of a chimpanzee (A-54) afflicted with experimental Creutzfeldt-Jakob disease. (×165.)

FIG. 2. Swollen nerve cell showing chromatolysis in the vacuolated cerebral cortex of a chimpanzee (A-59) afflicted with experimental kuru. (×400.)

FIG. 3. Vacuolated dendrite in the cerebral cortex of a chimpanzee (A-82) with experimental Creutzfeldt-Jakob disease. Note fragments of membranes (*arrows*) and finely granular material within the vacuole. SYN, synapse. (×30,000.)

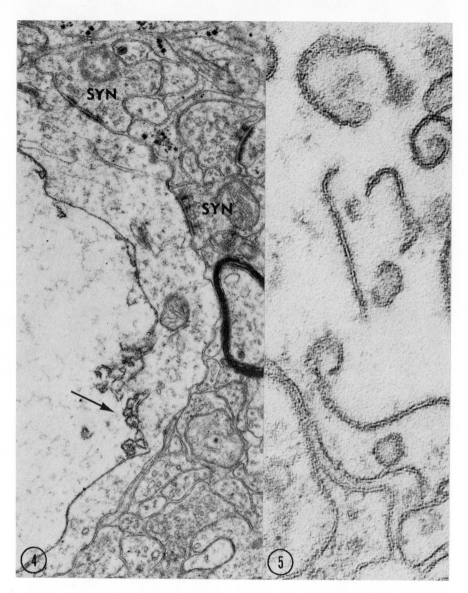

FIG. 4. Aggregates of curled fragments of membranes (arrow) at the margin of a vacuole within a dendrite in a chimpanzee (A-67) with experimental kuru. SYN, synapse. (×30,000.)
FIG. 5. Fragments of membranes at margin of a vacuolated neuronal process in chimpanzee (A-82) with experimental Creutzfeldt-Jakob disease. The abnormal membranes are slightly wider and more osmiophilic than normal plasma membranes at bottom of picture. (×150,000.)

DISCUSSION

The pathology of the gray matter in the transmissible spongiform encephalopathies consists of focal swelling and vacuolation of neurons in the absence of leukocytic infiltrates or other evidence of an immune response. Disrupted plasma membranes and aggregates of fragments of membranes are associated with the vacuolar alterations that lead to neuronal degeneration. Astrocytes in the vicinity of damaged neurons undergo similar hydropic changes and may fuse with nerve cells (Lampert et al., 1971), but in contrast to neurons they do not degenerate but react to injury by proliferation. Vacuoles are particularly prominent in dendrites that may reflect a predilection of the virus for postsynaptic endings or vacuolar degeneration secondary to changes in the neuronal perikaryon.

The properties of the infectious agents of scrapie, kuru, and Creutzfeldt-Jakob disease suggest a close association of the virus with membranes. The virus is susceptible to membrane-disrupting substances such as ether, periodate, urea, and phenol, but it is resistant to other procedures that usually destroy viruses such as UV and heat inactivation or exposure to acetylethylenamine, Formalin, RNAse, and DNAse (Gibbs and Gajdusek, 1974). Filtration experiments indicate that the scrapie virus measures about 20 to 30 nm, whereas the agent responsible for kuru and Creutzfeldt-Jakob disease has failed to pass through membranes with pores of 100 nm diameter. Tissue suspensions with high infectivity fail to show virus particles by electron-microscopy but always reveal abundant fragments of membranes. As emphasized in previous reports and demonstrated again in this chapter, the pathognomonic spongiform degeneration of neurons is associated with alterations of plasma membranes. Most conspicuous is the accumulation of curled fragments of membranes within and at the margin of intraneuronal vacuoles. Further studies are required to determine whether these unconventional viruses are indeed located within the abnormal membranes.

SUMMARY

The spongiform changes in the cerebral cortex of scrapie mice and of chimpanzees afflicted with experimental kuru and Creutzfeldt-Jakob disease were examined by electron microscopy. The pathognomonic findings consisted of swelling and vacuolation of neurons, particularly of dendrites. Fusion of swollen cells and processes occurred. The changes were associated with alterations of plasma membranes. Curled fragments of membranes accumulated at points of cell fusion and at the margin of vacuoles within dendrites. The abnormal membranes were wider and more osmiophilic than normal plasma membranes. These findings as well as other data on the nature of the atypical viruses of scrapie, kuru, and Creutzfeldt-

Jakob disease indicate that the infectious agents are closely associated with membranes and that alterations of neuronal membranes initiate the spongiform degeneration of neurons.

ACKNOWLEDGMENT

This work was supported by NIH grant no. NS 09053.

REFERENCES

Gajdusek, D. C., and Gibbs, Jr., C. J. (1973): Subacute and chronic diseases caused by atypical infections with unconventional viruses in aberrant hosts. In: *Perspectives in Virology, Vol. VIII: Persistent Virus Infection,* Edited by M. Pollard. Academic Press, New York.

Gajdusek, D. C., Gibbs, Jr., C. J., and Alpers, M. (1966): Experimental transmission of a kuru-like syndrome to chimpanzees. *Nature,* 209:794–796.

Gibbs, Jr., C. J., and Gajdusek, D. C. (1969): Infection as the etiology of spongiform encephalopathy. *Science,* 165:1023–1025.

Gibbs, Jr., C. J., and Gajdusek, D. C. (1974): Cell–virus interactions in slow infections of the nervous system. In: *The Neurosciences. Third Study Program,* edited by F. O. Schmitt and F. G. Worden. MIT Press, Cambridge, Massachusetts.

Lampert, P. W., Earle, K. M., Gibbs, Jr., C. J., and Gajdusek, D. C. (1969): Experimental kuru encephalopathy in chimpanzees and spider monkeys. *J. Neuropathol. Exp. Neurol.,* 28:353–370.

Lampert, P. W., Gajdusek, D. C., and Gibbs, Jr., C. J. (1971a): Experimental spongiform encephalopathy (Creutzfeldt-Jakob disease) in chimpanzees. Electron microscopic studies. *J. Neuropathol. Exp. Neurol.,* 30:20–32.

Lampert, P. W., Gajdusek, D. C., and Gibbs, Jr., C. J. (1972): Subacute spongiform virus encephalopathies. *Am. J. Pathol.,* 68:626–646.

Lampert, P. W., Hooks, J., Gibbs, Jr., C. J., and Gajdusek, D. C. (1971b): Altered plasma membranes in experimental scrapie. *Acta Neuropathol.,* 19:81–93.

Advances in Neurology, Vol. 12, edited by
G. W. Kreutzberg, Raven Press, New York
© 1975.

Dendritic Degeneration Following Hyperbaric Oxygen Exposure

J. D. Balentine

Department of Pathology, Medical University of South Carolina, Charleston, South Carolina 29401

INTRODUCTION AND BACKGROUND

Oxygen Toxicity

Exposure to excessive oxygen has long been known to be fraught with numerous detrimental effects since the early writings of Paul Bert in the nineteenth century (Bert, 1878). The nervous system is one of the more susceptible organ systems to the adversities of hyperbaric oxygen exposure. Acute central nervous system manifestations of oxygen toxicity have been well documented in man as well as in laboratory animals. Central nervous system (CNS) oxygen toxicity is especially a hazard above 3 to 4 atm of oxygen and may occur within less than 1 hr at that pressure. The principal manifestation consists of grand mal seizures, but may include focal motor seizures, constriction of visual fields, deafness, hyperacuity, changes of mood, and visual and auditory hallucinations (Behnke, Johnson, Poppen, and Motley, 1934; Donald, 1947). Inhibition of higher cortical function by high oxygen tensions has been observed in experimental animals (Bean and Wapner, 1943; L. Middaugh and J. D. Balentine, *unpublished observations*).

Biochemical data on oxygen toxicity have been abundant and persuasive in revealing profound and diverse effects on cellular function (Haugaard, 1968). High oxygen tensions inhibit over 42 enzymes (Davies and Davies, 1965), many of which are important in cellular respiration and energy production. In the CNS hyperoxia has not only resulted in inhibition of oxidative enzymes and ATP production but also in depletion of cerebral amines (Fairman, Mehl, and Meyers, 1971), possibly caused by inhibition of phenylalamine and tyrosine hydroxylases (Fisher and Kaufman, 1972), and interference with γ-aminobutyric acid metabolism (Wood, Watson, and Stacey, 1966).

Necrotic CNS Lesions of Hyperbaric Oxygenation

Selective neuronal necrosis of two basic patterns was observed by Balentine and Gutsche (1966) in rats paralyzed by 1-hr exposures, repeated on consecutive days, to 5 atm of oxygen. One pattern consisted of random necrosis of individual neuronal cell bodies within otherwise preserved regions of gray matter, affecting consistently the anterior medial horn cells of the entire spinal cord, the ventral cochlear nucleus, the nucleus of the spinal T5, and the superior olivary complex. The other pattern consisted of bilaterally symmetrical necrosis of nuclei involving supportive cells and their processes as well as neurons. The latter lesions consistently involved the globus pallidus and substantia nigra. The neocortex, corpus striatum, and hippocampus were spared, and the insensitivity of these areas to oxygen-induced necrosis has been confirmed by serial sectioning (Balentine, 1968).

Pathogenesis of the CNS Necrotic Lesions

Direct polarographic measurements of oxygen tensions in rats exposed to the same conditions of hyperbaric oxygen exposure resulting in the selective necrosis, reveal elevations of oxygen tensions in the oxygen-sensitive areas of the CNS and indicate that the necrotic lesions are probably associated with excessive tissue oxygenation (Ogilvie and Balentine, 1973, *in press*). These direct data are supported by the fact that ischemia protects the brain from the occurrence of the oxygen induced lesions (Balentine, 1968).

SUBCELLULAR CNS LESIONS OF HYPERBARIC OXYGENATION

Methods

In order to determine what subcellular events may be related to hyperbaric oxygenation, a model of exposure to oxygen insufficient to cause clinical manifestations of oxygen toxicity or necrosis was selected. After pilot studies were performed it was determined that a single 30-min exposure to 60 psig (approximately 5 atm) of oxygen would be suitable. Thirty-four female Sprague-Dawley rats weighing 150 to 200 g were subjected to this model of oxygen exposure and sacrificed at varying intervals after exposure: 30 min, 24 hr, 48 hr, 72 hr, 1 week, 2 weeks, and 30 days. The animals were fixed by perfusion with 1% paraformaldehyde and 2% glutaraldehyde in Millonig's phosphate buffer. Tissue from cervical anteromedial gray matter of the spinal cord, the neocortex, and substantia nigra was diced and postfixed in 2% osmic acid and embedded in Epon. Thick sections were stained with toluidine blue and thin sections with lead citrate and uranyl acetate. Comparable tissue from 18 anatomic control animals and 12 rats exposed to 60 psig of 5% oxygen in 95% nitrogen were similarly processed for electron microscopy. The ultrastructural findings in spinal cord gray matter along with further information on methodology are reported elsewhere in detail (Balentine, 1974).

Ancillary light-microscopic studies were also undertaken in order to ascertain the presence or absence of necrosis of neurons and to define better the anatomy of dendritic and axonal changes observed by electron microscopy. These consisted of coronally slicing portions of brain and spinal cord not processed for electron microscopy and embedding them in paraffin. Light-microscopic sections were cut from each block and stained routinely with hematoxylin and eosin. In addition, 24 more Sprague-Dawley female rats were exposed to the same model of oxygen exposure and sacrificed by perfusion with Susa's solution in a similar time sequence. Brains and spinal cords from these animals were cut coronally into 2 to 3-mm slices, which were embedded in paraffin. Routine sections from the blocks were stained with luxol fast blue and hematoxylin and eosin. The brain and spinal cord of four of these rats were serially sectioned on plastic filmstrip and stained with luxol fast blue, hematoxylin, and eosin. Serial sections of other selected paraffin- and Epon-embedded blocks from the animals studied by electron microscopy and from the ancillary study were obtained.

Because light-microscopic alterations of neurites, especially smaller

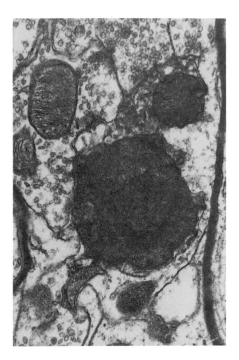

FIG. 1. Dense mitochondria in process interpreted as dendritic. Note larger mitochondrion, 0.94 μm in minimal diameter, with numerous haphazardly arranged cristae. Anterior horn gray matter of rat sacrificed 48 hr after a single 30-min exposure to 60 psig of oxygen. ($\times$34,000.)

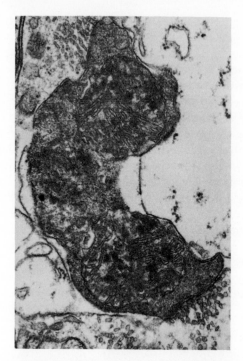

FIG. 2. Dendritic process with dense coarsely granular cytoplasm and mitochondria with dark matrices containing flocculent densities. Alterations indicative of dendritic degeneration. Anterior horn gray matter of rat sacrificed 48 hr after hyperbaric oxygen exposure. (×35,000.)

ones, were best observed in Epon-embedded thick sections, the model of hyperbaric oxygen exposure was repeated utilizing 13 rats for evaluation of the anatomic location of neuritic changes within the spinal cord gray and white matter. These animals were sacrificed after one of four intervals following oxygen exposure: 30 min, 24 hr, 72 hr, and 1 week. They were perfused with 1% paraformaldehyde in 2% glutaraldehyde followed by 4% paraformaldehyde and 5% glutaraldehyde. Six to eight 1 to 2-mm-thin coronal slices of the cervical enlargement of the spinal cord were postfixed in 4% paraformaldehyde in 5% glutaraldehyde and subsequently in 2% osmic acid. All fixatives were buffered with Millonig's phosphate buffer. The spinal cord slices were embedded in Epon. Two-μm-thick sections of entire cord cross sections were cut from each block and stained with toluidine blue.

An ultrastructural study of acid phosphatase activity in spinal cord gray matter following hyperbaric oxygen exposure has been undertaken to correlate lysosomal activity with the subcellular changes found (McKeever and Balentine, 1973).

Dendritic Degeneration

Abnormalities of dendrites were consistently found in the anterior horn gray matter of the spinal cords of experimental animals, especially in rats sacrificed from 30 min to 72 hr after oxygen exposure (Balentine, 1974). Dendritic mitochondria became dense and frequently enlarged with increased numbers and aberrant arrangement of the cristae (Fig. 1). Loss of architectural detail of other cytoplasmic constituents of the dendrites, which became coarsely granular and more electron-opaque, was commonly associated with the mitochondrial abnormalities. Small flocculent densities were observed in the mitochondria present within the dense granular dendritic processes (Fig. 2). The cytoplasmic abnormalities of the dendrites, interpreted as degenerative changes, were observed in the absence of necrosis of neuronal perikarya. Rarely dense dendrites containing aggregates of numerous neurofilaments were observed (Fig. 3), but no relationship of these filamentous changes to the other abnormalities noted has been established.

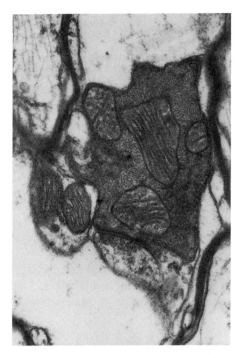

FIG. 3. Dendritic process containing numerous compacted 100-Å filaments seen in cross section. Normal mitochondria. Relationship of this change to dendritic degeneration shown in Fig. 2 is unknown. Anterior horn gray matter, 30 min after hyperbaric oxygen exposure. (×29,750.)

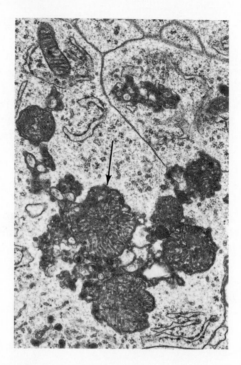

FIG. 4. Altered mitochondria and coarsely granular debris (arrow), interpreted as being of dendritic origin, engulfed by macrophage processes. Anterior horn gray matter, 1 week after hyperbaric oxygen exposure. (×18,000.)

The degenerating dendritic processes appeared to have disintegrated, releasing the abnormal mitochondria and debris into the extracellular space where they were engulfed and phagocytized by macrophages (Figs. 4–6). Autophagocytosis of abnormal dendritic mitochondria was also observed within dendrites and neuronal perikarya. Acid phosphatase activity has not been found in the degenerating dendrites, but was present within the lysosomes of the macrophages, intact dendrites, and neuronal perikarya involved in phagocytosis of the altered dendritic mitochondria and debris (McKeever and Balentine, 1973).

The coarsely dense dendritic changes associated with mitochondria abnormalities have been found frequently in the spinal cord gray matter and only rarely in the substantia nigra. No ultrastructural abnormalities of the neocortex were seen.

Axonal Degeneration

In oxygen-treated animals sacrificed from 24 hr to 30 days postexposure, abnormalities of axons were common. The most characteristic alterations

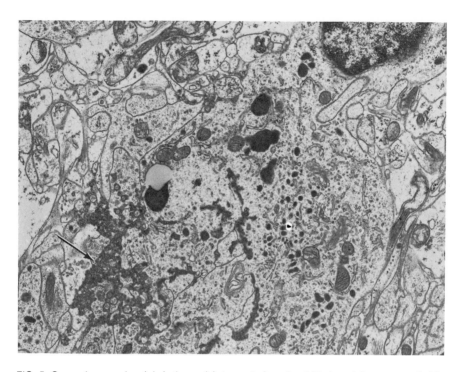

FIG. 5. Coarsely granular debris (*arrow*) interpreted as dendritic in origin, surrounded by macrophage processes. Note numerous dense core lysosomal granules in the cytoplasm of the macrophage. Anterior horn gray matter, 1 week after oxygen exposure. (×9,000.)

consisted of a loss of architectural detail with increased density of the axoplasm associated with mitochondrial changes similar to those noted in dendrites. Disappearance of axoplasm with the collapse of otherwise normal myelin sheaths was associated with the darkening of axoplasm. Breaking up of myelin sheaths into ovoids and vesicles was observed and considered to be secondary to axonal degeneration. The axonal changes affected small axons 1 to 2 μm in diameter, as well as larger axons. The ancillary thick-section study of whole cross sections of cervical cord revealed numerous degenerating axons in the anterior and anterolateral columns of the spinal cord white matter in addition to those in gray matter (Fig. 7). Axons in the posterior and lateral columns were affected to a lesser extent. In all of the white-matter columns the involved axons were those in close proximity to the gray matter with the peripheral white matter being spared. The axonal degeneration of oxygen toxicity has been associated with increased intra-axonal acid phosphatase (McKeever and Balentine, 1973) and heterophago-cytosis.

Axonal degeneration has been observed in both the anterior horn gray

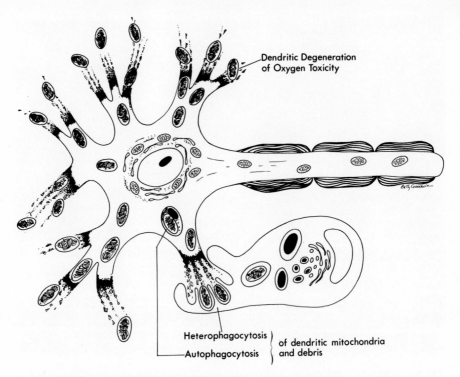

FIG. 6. Illustration of the nature of dendritic alterations induced by a single 30-min exposure to hyperbaric oxygen. Note enlarged dark mitochondria and the coarsely granular dendritic debris that are released from the altered dendrites and phagocytized by macrophages. Autophagy of abnormal mitochondria by otherwise normal dendrites also occurs.

matter (Balentine, 1974) and substantia nigra and, like the dendritic degeneration, was not associated with necrosis of neuronal perikarya.

DISCUSSION

The early postexposure period following hyperbaric oxygen exposure is characterized by dendritic degeneration of anterior horn cell in the presence of structurally intact neuronal perikarya (Fig. 6). The degenerative process is rapid in onset, being observed within 30 min following a single 30-min exposure to 60 psig of oxygen. Axonal degeneration is also observed following the same model of oxygen treatment; in the spinal cord, axons in the anterior gray horns as well as anterior lateral and posterior columns of white matter are involved. Both of these neuronal process degenerations occur in the presence of an intact blood brain barrier (Balentine, 1974) and in the absence of necrosis of neuronal perikarya. The time sequence of oc-

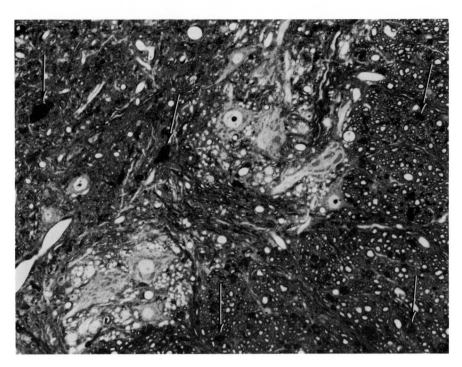

FIG. 7. Numerous degenerating axons (*arrows*) in anterior gray matter and anterior column of white matter. Portion of cross section of cervical spinal cord, 1 week after oxygen exposure. Epon-embedded section stained with toluidine blue. (×260.)

currence of the two changes indicate that dendritic precedes axonal degeneration, although there is considerable overlap 24 and 72 hr after oxygen exposure.

The enlarged dense mitochondria observed in the dendrites and axons in this study are similar to those observed in oxygen-exposed hepatic and alveolar cells by other investigators (Schaffner and Felig, 1965; Rosenbaum, Wittner, and Lenger, 1969). Because of the implication of mitochondria dysfunction in the biochemical toxicology of excessive oxygenation and the similarity of structural changes observed in various cells exposed to oxygen, the working hypothesis for the interpretation for the abnormalities found in neuronal cell processes in this investigation is that mitochondrial derangement within dendrites and axons leads to independent degeneration of these processes. However, the dendritic changes observed are in no way specific and are very similar to the retrograde degeneration of dendritic cytoplasm observed following experimental axotomy (Grant and Westman, 1968). If the hypothesis that the dendritic degeneration is related to mitochondrial oxygen toxicity is valid, it remains to be determined why the selective involvement of neuronal cell processes occurs. The dendritic alterations could be secondary to altered metabolism within the perikaryon or axon for which there is no reflected morphologic change.

The lack of finding ultrastructural abnormalities in the neocortex suggests that the dendritic degeneration of oxygen toxicity may be limited topographically. However, the light-microscopic observations of Epon-embedded spinal cords from experimental rats revealed that the axonal degeneration involved white matter much more than was anticipated and that lateral and posterior, as well as anterior, columns were affected. It may be that both axonal and dendritic oxygen induced degenerations are ubiquitous. Studies employing light-microscopic techniques are being undertaken to further assay the topography of the subcellular process degenerations in the CNS following hyperbaric oxygen exposure.

ACKNOWLEDGMENTS

This work was supported by U.S. Public Health Service Grant NS09837 from the National Institute of Neurological Diseases and Stroke, and by grants from the Medical University of South Carolina. Figures 1–5 are from material previously described (Balentine, 1974).

REFERENCES

Balentine, J. D. (1968): Pathogenesis of central nervous system lesions induced by exposure to hyperbaric oxygen. *Am. J. Pathol.*, 53:1097–1109.

Balentine, J. D. (1974): Ultrastructural pathology of hyperbaric oxygenation in the central nervous system: Observations in anterior horn gray matter. *Lab. Invest.*, 31:580–592.

Balentine, J. D., and Gutsche, B. B. (1966): Central nervous system lesions in rats exposed to oxygen at high pressure. *Am. J. Pathol.*, 48:107–127.

Bean, J. W., and Wapner, S. (1943): Effects of exposure to oxygen at high barometric pressure on higher functions of the CNS. *Proc. Soc. Exp. Biol.*, 54:134–135.

Behnke, A. R., Johnson, F. S., Poppen, J. R., and Motley, E. P. (1934): The effects of oxygen on man at pressures from one to four atmospheres. *Am. J. Physiol.*, 110:565–572.

Bert, P. (1878): *Barometric Pressure: Researches in Experimental Physiology*. Paris. Translated by M. A. Hitchcock and F. A. Hitchcock, 1943. College Book Co., Columbus, Ohio.

Davies, H. C., and Davies, R. C. (1965): Biochemical aspects of oxygen poisoning. In: *Handbook of Physiology, Vol. II: Respiration* edited by W. O. Fenn and H. Rahn, Sect 3, pp. 1047–1058.

Donald, A. W. (1947): Oxygen poisoning in man. *Br. Med. J.*, 1:667–672; 712–717.

Fairman, M. D., Mehl, R. G., and Myers, M. B. (1971): Brain norepinephrine and serotonin in central oxygen toxicity. *Life Sci.*, 10:21–34.

Fisher, D. B., and Kaufman, S. (1972): The inhibition of phenylalanine and tyrosine hydroxylases by high oxygen levels. *J. Neurochem.*, 19:1359–1365.

Grant, G., and Westman, D. (1968): Degenerative changes in dendrites central to axonal transections: Electron microscopic observations. *Experientia*, 24:169–170.

Haugaard, N. (1968): Cellular mechanisms of oxygen toxicity. *Physiol. Rev.*, 48:311–373.

McKeever, P., and Balentine, J. D. (1973): An ultrastructural study of acid phosphatase activity of rat ventral motor horn cells with observations on the effects of hyperbaric oxygen. *Lab. Invest.*, 29:633–641.

Ogilvie, R. W., and Balentine, J. D. (1973): Oxygen tensions in the deep gray matter of rats exposed to hyperbaric oxygen. Oxygen transport to tissue. *Advances in Experimental Medicine and Biology,* edited by H. I. Bicher and D. F. Bruley, 37A:299–304. Plenum, New York.

Ogilvie, R. W., and Balentine, J. D. (1975): Oxygen tensions in the gray matter of the spinal cord during exposure to hyperbaric oxygen at 5 atmospheres. *J. Neurosurg. (In press.)*

Rosenbaum, R., Wittner, M., and Lenger, M. (1969): Mitochondrial and other ultrastructural changes in great alveolar cells of oxygen adapted and poisoned rats. *Lab. Invest.,* 20:516–528.

Schaffner, F., and Felig, P. (1965): Changes in the hepatic structure in rats produced by breathing pure oxygen. *J. Cell Biol.,* 27:505–517.

Wood, J. D., Watson, W. J., and Stacey, N. E. (1966): A comparative study of hyperbaric oxygen induced and drug-induced convulsions with particular reference to γ-aminobutyric acid metabolism. *J. Neurochem.,* 13:361–370.

Advances in Neurology, Vol. 12, edited by
G. W. Kreutzberg, Raven Press, New York
© 1975.

Reversible Apical Swelling of Dendrites in the Cerebral Cortex of Cats During Respiratory Acidosis

W. Schlote, E. Betz, and H. Nguyen-Duong

Lehrstuhl für submikroskopische Pathologie und Neuropathologie, und Physiologisches Institut, Universität Tübingen, Liebermeisterstrasse 8, D-74 Tübingen, Federal Republic of Germany

The differential mode of reaction of cellular constituents of the cerebral cortex and even of parts of cells to various types of injury is a well-known phenomenon. It reflects different metabolic properties of cell types and of parts of cells. Selective swelling of apical parts of dendrites is an example of this type of alteration of nervous tissue. Swelling of apical dendrites in association with or without swelling of axonal terminals, of astrocytes, and of neuronal cell bodies has been observed in electron micrographs under various experimental conditions and in several human cerebral diseases (Table 1). Our studies of the effects of acidosis in the central nervous system

TABLE 1. *Swelling of apical, postsynaptic parts of dendrites in electron micrographs*

Disorder	Reference
Infantile spongiform degeneration (ISD) of the CNS	Gambetti, Mellman, and Gonatas (1969)
Infantile spongy cortical dystrophy in children caused by swelling of the postsynaptic dendrites	Kolkmann (1969); Ule (1968)
Experimental Creutzfeldt-Jakob disease in chimpanzees	Lampert, Gajdusek, and Gibbs (1971)
Experimental cobalt necrosis of rat brain	Fischer and Blinzinger (1968)
Experimental penicillin-induced epileptogenic lesion of the cerebral cortex of cats	Okada, Ayala, and Sung (1971)
Experimental Wernicke syndrome (thiamine deficiency) in pigeons and rats)	Ule, Kolkmann, and Brambring (1967)
Experimental methionine sulfoximine intoxication in rats	Ule (1968)
Experimental INH encephalopathy in ducks	Ule (1968)
Experimental 6-aminonicotinic acid, intoxication (Vitamin B_6 deficiency) in rats	Schneider (1970)
Experimental edema in virally induced brain tumors	Sipe, Vick, and Bigner (1972)
Brain edema in experimental NaCl intoxication in pigs	Deutschländer, Stavrou, and Dahme (1968)

of cats have shown reversible clear swellings of apical dendrites of the molecular layer of cerebral cortex as practically the only submicroscopic deviation from the normal state. Brief reports of the results in abstract form are already published (Schlote, Betz, Knebel, and Nguyen-Duong, 1970*a,b*).

METHODS

Neurophysiologic experiments

One group of 15 adult cats was narcotized with Nembutal (25 mg/kg) and artificially ventilated (Starling pump) for 1 hr with a mixture of 60 to 80% CO_2 and 40 to 20% O_2. The pO_2 was controlled by an oxytest device, the pCO_2 by ultrared absorption. The EEG and EKG were monitored continuously. In some cases, in addition, the aortal blood pressure was registered by a statham element. After 1 to $1\frac{1}{2}$ hr of high CO_2 respiration, in most cases, dysregulation of cardiac function occurred; the experiment was then terminated by ventilation with normal air and the animal awoke.

Biochemical Investigations

In a second series of experiments in five cats the skull was opened on both sides of the sagittal sinus and local cortical blood flow, extracellular local cortical pH, and local cortical pO_2 were recorded simultaneously. Arterial blood pressure, EEG, and the ECG were controlled during the gradually increased CO_2 concentration in the inspired air, which was maintained high for 1 hr. After this time during continued CO_2 inhalation we excised small pieces of cortical tissue with a special steel punch, cooled in liquid air (Schmahl, Betz, Dettinger, and Hohorst, 1966) and analyzed the concentration of ATP, ADP, creatine phosphate (Cr-P), creatine (Cr), lactate, and pyruvate of the cortical tissue with enzymatic–optic methods (Betz, Knebel, Neumann, and Nguyen-Duong, 1969).

Morphologic Observations

In a third group of seven animals, the same procedure was performed and after 1 hr of artificial high CO_2 ventilation, a biopsy of the suprasylvian gyrus was made by introducing two razor blades parallel to the course of the gyrus under an angle of 30°. After cutting the gyrus on both ends, the razor blades were elevated vertically, and the tissue was immediately placed in cacodylate-buffered 1% OsO_4 (pH 7.4) at 4°C. The tissue was further sectioned in slices of 2-mm thickness, perpendicular to the cortical surface, with dehydration in graded alcohols and embedding in Araldite. Semithin sections were stained by 1% toluidine blue in 1% sodium bicarbonate. Ultrathin sections were stained by a saturated alcoholic solution of uranyl acetate and by lead citrate (Venable and Coggeshall, 1965). The ultramicrotome was the LKB ultrotome III; the electron microscope was Carl Zeiss EM 9 S.

RESULTS

The alterations of cortical blood flow observed with increasing CO_2 concentration in the inspired air are reported by Betz et al. (1969). The A-V difference (between arterial blood and the blood in the sagittal sinus) became reduced after about 15 min of CO_2 inhalation. The EEG was gradually altered depending upon the percentage of CO_2 in the inspired air. It became isoelectric between 50 and 70% CO_2 in the inspired air, about 15 min after the beginning of CO_2 inhalation (Fig. 1). The cortical pH at the same time decreased from 7.2 to 7.3 down to 6.5 to 6.3. After 1 hr of high CO_2 ventilation, ATP and the ATP/ADP ratio in the cerebral cortex were not significantly altered when compared with controls, provided that normal cardiac function and arterial pressure were maintained (Fig. 2). A slight decrease of Cr-P and the Cr-P/Cr ratio was found, but sometimes these values were unchanged. The lactate concentration had increased; the lac/pyr relationship was insignificantly lower than the control values. In light and electron micrographs from the suprasylvian gyrus (Figs. 3 to 6), a spongiform porous texture of the molecular layer and of the middle layers of the cortex was evident in all cases. In the electron micrographs (Figs. 5 and 6), the pores corresponded to membrane-bound profiles, i.e., to cellular spaces. They contained swollen enlarged mitochondria. Quantitative estimation in electron micrographs revealed that 62% of the swollen cell processes were connected with presynaptic axon terminals (Fig. 7) and contained subsynaptic densities of normal

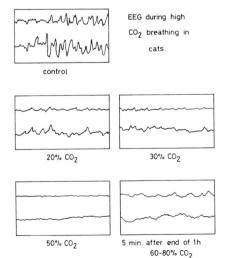

EEG during high CO_2 breathing in cats.

control

20% CO_2

30% CO_2

50% CO_2

5 min. after end of 1h 60-80% CO_2

FIG. 1. Bifrontal EEG reactions during and after high CO_2 ventilation in the cats of group 1.

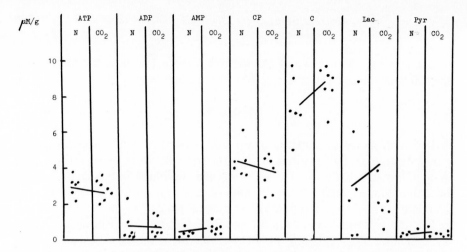

FIG. 2. Energy-rich phosphates and lactate–pyruvate after exposure to 70% CO_2 in the inspired air for 1 hr with arrest of the EEG in the cortex of cats of group 2 compared to normal values (N). From Betz et al. (1969).

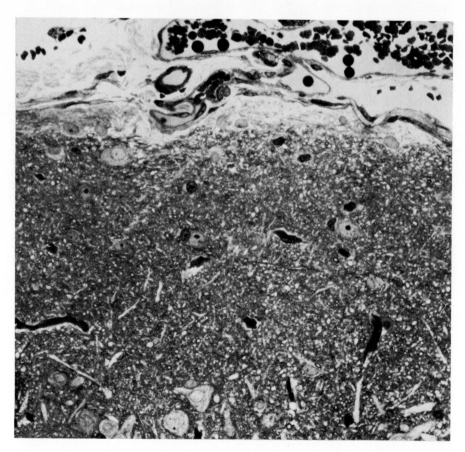

FIG. 3A. Semithin section from the molecular layer of the suprasylvian cortex of cats of group 3. Control. Toluidine blue staining. (×285.)

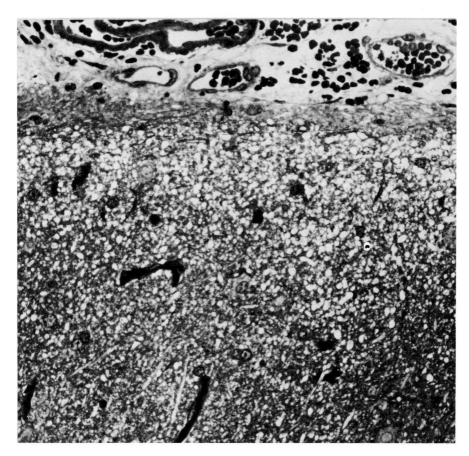

FIG. 3B. Semithin section from the molecular layer of the suprasylvian cortex of cats from group 3, after 1 hr of high CO_2 ventilation. Porous appearance of the neuropil. Toluidine blue staining. (×285.)

appearance. Therefore they were identified as postsynaptic dendrite apices, corresponding probably to the tips of apical and basal dendrites of pyramidal cells, situated in the middle layers of the cortex. It can be argued that most if not all of the enlarged cellular profiles were of dendritic origin, because the synaptic complex must not necessarily be seen in the plane of the section. The roundish shape of swollen profiles seems very characteristic of dendrites as compared to the irregular shaped electron-lucent profiles of swollen astrocytic processes seen, for example, in vaso-genic edema. Sections parallel to the course of the dendrites showed that the dendritic shafts adjoining the swollen tips were mostly intact; only occasionally were these parts also enlarged. All presynaptic terminals linked with the dendritic swellings were unchanged. Besides the synapses with swollen dendrite endings many normal axodendritic synapses were seen. The perikarya of nerve cells appeared to be generally darker than

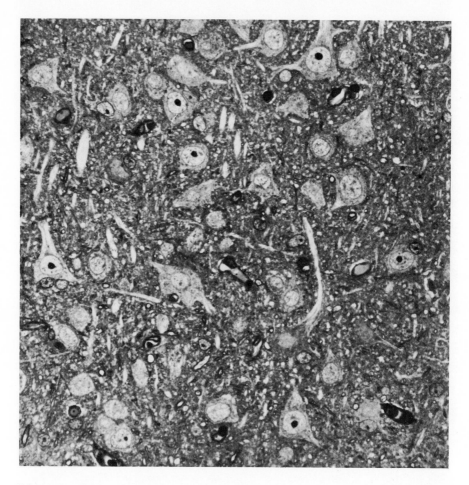

FIG. 4A. Semithin section from the IIIrd layer of the suprasylvian cortex. Control. Toluidine blue staining. (×285.)

in the controls, but there were no shrunken "dark neurons." The myelinated nerve fibers were intact. Endothelial cells of capillaries were unchanged. In the experiments as well as in the sham-operated controls with exposed cerebral cortex, within 1 hr some astrocytic processes were swollen. Enlarged dendrites could not be detected in the controls.

Some animals were allowed to recover. Within 3 to 5 min after termination of CO_2 ventilation and replacement by normal air, the electric activity of cerebral cortex was gradually restored and spontaneous respiration began. The behavior of the animals showed no striking alteration when they awoke. Cerebral biopsies performed 10 min after restoring of the normal EEG revealed clear dendritic swellings in approximately the same number and proportion as during the CO_2 ventilation. Cerebral biopsies made 8

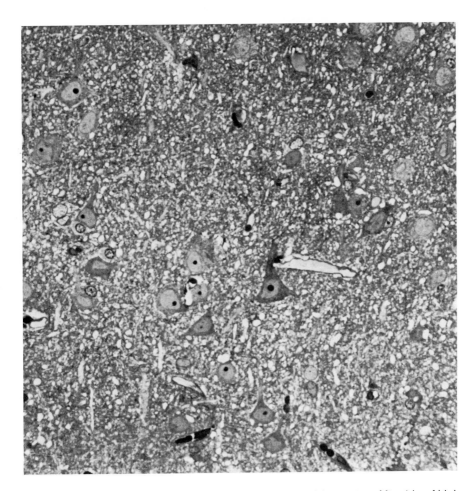

FIG. 4B. Semithin section from the IIIrd layer of the suprasylvian cortex. After 1 hr of high CO_2 ventilation. Porous appearance of the neuropil. Nerve cell perikarya are smaller and appear darker than in the control. Toluidine blue staining. (×285.)

and 10 days after the experiments showed a few swollen dendrites to be the only submicroscopic alteration of the tissue.

CONCLUSIONS

In contrast to the energetic insufficiency of cerebral tissue known to occur in hypoxia and ischemia (Lowry, Passoneau, Hasselberger, and Schulz, 1964), respiratory acidosis does not cause a marked decrease of energy-rich substrates of the cerebral cortex, but the EEG ceases independently of the tissue content of these compounds. The widespread

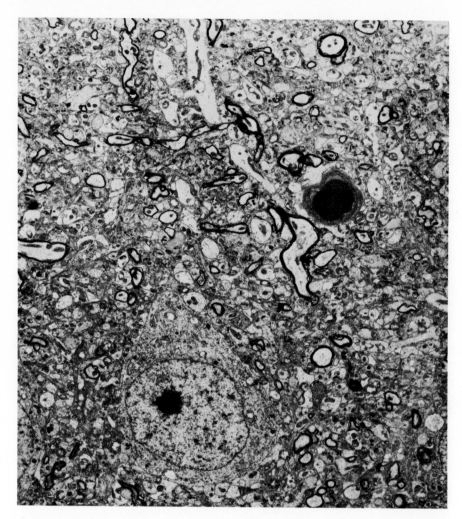

FIG. 5A. Ultrathin section from the IIIrd layer of the suprasylvian cortex. Control. (×3,600.)

focal clear swellings of postsynaptic dendrite apices evoked by 80% CO_2 ventilation and accompanied by an extracellular pH at the cortical surface in the range of 6.8 to 6.6 represents a nearly selective response of this part of the nerve cell to the modified state of energy metabolism during acidosis. According to Swanson (1969), the pH of the extracellular fluid of cerebral tissue is generally 0.3 lower than the pH of the surrounding medium. Hence, in the present investigation, a pH of 6.3 to 6.0 may actually be present during respiratory acidosis in cortical tissue in which the dendritic swellings develop. The near-normal content of energy-rich compounds indicates that the energy production during respiratory acidosis is not

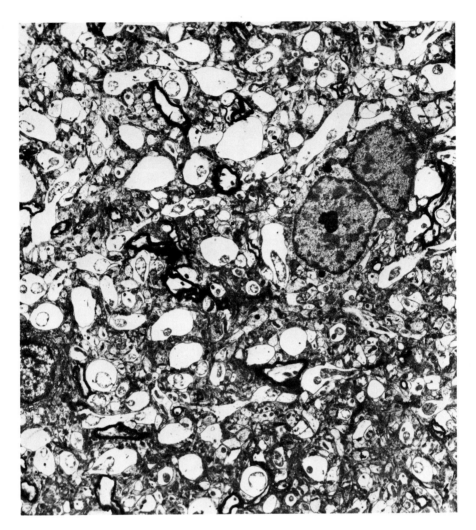

FIG. 5B. Ultrathin section from the IIIrd layer of the suprasylvian cortex. After 1 hr of high CO_2 ventilation. Swollen round cell profiles are abundant in the neuropil. ($\times 3,600$.)

significantly altered. But this may hold true only for the bulk of the tissue, whereas differences may exist between different parts of the cell. The severely swollen mitochondria in the clear dendritic swellings indicate a disorder of energy metabolism. Locally increased lactate production establishing an osmotic gradient could well be one of the factors leading to the electron-lucent swellings. The absence of accompanying swelling of astrocytes favors the view that they are not, or not only, caused by inhibition of Na^+, K^+-stimulated adenosine triphosphatase, i.e., by dysfunction of the sodium pump. In experimental ouabain intoxication of the brain,

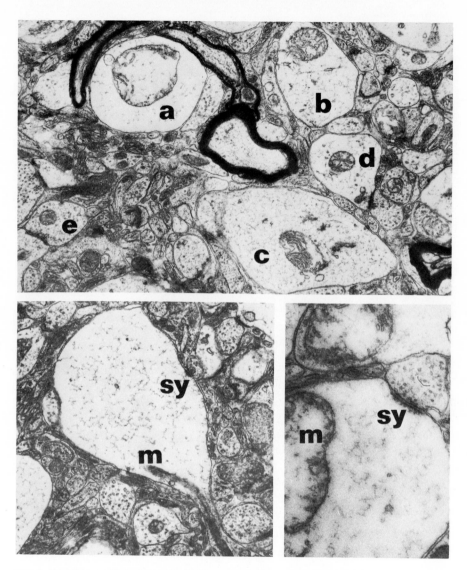

FIG. 6. Ultrathin sections from the IIIrd layer of the suprasylvian cortex after 1 hr of high CO_2 ventilation. (*Top*) Clear profiles, a–c, contain enlarged, vacuolated mitochondria. Axodendritic synapse attached to profile d. Myelinated nerve fiber deformed by swollen profile a. (×16,660.) (*Bottom, left*) Swelling of dendrite tip with synapse, sy, the adjoining dendrite shaft appearing normal with tangentially sectioned mitochondrion, m. (×24,500.) (*Bottom, right*) Swelling of dendrite with normal subsynaptic density, sy, and adjoining normal presynaptic terminal. Enlarged mitochondrion, m, in the dendrite. (×31,500.)

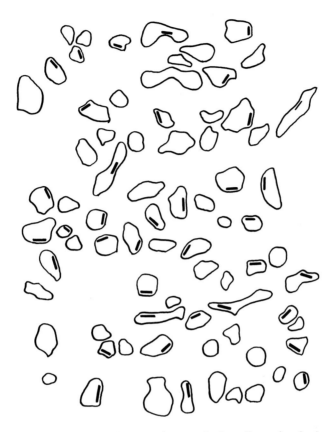

FIG. 7. Tracing from montage of electron micrographs from the molecular layer of supra-sylvian cortex after 1 hr of high CO_2 ventilation, as used for quantitative estimation of synaptic sites on membrane-bound clear profiles. Synapses were identified by attached presynaptic terminals and by subsynaptic densities at the opposite place inside the clear profiles. Identified synaptic sites are indicated by bars, i.e., subsynaptic densities.

excessive swelling of astrocytes and swelling of presynaptic axon terminals is the main finding, whereas dendritic enlargements are rare and of minor degree (Cornog, Gonatas, and Feierman, 1967; Tanaka, 1969). By comparing our results to the electron-microscopic alterations of brain tissue in experimental hypoxia and ischemia, an entirely different pattern of structural alterations (Nunes, Hossmann, and Farkas-Bargeton, 1973) appears, corresponding in this condition to the rapid decrease of energy-rich compounds. Surprisingly, in a study of the effect of acute hypoxia and hypercapnia on the CNS Bakay and Lee (1968) did not mention dendritic swellings, but it is not clear whether the tissue pH achieved was as below, as in our experiments. The only other condition evoking a nearly selective swelling of dendrite apices is the penicillin-induced epileptogenic lesion produced by applying penicillin solutions locally to the exposed cerebral cortex of cats (Okada, Ayala, and Sung, 1971). The pathogenesis of this type of lesion is unknown.

Concerning the correlation between morphology and electrophysiology in our experiments, it may be pointed out that no direct reciprocal temporal correlation exists between them. The dendritic swellings persist during an unknown period of time after normalization of the EEG, indicating the slower restitution of morphologic than of biochemical alterations. Keeping in mind that the postsynaptic bars of the synapses seem not to be altered structurally in the electron-lucent dendrites and that many synapses remain intact, it can be understood that electrophysiologic activity is rapidly restored.

Clear swellings of the dendrite apices as evoked during respiratory acidosis, which give a porous appearance to the cerebral cortex in light-microscopic preparations (dendritogenic status spongiosus), represent a selective but nonspecific reaction of this special part of the nerve cell, indicating its selective vulnerability. Further investigations are necessary to elucidate the nature of underlying peculiarities of metabolism, membrane composition, and permeability of the terminal arborizations of cortical dendrites.

REFERENCES

Bakay, L., and Lee, I. C. (1968): The effect of acute hypoxia and hypercapnia on the ultrastructure of the central nervous system. *Brain,* 91:697–706.

Betz, E., Knebel, U., Neumann, L., and Nguyen-Duong, H. (1969): Effects of high concentrations of CO_2 on cerebral metabolism and EEG activity. In: *Cerebral Blood Flow,* edited by M. Brock, C. Fieschi, D. H. Ingvar, N. A. Lassen, and K. Schürmann. Springer-Verlag: Berlin, Heidelberg, New York.

Cornog, J. L., Gonatas, N. K., and Feierman, J. R. (1967): Effects of intracerebral injection of ouabain on the fine structure of rat cerebral cortex. *Am. J. Pathol.,* 51:573.

Deutschländer, N., Stavron, D., and Dahme, E. (1968): Elektronenmikroskopische und histochemische Hirnbefunde bei der Kochsalzvergiftung des Schweines. Ein experimenteller Beitrag zur Hirnödemfrage. *Verh. Dtsch. Ges. Pathol.,* 52: 264–269.

Fischer, J., and Blinzinger, K. (1968): Vorkommen von Glykogen in geschwollenen Dendriten bei experimenteller Kobaltnekrose des Rattengehirns. *Virchows Arch. (Zellpathol.),* 1:201–210.

Gambetti, P., Mellmann, W. J., and Gonatas, N. K. (1969): Familial spongy degeneration of the c.n.s. (van Bogaert-Bertrand disease). An ultrastructural study. *Acta Neuropathol.,* 12:103–115.

Kolkmann, F. W. (1969): Die spongiösen Dystrophien des ZNS im Kindes – und Erwachsenenalter. Habilitationsschrift, Heidelberg.

Lampert, P. W., Gajdusek, D. C., Gibbs, C. J. (1971): Experimental spongiform encephalopathy (CJD) in chimpanzees. Electron microscopic studies. *J. Neuropathol. Exp. Neurol.,* 30:23.

Lowry, H. O., Passonneau, J. O., Hasselberger, F. X., and Schulz, D. W. (1964): Effect of ischemia on known substrates and cofactors of the glycolytic pathway in Brain. *J. Biol. Chem.,* 239:18.

Nunes, A., Hossmann, K., and Farkas-Bargeton, E. (1973): Ultrastructural and histological investigation of the cerebral cortex of cat during and after complete ischemia. *Acta Neuropathol.,* 26:329.

Okada, K., Ayala, C. F., and Sung, J. H. (1971): Ultrastructure of Penicillin-induced epileptogenic lesion of the cerebral cortex in cats. *J. Neuropathol. Exp. Neurol.,* 30:348.

Schlote, W., Betz, E., Knebel, U., and Nguyen-Duong. H. (1970*a*): EEG-Veränderungen und Dendritenschwellung bei schwerer respiratorischer Acidose. *Pfluegers Arch.,* 316: (3/4), R74.

Schlote, W., Betz, E., Knebel, U., and Nguyen-Duong, H. (1970*b*): EEG-Veränderungen und Dendritenschwellung bei schwerer respiratorischer Acidose. *Wien. Klin. Wochenschr.,* 82:667.

Schmahl, F. W., Betz, E., Dettinger, E., and Hohorst, A. J. (1966): Energiestoffwechsel der Grosshirnrinde und Elektrencephalogramm beim Sauerstoffmangel. *Pfluegers Arch.,* 292: 46–59.

Schneider, H. (1970): Schädigung der Formatio reticularis durch den Antimetaboliten 6-Aminonikotinsäureamid. VI. *Congres Internationale de Neuropathologie.* Masson, Paris.

Sipe, J. C., Vick, N. A., and Bigner, D. D. (1972): Grey matter edema: The marginal zone of autochthonous virally-induced gliomes. *J. Neurol. Sci.,* 17:185–191.

Swanson, P. D. (1969): pH effects on the metabolic properties of isolated cerebral tissues. *Neurology,* 19:289.

Tanaka, R. (1969): Electron microscopic study of ouabain-induced edematous brain. *Brain Nerve* (*Japan*), 21:853–868.

Ule, G. (1968): Feinstruktur der spongiösen Dystrophie der grauen Substanz. *Verh. Dtsch. Ges. Pathol.,* 52:142–155.

Ule, G., Kolkmann, F. W., and Brambring, P. (1967): Experimentelle elektronenmikroskopische Untersuchungen zur formalen Pathogenese der Wernickeschen Encephalopathie. *Klin. Wochenschr.,* 45:886–887.

Venable, J. H., and Coggeshall, R. (1965): A simplified lead citrate stain for use in electron microscopy. *J. Cell Biol.,* 25:407–408.

SUBJECT INDEX